LEGAL and ETHICAL CONSIDERATIONS
for Dental Hygienists and Assistants

Vist our website at www.mosby.com

LEGAL and ETHICAL CONSIDERATIONS

for Dental Hygienists and Assistants

JUDITH A. DAVISON, J.D., R.D.H.

Attorney at Law
Windham, Maine

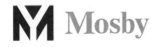

M Mosby

A *Harcourt Health Sciences Company*
St. Louis   Philadelphia   London   Sydney   Toronto

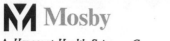

Mosby

A *Harcourt Health Sciences Company*

Editor-in-Chief: John Schrefer
Acquisitions Editor: Penny Rudolph
Developmental Editor: Angela Reiner
Project Manager: Patricia Tannian
Production Editor: Steve Hetager
Design Manager: Gail Morey Hudson
Cover Design: Teresa Breckwoldt

Mosby, Inc.
A Harcourt Health Sciences Company
11830 Westline Industrial Drive
St. Louis, Missouri 63146

Printed in the United States of America

ISBN 1-55664-422-1

00 01 02 03 CL/FF 9 8 7 6 5 4 3 2

To
FRED

Preface

Long after you have forgotten radiology and dental materials, long after you have retired as an active member of the dental health profession, you will still live with the *law*. You will live with the law in every facet of your life, including the mortgage on your home, credit cards, marriage, divorce, and insurance of all kinds. Every profession has interaction with the law. *Legal and Ethical Considerations for Dental Hygienists and Assistants* is an attempt to show the relationship between the law and the dental health professions.

This is not a law book. It is meant to be a guide to help the dental professional to practice within the law. Should you find yourself in a legal dilemma, nothing takes the place of an attorney who is licensed to practice law in the state in which you reside.

The law is complex and flexible. As a result, there is no way to make it simplistic. Although this book contains many definitions and examples, in many situations even a definition will not simplify the law. In part, it is complex because state and federal laws, rules, and regulations are imposed on health professionals. Because the law is flexible, there are no black and white answers to most legal problems. The law discussed here is constantly changing. Legislatures amend statutes with regularity; therefore, state and federal laws often do not remain in the form in which they were originally passed. Lawsuits produce case law to provide guidelines for future court decisions. Often we are required to change our behavior to conform to the newly decided case law. It is difficult to predict exactly what legal principles will change and in what direction. Each lawsuit has its own particular set of facts, witness testimony, expert testimony, jury, and judge. The law is, therefore, interpreted to adjudicate each current set of circumstances before the court. A lawsuit based on a specific set of facts and decided by a court of law in one state may result in a different decision by a court of law in another state. In addition, a final decision of one court can be applied differently in other court decisions. It is therefore difficult to predict with certainty what the law requires in all circumstances.

Since medical and dental laws are constantly changing, many of the cases discussed in this book may be overturned in part or in whole by other court decisions. These cases are included to demonstrate how courts handle specific issues relating to dental or medical care, not to give specific legal advice.

There are also no black and white answers to ethical dilemmas. Each of the dental professions has a professional code of ethics to guide it. However, in many instances we are left to our own devices, as ethics is more subjective than the law. In many given circumstances we must act or react as individuals, keeping in mind what the law requires, as well as what we believe is right for ourselves and all others involved.

Each section of this book consists of three chapters, with the exception of Section II, which contains six chapters, and the last section, which consists of a discussion relating to changing the law. For each group of three chapters, I have included a case study with study questions. I hope that these materials will help you to apply information found in the chapters to the dental office setting. There are also responses from other professionals to these case studies, so that the reader may gain more than one point of view. These professionals include attorneys, dentists, educators, dental assistants, dental hygienists, and persons who belong to more than one of these professions, so that many perspectives are available. For instance, the case study responses to the second case study in Section II are by an attorney, a dentist, a dental assistant/office manager, and a dental hygienist. There are fewer responses to other case studies, but each has more than one view. The answers to the questions at the end of each section are those of the author.

Most cases reported in this book refer primarily to the doctor or dentist as opposed to the dental hygienist or dental assistant. This is because an illegal act committed by a dental hygienist or dental assistant is attributable to his or her employer in most cases. However, the cases reported are applicable to all dental health professionals.

My hope is that after reading this book you will be better informed, and as a result become a more prudent and a more confident dental professional

Judith A. Davison

Acknowledgments

I would be remiss if I did not acknowledge those individuals who gave of their time, energy, and knowledge to assist in this endeavor. My sincere thanks to Christina Corbin-Price, Marilyn Cortell, Carolyn Hartnett, Joan Leland, Laurence Minott, Morris Robbins, Jonathan Shapiro, Geoffrey Wagner, and Frederick Williams, who wrote responses for the case studies. Each of you gave me the needed support to make this book possible.

My gratitude to Emma Montgomery, for her invaluable assistance; Cathy Turbyne, who graciously shared materials from her business, Turbyne & Associates; Pro Dentec, for the generous offer of its materials; and Kathryn Murray, who spent many hours assisting with legal research.

My special thanks to Mosby, Inc., and its staff, in particular Penny Rudolph, Angie Reiner, and Steve Hetager, who made special efforts to ensure that this book became a reality.

Excerpts from the following books appear with the kind permission of the copyright holders: *Community Health Today*, Allyn & Bacon; *The Health Robbers: A Close Look at Quackery in America*, Prometheus Books; *Dental Clinics of North America*, W.B. Saunders.

Judith A. Davison

Biographies of Case Study Contributors

Frederick D. Williams is an attorney at law and a member of the New York and Maine state bars. He is a sole practitioner and has for the past 26 years focused primarily on corporate law, real estate, probate, and family matters. He received his bachelor of science degree from the College of the City of New York and his juris doctorate degree from New York Law School. For 15 years, Mr. Williams taught business law at St. Joseph's College, Windham, Maine, as an adjunct professor. In the past he has been president of the Cumberland County Bar Association and has served on the Town Council of Windham, Maine. He also served as a member of the Board of Directors of Westbrook Community Hospital and is a member of the Board of Corporators of Maine Medical Center.

Carolyn A. Hartnett graduated from The Forsyth School for Dental Hygienists, and received her baccalaureate degree from Keene State College and her master's degree in education from the University of New Hampshire. Currently she is the Department Head of the Dental Auxiliaries Department at New Hampshire Community Technical Institute, in Concord, New Hampshire. She has taught courses in dental materials and periodontics. At present, she teaches dental hygiene theory to freshmen students and ethics and jurisprudence to seniors. She also instructs in the dental assistant clinical courses as well as the freshmen and senior dental hygiene clinics.

Laurence P. Minott, Jr., graduated from Lincoln Academy, Newcastle, Maine, in 1964 and immediately enlisted in the U.S. Coast Guard. During the next 22 years, among other things, he served as a dental technician. He completed a bachelor of arts degree at Marshall University, Huntington, West Virginia. Mr. Minott graduated from Suffolk University Law School, Boston, Massachusetts. He practiced law for a short time as an associate at the law offices of Lowell D. Weeks. Then, in 1988, he opened his own practice and worked as a solo practitioner until joining the law firm of Sawyer, Sawyer & Minott in the summer of 1992. He is currently the managing partner of the firm.

Joan Leland has been a dental office manager for seven years and also operates a billing service business from her home. She attended college at Mount Ida Junior College, Newton, Massachusetts, where she studied dental assisting and office management. After college Ms. Leland moved to Connecticut, where she worked as a dental assistant for the next three years. She then accepted a position with Connecticut General Life Insurance Company as a field claim examiner. It was here that she took classes in processing both medical and dental claims. When Ms. Leland moved to Maine in 1988, she became a claims processor for National Employee Benefit Services for the following four years, until she accepted her current position as a dental office manager, which she has held for the last seven years. This past year, Ms. Leland fulfilled her dream of having her own business and is currently providing billing services for businesses in the greater Portland area.

Geoffrey W. Wagner, is a practicing dentist in Falmouth, Maine, where his offices have been for the last 16 years. Although Dr. Wagner is a general dentist, his interests focus heavily on pediatric, handicapped, and hospital dentistry. Previously, he had completed a general practice residency at the Maine Medical Center in Portland, Maine, after graduation from The University of Iowa College of Dentistry in 1981. During his time in Portland, Dr. Wagner has served as part-time dental hygiene clinical faculty member at Westbrook College, Department of Dental Hygiene, as a member of the executive committee of the Maine Dental Association, and as a board member and clinical advisor for the Head Start program.

Marilyn Cortell received her associate's degree in dental hygiene from Middlesex Community College, Bedford, Massachusetts, and her bachelor and master of science degrees from Lesley College, Cambridge, Massachusetts. She has been actively involved in the profession of dental hygiene since 1977 and has served as vice president, president-elect, and president of the Massachusetts Dental Hygienists' Association. At the end of her presidential term Ms. Cortell received the Governor of the State of Massachusetts Outstanding Leadership Award along with an appointment to the American Dental Hygienists' Association's Council on Public Relations, where she served a one-year term. Ms. Cortell continues to work and teach in the profession of dental hygiene and is currently a member of the editorial board of *RDH* magazine.

Morris L. Robbins completed his D.D.S. degree at The University of Tennessee and a fellowship in pathology with the U.S. Public Health Service. He is licensed to practice dentistry in Tennessee and Florida. After completing his fellowship, he joined the faculty of The University of Tennessee College of Dentistry. He achieved the positions of Associate Professor and Assistant Chairman of the Department of Oral Diagnosis with tenure in 1978. He then was selected as chair of the Department of Dental Hygiene in the College of Allied Health Sciences. He was named Assistant Dean for Clinical Affairs in the College of Dentistry in 1982, and then Associate Dean in 1986. Dr. Robbins has chaired many college and campus committees, co-authored a book on oral pathology, published over twenty scientific articles, and lectured nationally and internationally. He is active in organized dentistry, serving as president of the Memphis Dental Society, and as president-elect of the Tennessee Dental Association for 1998-1999. He has chaired various committees for the state dental association, as well as serving as a consultant to the American Dental Association. Dr. Robbins is the recipient of the St. George Award from the American Cancer Society and The University of Tennessee Alumni Public Service Award.

Christina Corbin-Price holds an associate of science degree in dental hygiene and a bachelor of science degree in business management from Westbrook College, Portland, Maine. She has practiced dental hygiene for the past 16 years and has held many positions within the Maine Dental Hygienists' Association's Executive Board. She has taught in various clinical settings. Ms. Corbin-Price practices full time as a dental hygienist and is co-owner of Davison, Price & Associates, a business that provides consulting and educational services relating to dental ergonomics. Ms. Corbin-Price recently received the Dental Hygienist of the Year Award from the Maine Dental Hygienists' Association.

Jonathan Shapiro is a director with the labor and employment law firm of Moon, Moss, McGill, Hayes & Shapiro, P.A. Mr. Shapiro concentrates his practice in the areas of employment, labor, and employee benefits law and litigation on behalf of management. He has represented management before federal and state courts and administrative agencies throughout New England, the Mid-Atlantic region, and the Midwest on a wide variety of labor and employment issues, including the defense against wrongful termination, discrimination, and collateral tort claims. Mr. Shapiro regularly counsels employers in New England, New York, New Jersey, Illinois, Maryland, Pennsylvania, Texas, and Virginia on a broad range of business and employment matters, including designing and implementing personnel policies and practices, overseeing the hiring and termination of employees, negotiating severance packages for senior executives, conducting internal corporate audits and investigations, and safeguarding corporate property and information. Mr. Shapiro has developed particular expertise in representing and advising employers in the health care industry, including health management organizations and other health benefits companies, management service organizations that provide management and administrative services to medical practice groups, and medical providers and practice groups. Mr. Shapiro is a graduate of McGill University in Montreal, Quebec, and the Duke University School of Law. He has been admitted to practice in Maine, Massachusetts, New York, and the District of Columbia.

Contents

List of Cases Cited

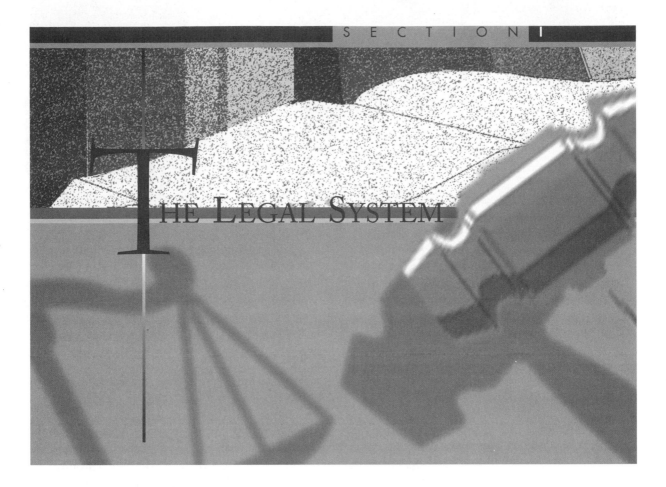

SECTION I

THE LEGAL SYSTEM

SECTION OUTLINE

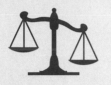

CASE STUDY

Mr. Silas Burton, 67 years old, resides in Smith, Ohio. Mr. Burton has a maxillary partial denture that relies on tooth #3 as an anchor tooth. On May 2, tooth #30 became painful to pressure, and Mr. Burton was unable to chew food on the right side of his mouth. By the next morning the entire area was causing severe pain. The right side was extremely edematous. Mr. Burton ingested two aspirins to relieve the pain and reduce the edema. The pain and edema persisted. On May 9, he went to Dr. James Albright, his dentist, located in Brown, Indiana. Although the office was extremely busy, Ms. Jean Casey, R.D.H., seated Mr. Burton in Dr. Albright's operatory. She administered local anesthesia in the maxillary right quadrant and informed Dr. Albright that the patient was anesthetized and awaiting treatment. Dr. Albright rushed into the room, washed his hands, and proceeded to extract tooth #3. Still in pain on May 13, Mr. Burton returned to Dr. Albright's office because the right side of his face was still edematous. After examination, Dr. Albright realized that he had extracted the wrong tooth and told Mr. Burton how sorry he was.

As Dr. Albright initiated extraction of tooth #30, Mr. Burton stopped breathing and became cyanotic. Ms. Sara Smythe, C.D.A., immediately administered CPR. She was not certified to administer CPR, but recalled how to do it from her Girl Scout days. An ambulance transported Mr. Burton to the hospital. After recovery, Mr. Burton went to Dr. Halper for the extraction of tooth #30 and fabrication of a new partial at a cost of $5,000. Then Mr. Burton acquired the services of an attorney. He directed the attorney to sue Dr. Albright, Ms. Casey, and Ms. Smythe in the Ohio Supreme Court for $1,000,000. Also, he reported the incidents to the Ohio Board of Medical Examiners.

Ms. Smythe had been a dental assistant for many years and was a valuable employee. She had been employed by Dr. Albright for the past ten years and was familiar with all procedures utilized routinely in the office. One day Dr. Albright explained to Ms. Smythe that an emergency patient had just been seated in the next operatory and that she was to finish the appointment for the patient currently in his dental chair. Dr. Albright had just completed preparations for teeth #19 and #20. Flattered that the doctor thought so highly of her skills, Ms. Smythe completed both restorations.

While Ms. Casey was waiting for her next patient to arrive, she observed the receptionist placing cash received from a patient into an envelope. The receptionist placed the envelope in a location different from where checks for deposit were kept. Later, Ms. Casey checked the computer and found no documentation of payment in the patient's record.

The first issue to arise is whether Ms. Casey, a registered dental hygienist, acted within the scope of her authority. We have no way to resolve this issue without a thorough review of the Dental Practice Act of Indiana. Many states permit a dental hygienist to administer local anesthesia. In many states a dental hygienist may administer local anesthesia if it is done in his or her capacity as a dental hygienist. For example, were Ms. Casey to administer local anesthesia in order to prepare a patient for an extraction by the dentist, then it would be my opinion that such an act would be prohibited. However, were Ms. Casey to administer local anesthesia in order to perform a scaling, such an act would not be prohibited in those states where such activity is permissible. Again, we must look to the Dental Practice Act of the particular state, since each Act defines the scope of practice for dental hygienists.

In extracting the wrong tooth, Dr. Albright was negligent; he violated the standard of care due his patient. As will be pointed out in later chapters, dealing with the subject of torts, Dr. Albright owed a duty to his patient and he breached that duty. As a consequence, the patient has an action in tort wherein he may sue Dr. Albright for injury, pain and suffering, and other related costs. This type of tort presents several questions. Did Dr. Albright examine the patient's record, the x-rays, or the patient himself prior to performing the extraction? Did he have a duty to do so? Of course!

Notwithstanding the fact that Ms. Smythe was not certified to perform CPR, there would appear to be no liability unless it can be shown that she acted in a reckless manner and thereby caused injury to Mr. Burton. There is no question that if Mr. Burton had suffered injury as a result of the improper administration of CPR, both Ms. Smythe and Dr. Albright would be liable (respondeat superior). If we assume that all personnel on Dr. Albright's staff were certified,

except for Ms. Smythe, then it would be incumbent upon Dr. Albright to appoint either himself or one of his staff to administer CPR when and if the need arose. As to whether Ms. Smythe was acting within the scope of her authority in completing the restorations, we would need to examine the Indiana Dental Practice Act, as this is a legal function for dental hygienists and dental assistants in some states.

I cannot detect from the facts that Dr. Halper acted in a manner inconsistent with the requisite standard of care. However, the question as to whether Dr. Halper secured a medical history of Mr. Burton or performed a thorough examination, including x-rays, begs an answer. In short, did he or did he not follow standard procedure prior to and during the extraction process?

The Ohio Board of Medical Examiners cannot entertain Mr. Burton's complaint. The state board of dentistry should entertain complaints regarding members of the dental profession, and it must be in the state that granted the license. Usually the correct procedure dictates taking complaints regarding dental professionals to the state board of dentistry in the state in which the dentist is licensed to practice, prior to initiating any court action. The general rule is that a complainant must exhaust all administrative remedies available prior to initiating litigation. In this particular situation the Indiana Board of Dentistry should be notified, since Dr. Albright's practice and license are in Indiana, not in Ohio, where Mr. Burton resides.

Initial litigation must proceed in a court of trial jurisdiction. A court of appellate jurisdiction cannot entertain a trial. Since the parties are not residents of the same state, litigation could be initiated in the United States District Court for that particular district (where either of the parties resides), because of diversity of citizenship. There is, however, a minimum monetary requirement to file a case in the U.S. District

RESPONSE TO CASE STUDY—cont'd

Court. The monetary claim requesting damages must be reasonable and commensurate with the injury suffered. In the event Mr. Burton, a resident of Ohio, files his lawsuit in U.S. District Court in Ohio, Dr. Albright has the right to request a change of venue to the U.S. District Court in Indiana, since that is his residence and also the situs where the alleged injury occurred. The court will weigh all factors in determining whether to change the venue.

Ms. Casey has an ethical and legal predicament regarding the receptionist's handling of Dr. Albright's money. Should she report the incident? If so, to whom? Is the receptionist acting on her own, or was she directed to handle the finances in this manner? Ms. Casey is also faced with a criminal issue. Who should be prosecuted under criminal law? Ms. Casey must do what her own ethical standards dictate, but, more important, she must consider the crime of "misprison," having knowledge of the commission of a crime and failing to reveal it to the proper authorities. This of necessity must be Ms. Casey's first consideration.

RESPONSE TO CASE STUDY

Carolyn A. Hartnett, C.D.A., R.D.H., M.Ed.

The series of events that is described in the case study could easily take place in any dental office where there is little communication among staff and with patients. In this case it is unclear whether principles of ethics and jurisprudence are known in theory, but, at the least, their application gets lost as the pace gets frantic and crisis management takes over.

The happenings in Dr. Albright's office are a clear example of this. A variety of violations of both the ethical and legal principles of health care management and treatment can be noted, and these transgressions occur in the judgment and in the actions of each member of the practice. Since Ms. Casey, the registered dental hygienist, initiated Mr. Burton's treatment, the problems started there. In her eagerness to relieve Mr. Burton of his pain and to help out her busy employer, Ms. Casey showed very poor judgment in the crisis management of this patient. She was delinquent in her assessment of the patient in both the areas of taking a medical history and obtaining instructions from the dentist for the use of radiographs for diagnostic purposes. She was delinquent in her treatment of the patient for diagnosing and performing functions beyond the legal scope of dental hygiene practice.

Although Ms. Sara Smythe, the certified dental assistant, does not play as large a role in the treatment of Mr. Burton as Ms. Casey does, there are issues surrounding her decision to perform CPR. Certainly, it would have been more ethically correct for her to keep up her certification, but if she had not, there were better-qualified staff to handle this function. Her willingness to perform functions asked of her by Dr. Albright, as described later in the case, clearly indicates that she, like Ms. Casey, is agreeable to performing tasks well beyond her legal scope of practice.

As Ms. Casey observed, the financial accounting that goes on behind the desk is a real legal problem. Because the person who collects the moneys is the same person who is independently responsible for the bookkeeping, there are few checks and balances on the recording of each transaction. Income tax evasion can easily become a reality.

RESPONSE TO CASE STUDY—cont'd

Throughout the case study, the person who must obviously accept the most blame is the dentist. As written in most state practice acts, all dental auxiliaries work under the license of the dentist. Dr. Albright is the person who has illegally delegated functions to his hygienist and assistant. He is ultimately responsible for keeping accurate books and submitting proper income figures. As a lawsuit ensues, he is the one that must accept the most liability.

In addition to illustrating the unsound decisions and actions of each participant in Dr. Albright's office, this case clearly shows the impact of each person's role on that of the other people in the office. When ethical and legal principles are not followed, more than just the patient is affected. The effects snowball, and everyone becomes at risk. Many conclusions can be reached by studying this case, including the obvious importance of each member of the dental team carrying his or her own liability insurance.

CASE STUDY QUESTIONS

1. Did Ms. Casey exceed her authority? If so, how?
2. Did Ms. Smythe exceed her authority? If so, how?
3. Did Dr. Halper provide competent dental health care to Mr. Burton?
4. Is the Ohio Board of Medical Examiners the proper body to receive Mr. Burton's complaint?
5. Is the Ohio Supreme Court the proper court to take Mr. Burton's litigation? If not, name the proper court.
6. What must Mr. Burton's attorney do to secure personal jurisdiction of Dr. Albright?
7. In preparation for trial, is Mr. Burton entitled to copies of his dental records and procedures utilized by Dr. Albright in his treatment of Mr. Burton? If so, what method should be used to obtain them?
8. Is Dr. Albright entitled to a jury trial if Mr. Burton objects to a jury trial?
9. Could Dr. Albright, Ms. Casey, and Ms. Smythe lose their professional licenses? If so, by whose authority?
10. What ethical considerations does Ms. Casey have in regard to the dental receptionist's mishandling of money?

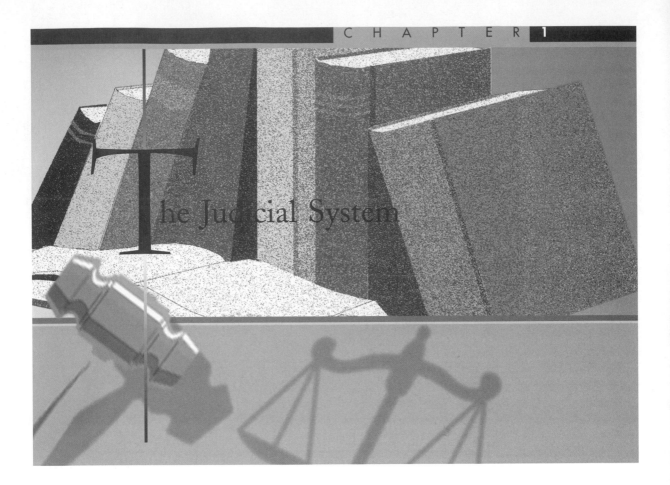

The Judicial System

LEARNING OUTCOMES

After reading this chapter, you should be able to:
- Identify the sources of law.
- Describe the federal court system.
- Describe the state court system.
- Find case law or statutory law sources.

KEY WORDS

ADJUDICATE
APPELLATE JURISDICTION
ARRAIGNMENT
CITATION
CIVIL JURISDICTION
COMMON LAW
CRIMINAL JURISDICTION
DIVERSITY OF CITIZENSHIP

FELONY
JUDICIAL CIRCUIT
LITIGANTS
MISDEMEANOR
PROBATE
QUASIJUDICIAL
STATUTES
TRIAL JURISDICTION

Ignorance of the law is not an excuse! If this statement is true (and it is), what does it mean and why is it true? Generically, law is a body of rules of action or conduct, prescribed by a controlling authority and having binding legal force.[1]

Most lawyers tend to view law as the cumulative sum of regulations and rules used in the governing of a society. Based on customs, requirements, and needs of a society, law is dynamic and flexible, not static. These characteristics will become evident in subsequent chapters. Law is a composite of federal and state statutes, procedures, and regulations, court decisions, rulings of governmental administrative agencies, and presidential edicts or executive orders.

Generally, law refers to rules made by humans, regulating social conduct in a legally binding and formal manner. Laws are derived from two sources:

1. Legislative enactments (statutes or statutory law)
2. Judicial decisions (interpret legal issues raised in court by **litigants** to a dispute and are collectively referred to as **common law)**

THE COURT SYSTEM

A dual system of courts, federal and state, makes the American legal system unique. The founding fathers provided one federal court, the U.S. Supreme Court. As required, lesser federal courts were established by Congress.

Because the Constitution did not prohibit them from doing so, the states have created courts to resolve disputes arising out of their legislative enactments, rules, and regulations. Judgments and decrees of the state courts may not take priority over those of the federal courts. State court decrees and judgments are enforced by the courts of their sister states.

The federal system of courts (Figure 1-1) consists of the following:

1. *United States Supreme Court.* The Court has nine justices with jurisdiction of an appellate nature. Decisions cannot be overturned by another court, but can be changed by congressional legislation or subsequent Supreme Court decisions. The Court accepts only cases it chooses to hear.
2. *United States Courts of Appeals.* These courts have appellate jurisdiction only.
3. *United States District Courts.* District courts have trial jurisdiction only. A U.S. District Court may accept a case if the issues involve federal law or the parties have **diversity of citizenship** (e.g., a dentist who is a resident of Texas is suing a New York business for shipping defective dental equipment). Damages alleged by a plaintiff must be no less than $75,000 in order for a case to be accepted by the court.
4. *United States Bankruptcy Courts* and *United States Tax Courts.* Both are parts of the United States District Courts.

The states' court systems (Figure 1-2) vary in makeup, generally consisting of the following:

1. *State supreme court.* This court has appellate jurisdiction only.
2. *State superior courts.* These courts have **trial, appellate, civil,** and **criminal jurisdiction.** A monetary restriction is usually associated with the jurisdic-

---

[1]*United States Fidelity and Guaranty Co. v. Guenther,* 281 U.S. 34 (1930).

LITIGANT

A party to a lawsuit.

COMMON LAW

Judge-made law or law based on court decisions.

DIVERSITY OF CITIZENSHIP

One of the criteria for jurisdiction of federal courts; the situation that exists when one party to the lawsuit is a citizen of one state and the other party is a citizen of another state or country.

TRIAL JURISDICTION

Authority of a court to hear cases only at the trial stage (as opposed to appellate jurisdiction)

APPELLATE JURISDICTION

Authority of a court to hear only cases that are on appeal, in order to review and revise judicial decisions of lower courts.

CRIMINAL JURISDICTION

Authority of a court to hear only criminal cases.

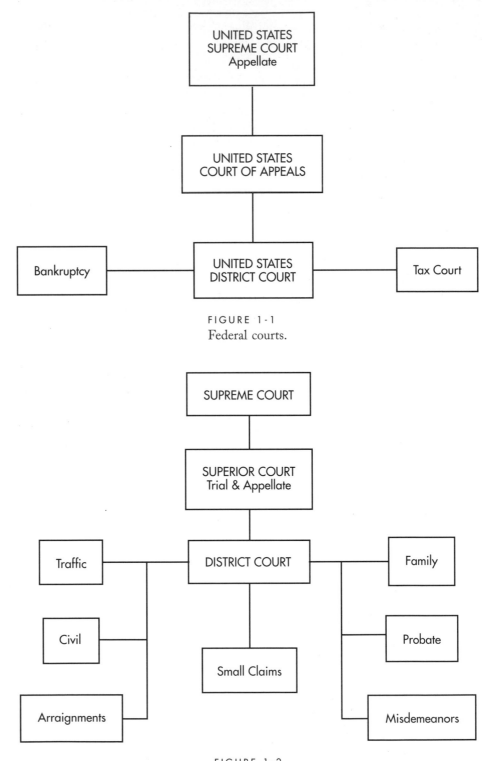

FIGURE 1-1
Federal courts.

FIGURE 1-2
State courts.

tion of these courts. An administrative court that would entertain civil actions only may be associated with a superior court. **Felonies** would be handled in the criminal division of a superior court.

3. *State district courts.* These courts have trial jurisdiction. Traffic cases, **probate,** family matters (divorce), **arraignments** for felonies, small claims, juvenile cases, and criminal **misdemeanors** would be handled. A maximum limit on the amount of money involved in a dispute varies from state to state in district courts. If a state's monetary limit is reached, the case must be initiated in a state superior court.

Generally, if a lawsuit is filed in state court against a dental health care provider, the action would be initiated in the state district court. However, if the damages claimed are in excess of the state's limit, the action would be initiated in the state superior court. After trial and if an appeal is appropriate, the case would go to the next level of appeal. Decisions from state district court would be appealed to state superior court, and decisions from state superior court to the state supreme court. (Dissatisfaction with a decision is not a basis for appeal.)

FINDING THE LAW
Statutes

As stated earlier, ignorance of the law is not an excuse. It only makes sense that we should know the law as it pertains to our needs in life. However, we must first know how and where to find the law. When we speak of the law, we are referring to **statutes.** Statutes are laws written by federal and state legislatures. Federal statutes are contained in the United States Code. The United States Code categorizes statutes by title, number, and name. For instance, Title 42 of the U.S. Code is The Public Health and Welfare. Regulations are rules written by administrative agencies (such as the federal Food and Drug Administration, FDA) to assist in executing the law. Federal regulations can be found in the Code of Federal Regulations (CFR). If you are searching for a specific agency's body of regulations, the CFR has an alphabetical list of agencies, which is printed in the back of each volume. Some states have their regulations in an administrative code and others in manuals. States organize their statutes by topic, number, or title. The state dental laws are examples. The Dental Practice Act of Wyoming begins with 35-15-101 and ends with 35-15-130. The Rules and Regulations are Chapters I to IX. In Maine, the state dental laws are found under Title 32 (Professions and Occupations), Chapter 16 (Dentists and Dental Hygienists), Subchapter 1 (General Provisions). (See Appendixes H and I.)

The easiest place to start searching for law is in the public library. Federal statutes and often state and local statutes can be located in the reference section in the majority of large public libraries. Librarians are usually helpful in providing assistance in searching for any specific law. For court cases or agency rulings (such as those of the Equal Employment Opportunity Commission) it will be necessary to locate a law library. Court "reports," which are free and open to the public, can be found in most county courthouses. Law school libraries are usually available to the public also.

FELONY

Any offense punishable by death or by imprisonment for at least one year.

PROBATE

Generally, a court established to administer estates of deceased individuals, adoptions, and name changes.

ARRAIGNMENT

Pretrial procedure whereby an accused individual is brought before a court to answer (guilty or not guilty) to a criminal charge in an indictment or information.

MISDEMEANOR

A crime punishable by less than a year in prison; a violation of the law that is less than a felony.

STATUTES

Laws enacted and written by federal or state legislatures.

Secondary Sources

Secondary sources include books and articles, such as:

1. Indest G, Egolf B: Is medicine headed for an assembly line? *Business Law Today* 6(6):32, July-August, 1997.
2. Cohen M, Berring R, Olson K: *Finding the Law*, ed 10, St Paul, 1995, West Publishing.

Secondary sources often contain citations for relevant state or federal case law or statutes. They are frequently a good way to begin your research and provide a guide to extending your search.

Primary Sources

Primary sources include state and federal laws (statutes) and cases (published decisions of state and federal courts). First, find the statute that pertains to your case and then the court case that interprets that statute. Generally, state cases reported are those of the state supreme court. On the federal level, cases reported are those decided by the United States Supreme Court and the federal appellate courts (i.e., U.S. Courts of Appeals).

When deciding the questions of law before them, judges often look to findings and conclusions of other, previously decided cases. Case law establishes precedents for later cases to follow. In the same jurisdiction, a lower court must follow the rule of law from a higher court in a like case. If a decision must be followed, it is "binding." If a decision is not binding, it is "persuasive" authority. Written judicial opinions refer to preceding cases that involve similarities or differences regarding points of law. Federal decisions vary in the weight they are given by judges deciding other cases. The most persuasive decisions, of course, are those of the highest court, the United States Supreme Court. United States Supreme Court decisions supersede all other court decisions (state and federal). Second in the hierarchy are the federal courts of appeals. Decisions of the federal appeals courts are given more weight within the courts' own **judicial circuits.** Therefore, you would want to find a decision from within the judicial circuit in which you reside. There are thirteen U.S. Courts of Appeals, eleven circuits (each with three or more states), and the District of Columbia Circuit and the Federal Circuit (Figure 1-3). The lowest level consists of decisions from the federal district courts. You would want to look for cases decided in the federal district in which you reside.

JUDICIAL CIRCUIT

One of thirteen judicial divisions in the United States (see Figure 1-3).

Researching the Law

Researching state law is similar to researching federal law, with three levels of courts. The most authoritative decisions are those from a state's supreme court or supreme judicial court; next are those from the state's appellate courts, and, finally, those from the state's trial courts.

Much legal research can now be accomplished on the Internet. Two major computer services provide legal research, Westlaw and Lexis-Nexis. These can be very expensive and are usually utilized by attorneys. There are many additional online sites, such as Lawyer's Weekly, where legal information is available.

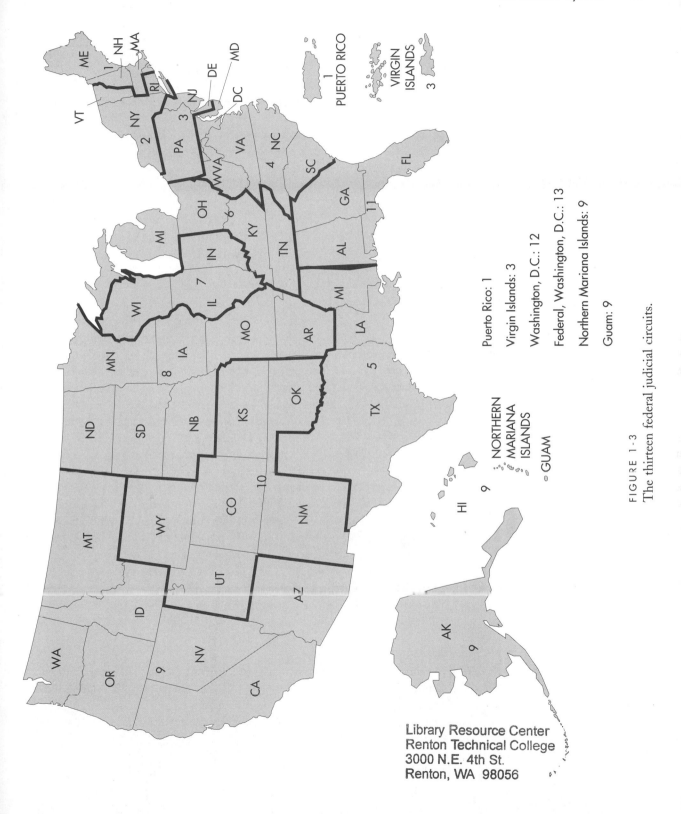

FIGURE 1-3
The thirteen federal judicial circuits.

Puerto Rico: 1

Virgin Islands: 3

Washington, D.C.: 12

Federal, Washington, D.C.: 13

Northern Mariana Islands: 9

Guam: 9

As a nation, we are a "common law" country. This means that the law of the nation must be seen as an evolving body of court decisions made by judges on the basis of cases they hear, which have the effect of law and are binding upon us. Accordingly, printed judicial opinions are considered a primary source of the law because they represent the law. Statutes are also a primary source, as they are also authoritative and binding.

Administrative law is a third important source of law. Agency regulations are similar in form to statutes but frequently more detailed. Agencies conduct hearings to address individual grievances or **adjudicate** particular disputes, and thus they act in a **quasijudicial** capacity. (See Finding the Law, supra.)

Often there is a need to research a court case on the basis of the subject matter. The most comprehensive case digest system is the West Publishing Company's key number system, whereby the reported cases are arranged alphabetically by subject classification. All cases are published in chronological order.

Citations

In order to find cases, we must first understand the components of a **citation,** the name given to a case, and where it is reported. There is a uniform system of citation, which includes the names of the parties, the volume number, where the case is reported, the page number, and the year of the opinion.

This is true whether you are researching federal law or state law. For federal law, if the case is decided by the United States Supreme Court, it can be found in either *United States Reports* (U.S.) or the *Supreme Court Reporter* (S.Ct.). If the case is a federal case decided by a lower federal court, it can be located in the *Federal Reporter* (F.3d). Cases may be located in either F., F.2d, or F.3d series. F.3d is where current law is located. Federal cases are also found in the *Federal Supplement* (F. Supp.).

For instance, consider the case of *Meritor Savings Bank v.* (versus) *Vinson*, 477 U.S. 57 (1986). This is a case between two parties, as opposed to the government and a party; therefore, it is a civil case, and it was decided by the United States Supreme Court in 1986. It may be found in the 477th volume of *United States Reports* (U.S.) at page 57.

Abraham v. Exxon Corporation, 85 F.3d 1126 (5th Cir. 1996), is a federal civil case decided by the Fifth Circuit Court of Appeals in 1996. It may be found in the 85th volume of the *Federal Reporter*, third series, at page 1126. This case was not appealed to the United States Supreme Court.

State Reports

States usually publish their own official state reports. All published state court decisions can be located in the West Reporter System. The country is divided into seven regions. All decisions of a state's supreme and appellate courts are published in its regional reporter. There are first and second series for the reporters in all regions. These regions and reporters are as follows:

1. A. and A.2d *(Atlantic Reporter)* includes court decisions from Connecticut, Delaware, the District of Columbia, Maine, Maryland, New Hampshire, New Jersey, Pennsylvania, Rhode Island, and Vermont.

ADJUDICATE

To make a final determination of issues through court action; to settle by judicial decree.

QUASIJUDICIAL

Relating to judicial action of an administrative officer or body (such as the board of dental examiners) rather than a judge.

CITATION

A reference to legal authority, such as reported case law or statutes.

2. N.E. and N.E.2d *(Northeastern Reporter)* includes court decisions from New York, Illinois, Indiana, Massachusetts, and Ohio.

3. N.W. and N.W.2d *(Northwestern Reporter)* includes court decisions from Iowa, Michigan, Minnesota, Nebraska, North Dakota, South Dakota, and Wisconsin.

4. P. and P.2d *(Pacific Reporter)* includes court decisions from Alaska, Arizona, California, Colorado, Hawaii, Idaho, Kansas, Montana, Nevada, New Mexico, Oklahoma, Oregon, Utah, Washington, and Wyoming.

5. S.E. and S.E.2d *(Southeastern Reporter)* includes court decisions from Georgia, North Carolina, South Carolina, Virginia, and West Virginia.

6. S.W. and SW.2d *(Southwestern Reporter)* includes decisions from Arkansas, Kentucky, Missouri, Tennessee, and Texas.

7. S. and S.2d *(Southern Reporter)* includes decisions from Alabama, Florida, Louisiana, and Mississippi.

8. Cal. Rptr. *(California Reporter)* includes appellate decisions from California, and N.Y.S. *(New York Supplement)* includes appellate decisions from New York.

For instance, *Bundy v. State of Florida*, 471 S.2d 9 (1985), is a Florida case. Since the state of Florida is a party, we know that this is a criminal case in which Bundy is appealing a decision (conviction) that was in favor of the State of Florida in the lower court. It may be found in volume 471 of the *South Second Reporter* at page 9. The case was decided in 1985.

State v. Hoffman, 733 P.2d 502 (Utah 1987), is a criminal case decided in 1987 in the state of Utah. It can be found in the 733rd volume of the *Pacific Second Reporter* at page 502.

American Law Reports

Annotations on specific legal topics are contained in *American Law Reports*, known as ALR. Annotations on United States Supreme Court decisions are contained in *United States Supreme Court Reports* and *Lawyer's Edition*. Each has its own citation system. For example, *U.S. v. Cores*, 356 U.S. 405, 2 L. Ed.2d, 873 (1958), is a federal criminal action decided in 1958. It can be found in the 356th volume of *United States Reports* at page 405. It can also be found in volume 2 of the *Lawyer's Edition, Second Reporter,* at page 873.

Additional Sources

Additional secondary sources for legal research are legal encyclopedias, *American Jurisprudence* (cited as Am. Jur.), and *Corpus Juris Secundum* (cited as C.J.S.). Material in encyclopedias is organized by subject matter alphabetically. Another resource is the West Digest System, which publishes case summaries. These summaries are arranged by topic. There are federal and state digests. Each topic includes citations for pertinent statutes or case law.

Law review articles, written by lawyers, law professors, and law students, contain information on a variety of legal topics. Law review articles are often cited in other publications. Citations for law review articles are similar to citations for case law. An example would be 65 Temp. L. Rev. 459 (1992). If we looked in volume 65 of the *Temple Law Review*, at page 459, we would find an article by W. John Thomas entitled "The Medical Malpractice 'Crisis': A Critical Examination of a Public Debate," published in 1992.

Changes in Statutes

Finally, the law is constantly changing, and you will need to know whether your research has produced current law. Changes in a statute are found in the back of the book in which you find the statute. The back of the book contains a pocket that holds "pocket parts," which provide all updates on the statutes found in that particular volume. Case law is updated daily. Shepard's Citation System provides such information for case law. Shepard's lists every reference to a particular case. By utilizing this system, you can find cases that agree with the findings in the case you are researching or cases that disagree in part or in whole with the case you are researching.

Helpful Sources for Reading Legal Documents

Reading legal documents is like reading dental documents; to the lay person, both are like reading a foreign language. By now you have mastered the basics of dental terminology. However, a law dictionary is an essential resource when you are researching the law. *Black's Law Dictionary* is probably the most used law dictionary. It contains definitions of legal terminology, an extensive table of abbreviations used in legal publications, and a reprint of United States Constitution. West Publishing Co. publishes *Black's*. Another publication that may be of assistance in clarifying legal terminology is *Legal Thesaurus*, by William C. Burton, published by Macmillan Publishing Co.

Common Terms: Infra versus Supra

The terms *infra* and *supra* are used frequently in legal documents or legal citations. Infra ("below") refers to a section of the reading that has not yet been mentioned but is within the writing. Supra ("above") is the opposite; it refers to a preceding section of the reading, such as a citation. For example, if a reference has been made in a text to the case *Jones v. Smith*, 243 U.S. 15, and a later reference is made to the same case, it is sufficient to state "see *Jones*, supra," as opposed to giving the entire citation.

Also, when sections of a particular writing are referred to in a text, the proper designation for a section is § and the plural (sections) is referred to as §§.

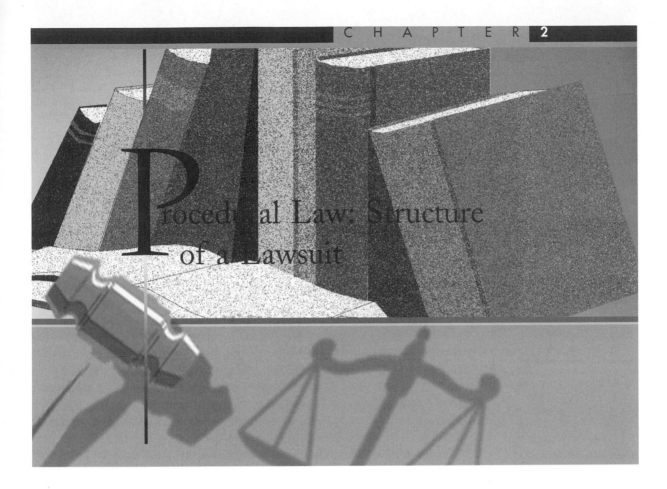

Procedural Law: Structure of a Lawsuit

LEARNING OUTCOMES

After reading this chapter, you should be able to:
- Describe general procedures followed in a lawsuit.
- List three means of discovery.
- Determine when it is appropriate to appeal a court's decision.
- Explain what summary judgment is, and recognize when it is granted.

KEY WORDS

AFFIDAVIT
AFFIRMATIVE DEFENSE
ALLEGATION
ANSWER
APPEAL
APPELLATE REVIEW
CAUSE OF ACTION
COMPLAINT
CONFLICT OF INTEREST
CONTEMPT OF COURT
DEFENDANT
DEPOSITION
DISCOVERY
IMPANEL
INTERROGATORIES
JUDGMENT
JURISDICTION
LONG ARM STATUTES
MOTION

NOTICE
PARTY
PERSONAL JURISDICTION
PLAINTIFF
PLEADINGS
PREEMPTORY CHALLENGE
PRIMA FACIE CASE
PROCESS
REQUESTS FOR ADMISSIONS
SANCTIONS
STATUTE OF LIMITATIONS
SUBJECT MATTER JURISDICTION
SUMMARY JUDGMENT
TERRITORIAL JURISDICTION
TORT
TRIAL
VENUE
VOIR DIRE

An injured **party,** or **plaintiff,** determines that he or she has a **cause of action** against another individual, or **defendant.** This determination is based on the facts of the situation and the rights and duties of each party. A lawsuit is initiated to resolve the controversy between the parties. Rules of procedure have been established to ensure orderliness and fairness. The plaintiff or the defendant may be an individual, a corporation, a partnership, or another legally recognized entity.

JURISDICTION

For a final judgment of the court to be valid, the parties must have adequate notice, the court must have territorial jurisdiction over the parties, and the court must have jurisdiction over the subject matter of the lawsuit as well as personal jurisdiction of the parties.

Notice

Notice is provided by service of process. Service of process occurs when a summons orders the defendant to appear in court at the risk of losing a judgment by default. Under most rules of court (state and federal) the summons must be delivered with a copy of the complaint. The clerk of court issues the summons, which may be served on an individual in several ways: it may be served by sheriff (state court) or by U.S. marshall (federal court), and it may be served personally or left at the home of the defendant. Mailing these documents is becoming more popular in civil matters.

Territorial Jurisdiction

Territorial jurisdiction is determined by a body of rules that operate between states to determine the authority of the courts in the respective states. If the basis of a lawsuit and the parties to that lawsuit are all from one state, territorial jurisdiction is not an issue.

Historically, a state court could have **jurisdiction** only if the person or thing involved in litigation was within the borders of the state. States now have **long arm statutes** to gain jurisdiction over individuals outside their borders. Out-of-state businesses are subject to the jurisdiction of the courts of states in which they do business.

A state court cannot render a **judgment** over a controversy involving land in another state, as the court would have no way to enforce its decree with respect to the land. The principle of **personal jurisdiction** requires the court to have authority to determine rights and duties of the parties, including the power to bind the parties personally. Personal jurisdiction is obtained by one of the following:

1. Service of **process** upon a resident
2. Service upon a nonresident while he or she is in the state
3. Service by certified mail in certain civil cases
4. The defendant's consent to jurisdiction if the court has no personal jurisdiction

Subject Matter Jurisdiction: State Courts

The proper state court in which to bring a lawsuit must be determined by the subject matter of the controversy. Most states have several levels of courts (see Figure 1-2, p. 8). **Subject matter jurisdiction** for each type of court is defined by statute and varies from state to state; it is often determined on the basis of the type of legal issue involved or the amount of money in question (amount of damages claimed).

Subject Matter Jurisdiction: Federal Courts

The federal courts are restricted by the U.S. Constitution to hearing very specialized cases (such as controversies over patents) or cases presenting issues under the U.S. Constitution, federal laws, or treaties. Federal courts also have jurisdiction over cases involving citizens of different states and involving a certain amount of money. Both criteria must be met: diversity of citizenship (plaintiff and defendant must reside in different states) and the amount of money in controversy must be at least $75,000.

VENUE

After identifying the proper court, the plaintiff must determine **venue,** or the proper place or location within the state to bring the lawsuit (i.e., county or municipality). For example, if subject matter jurisdiction dictates that a district court will hear the case, the district court of which county in the state will hear the case must then be determined. Venue is determined by one or more of the following:

1. Location of the subject matter
2. Residence of one of the parties
3. Location of the defendant's place of business
4. Where the cause of action arose
5. Where the plaintiff chooses

The defendant may request a change of venue.

PLEADINGS

Generally, **pleadings** are the **complaint** by the plaintiff and the defendant's answer. The plaintiff's lawyer files a complaint with the proper court. The complaint and a summons (notice to the defendant) are served on the defendant. The law prescribes various methods by which these documents may be served. The usual procedure is in person or by mail in certain civil actions. The plaintiff's complaint must state a valid claim under the law for which the law permits recovery, or the complaint is defective and may be objected to by the defendant.

In addition, the facts of the case must be sufficient to satisfy the requirements of the rule of law. The complaint should set forth alleged facts to support the claim. The complaint must allege adequate facts regarding the claim to set forth a **prima facie case** (i.e., the facts alleged would permit the plaintiff's recovery absent a defendant's affirmative defense). The court will permit the plaintiff to amend the complaint in response to the defendant's objections. The defendant must answer

---

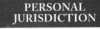

LONG ARM STATUTES

State statutes that enable a state court to gain personal jurisdiction, for limited purposes, over a business or individual who is a nonresident.

JUDGMENT

The official decision of a court.

PERSONAL JURISDICTION

The authority of a court over a person (defendant), as opposed to jurisdiction of a court over the person's property.

PROCESS

In law, a summons and a complaint and related documents served upon a defendant in a lawsuit.

SUBJECT MATTER JURISDICTION

Authority of a court to hear cases of a particular type or cases relating to a specific subject matter. For instance, bankruptcy court has the authority to only hear bankruptcy cases.

VENUE

Geographical location where a trial is held.

PLEADINGS

Claims and defenses formally made by parties of a lawsuit. Examples would be complaints and answers (see Figures 2-2 and 2-3).

COMPLAINT

A claim for relief that initiates a lawsuit.

PRIMA FACIE CASE

A lawsuit in which facts or evidence can be judged from first sight, unless disproved by some other contradictory evidence.

the complaint by alleging specific admissions, denials, and defenses to the plaintiff's complaint. The defendant may admit certain facts made in the complaint and deny others. If facts are not denied, they will be held as admissions. The defendant may also allege affirmative defenses. An **affirmative defense** is a new matter, not stated by the plaintiff in the complaint, that may be proved to avoid a claim. In such a case, even if the allegations in the complaint were true, the plaintiff would not prevail, because of the affirmative defense. Affirmative defenses must be pleaded in the defendant's answer. An example of an affirmative defense would be the lack of personal jurisdiction over the defendant. The plaintiff could, then, raise issues concerning defects in the defendant's answer. Another affirmative defense would be the **statute of limitations,** which does not allow legal action to be initiated unless it is done within a specific time period. That time period is measured from the time the cause of action arose to the filing of the complaint.

DISCOVERY

After the pleading process is complete, **discovery** begins. Discovery permits both parties (the defendant and the plaintiff) to know as many facts relating to the dispute as possible. Each has an opportunity to question the opposing party and all witnesses prior to trial. A number of discovery devices are utilized, primarily oral examination and written questions directed to a party or a witness.

Deposition

A **deposition** is the testimony that results from the oral examination of a witness, under oath, out of court. A court reporter records the proceedings. A party may have its lawyer present during the deposition. The party being deposed is subject to examination and cross-examination by the opposing party. Depositions are taken to obtain information and are generally not admissible at trial. An exception may be made in the event of the death of the witness deposed.

Interrogatories

Interrogatories are written questions from one party to another that require written responses. Interrogatories may be addressed only to a party (plaintiff or defendant) to the action. The party must answer or object to each interrogatory within a specified time. A more complete answer may be required if the response is evasive or incomplete. Interrogatories must be under oath and signed.

Requests for Admissions

Requests for admissions are requests made by one party to the other to admit facts that are not in doubt. The responding party may admit or deny each fact. If a fact is denied and then proved to be true in court, the party denying could be liable for the cost of proving the alleged fact.

Inspection of Real Evidence

Real evidence in possession of one party may be inspected, copied, tested, or sampled by the other party. For instance, if a patient's dental treatment is at issue, the dental record is real evidence.

Medical Examinations

If the physical or medical condition of a party is an issue, the court may order that party to submit to an examination by experts employed by other parties or the court.

Scope of Discovery

Discovery may extend to all information that is relevant to the subject matter of the lawsuit, whether or not it is admissible in court. Certain information is protected against disclosure and is said to be privileged (e.g., communication between spouses, physician-patient communication).

Sanctions

Failure to comply with a court order to answer a discovery request may result in a finding of contempt of court against the noncomplying party. **Contempt of court** may result in incarceration and/or the imposition of fines, costs of court, and expenses of the other party.

PRETRIAL CONFERENCE

Just before **trial,** a pretrial conference is held. Attorneys for each party meet with the judge to decide what issues remain for trial and whether a settlement prior to trial is possible.

The Seventh Amendment to the U.S. Constitution gives everyone the right to a jury trial (as opposed to trial by a judge), and in many types of cases either party may choose a jury trial. A party must demand a jury trial, or the right is waived.

SUMMARY JUDGMENT

"Summary judgment shall enter, if when viewing the evidence in the light most favorable to the non-movant, the court determines that there is no genuine issue of material fact and the movant is entitled to judgment as a matter of law."[1]

A written **motion** for **summary judgment** may be made by either party prior to or during trial. A motion for summary judgment alleges that a fact is true that would decide the case in favor of the moving party. If the opposing party does not file a counter-motion and if the judge finds for the first party, he or she will grant summary judgment for that party and the lawsuit is ended without the expense of a full trial.

Summary judgment is granted when there is "no genuine issue of fact and, on the basis of the undisputed facts, the movant is entitled to judgment as a matter of law." This is the rule of evidence as stated in the Federal Rules of Evidence, Rule 56. (Note that the quote from the Kodak case, supra, is a judicial interpretation of this rule. Case law generally consists of interpretations of laws, rules, and regulations.) A motion for summary judgment must be in writing and may be based on admissions made by the parties in the pleadings, answers to interrogatories, or depositions. **Affidavits** of personal knowledge of facts are also admissible.

REQUESTS FOR ADMISSIONS
Requests for written statements of fact presented to an adverse party. That party must admit or deny these statements (see Figure 2-5).

SANCTIONS
Penalties imposed for violating the law or failure to comply with a court order.

CONTEMPT OF COURT
Any act designed to obstruct the administration of justice.

TRIAL
A court's examination of facts and resolving of issues between parties to a lawsuit (criminal or civil).

MOTION
An application to a court or judge in order to obtain a rule or order directing an act to be done in favor of the applicant.

SUMMARY JUDGMENT
A motion made by either party to a lawsuit that may be granted by the court when there is no real issue of fact and the moving party is entitled to judgment.

AFFIDAVIT
A written statement of facts made under oath.

---

[1]*Eastman Kodak Co. v. Image Technical Services, Inc.*, 504 U.S. 451 (1992).

VOIR DIRE

A process by which the court examines jurors or witnesses to determine their ability to participate in the trial.

CONFLICT OF INTEREST

The situation that exists when there is discord between an individual's public duty and his or her private monetary interest.

PREEMPTORY CHALLENGE

The privilege or right of each party to a lawsuit to request deletion of specific jurors during jury selection, without having to give a reason.

IMPANEL

To accomplish the entire process of jury selection, to final selection of those jurors who will sit for a specific case.

APPEAL

To submit a lawsuit to a superior court or an appellate court to review the decision of a lower trial court or administrative agency.

APPELLATE REVIEW

Review of a lower court's proceedings by an appellate court.

If evidence shows a genuine issue as to any material fact, the motion for summary judgment must be denied. Summary judgment may be granted in part—that is, on a specific claim or issue.

TRIAL

Cases are tried before a jury if a jury trial is requested by either party. Some cases are tried before a judge or judges only. Jury selection is conducted by the lawyers and/or the judge and is called a **voir dire** examination. The selection of specific jurors can be challenged if there is a **conflict of interest,** or a few may be disqualified for any reason, which is called a **preemptory challenge.** After completion of jury selection, the jury is said to be **impaneled.**

The attorney for each party presents opening statements that describe the case and explain what he or she will attempt to prove. The attorney for the plaintiff begins by presenting his or her case-in-chief. The plaintiff has the burden of proving the statements made in the complaint. The burden of proof required by law must be met on each element necessary to prove the claim. In civil cases that burden is usually "preponderance of the evidence," meaning that the evidence is more convincing than the evidence presented by the other party. In criminal cases the burden of proof is "beyond a reasonable doubt," as criminal cases have more serious implications. If a defendant is found guilty of a criminal offense, the punishment may be incarceration or, in some instances, the death penalty.

The plaintiff presents witnesses and other evidence to prove his or her case. The defendant then cross-examines the witnesses. Next, the defendant presents his or her case-in-chief by attempting to prove his or her defenses. The plaintiff has an opportunity to cross-examine the witnesses for the defense.

Both parties have an opportunity to make concluding statements after all witnesses and evidence have been presented. Here, each point favorable to its case and unfavorable to the opposing party is presented. The plaintiff has the last statement or closing argument. The judge will provide instructions to the jury as to issues of law, burdens of proof, and so forth. The jury deliberates and makes a decision, and the court then renders a final judgment. **Appeals** may be made after final judgment.

APPELLATE REVIEW

An appellate court reviews the case for errors that may have affected the outcome of the judgment. The appellate court does not retry the case, but may reverse the trial court's decision or send the case back to the trial court to be retried if it finds an error in law or inadequate evidence to support the trial court's finding. The appellate court will consider objections of the parties only if those objections were made during the trial court proceedings. After an appeal is accepted by an appellate court, the trial court has no further jurisdiction of the case.

REVIEW OF STRUCTURE OF A LAWSUIT

A lawsuit is the process by which a court resolves conflicts among people over a specific matter. Procedural problems within that lawsuit can be complex. This chapter explains some of these complexities. Perhaps an example of a specific case will clarify the process.

Let us say that Dr. Bill Allen, who resides in Fremont, California, purchases dental equipment from the local dental equipment dealer, Fremont Dental, owned by Jack Bailey. ABC Dental, a Massachusetts corporation whose manufacturing plant and principal place of business are in Medford, Massachusetts, manufactured the equipment.

While Dr. Allen is using the high-speed handpiece, the equipment malfunctions, causing a fire in the operatory and badly injuring him.. It is obvious to Dr. Allen that his injuries are a result of this defective equipment; however, neither Fremont Dental nor ABC Dental will assume responsibility. What does Dr. Allen do to bring a lawsuit to recover for his damages?

Dr. Allen's first step would be to find an attorney who will investigate the facts and act on Dr. Allen's behalf. In this case the attorney would look to the law of contracts, since there was a contractual relationship between Dr. Allen and Fremont Dental, and to the law of **torts,** since there may be negligence or strict liability involved, to determine if either Fremont Dental or ABC Dental has a legal responsibility to pay Dr. Allen for his injuries. Dr. Allen bought the equipment from Fremont Dental, so there is a sales contract between the two parties. Was the equipment defective? And if it was, what are the damages? Do damages include the price of the equipment, Dr. Allen's physical injuries, and other expenses? Did ABC Dental have a duty to Dr. Allen?

After Dr. Allen's attorney researches the accident, he informs Dr. Allen of the following:

1. Fremont Dental had a contractual duty to Dr. Allen to deliver equipment to him that was free from defects.
2. Fremont Dental breached its contractual duty. Therefore, Fremont Dental is legally responsible for the cost of the equipment and Dr. Allen's injuries.
3. ABC Dental had a duty under the law of torts to provide Dr. Allen with equipment free from defects.
4. ABC Dental breached its duty to Dr. Allen and is legally responsible for the cost of the equipment and Dr. Allen's injuries.

TORT

A civil wrong or injury, other than a breach of contract, for which the plaintiff is compensated monetarily (should the plaintiff prevail) for the unreasonable harm he or she has sustained. An example of such a wrong is negligence (see Chapter 4).

Jurisdiction

The first issue that needs to be addressed is jurisdiction. Can Dr. Allen obtain jurisdiction over Fremont Dental and/or ABC Dental? Generally, a company located within a state is subject to the jurisdiction of the courts of that state. The state of California has jurisdiction over Fremont Dental. But what about an out-of-state business such as ABC Dental? Most states have statutes that authorize out-of-state service of process under specific conditions. In this case ABC Dental was doing business in California; therefore, it is subject to the jurisdiction of the California courts.

The next issue to be addressed is which court in California has jurisdiction over the subject matter of the lawsuit. We look first to the trial courts. Dr. Allen should estimate his total damages to determine which trial court should hear the case. If

Dr. Allen's injuries cost him more than the amount allowed in district court, his action would be filed in superior court.

Dr. Allen, through his attorney, would draw up the complaint or statement of claim or allegations against the defendants. In the complaint Dr. Allen would describe who he is, who the defendants are, what happened to him, and why he believes he is entitled to recover a judgment against the defendants. Before filing the complaint, Dr. Allen must determine venue. Since each county has a superior court, in which county should the complaint be filed? Generally, the proper county is where the defendant resides. Since Jack Bailey is the owner of Fremont Dental, he would be the defendant and the county in which he resides would determine venue. The complaint is then filed with the clerk of the superior court. A summons is then served on the defendants to notify them of the suit. The summons is served with a copy of the complaint.

In this case, when the complaint is filed, Dr. Allen must also give the clerk a summons, containing the names of the parties and a notice to the defendants that they must come and defend themselves in court. Since there are two defendants, two copies of the complaint and summons for each defendant are necessary. The clerk puts the court's seal on the summons, making it official notice. Dr. Allen must now hire a process server to make service of the summons and complaint on the defendants. The process server would go to Fremont Dental and personally hand Mr. Bailey a copy of the summons and a copy of the complaint. The process server then endorses the back of the original summons to indicate that service was made and returns it to the court. This is called "return of service." If this process is done properly, the court acquires jurisdiction over Mr. Bailey. Mr. Bailey then contacts his attorney, who will respond with a defense of this action. What about ABC Dental? Its place of business and incorporation is in Massachusetts. In this case, copies of the summons and complaint would be sent to the Massachusetts Secretary of State with directions to deliver the documents to ABC Dental. (Some states require that the plaintiff obtain a court order directing that a substitute service be made to the corporation). The California superior court would obtain jurisdiction over ABC Dental if this procedure were completed properly.

Pleadings

ANSWER

The formal written statement made by a defendant giving the grounds for his or her defense.

Fremont Dental and ABC Dental will then submit an **answer,** a pleading responding to factual matters in the plaintiff's claim. There are various defenses that either may raise. The following are a few common considerations in developing a defense to a lawsuit. First, the complaint must state a claim that, if proved in court, would entitle the plaintiff to recover damages. In this case, the law of torts recognizes that a manufacturer of goods is liable for damages to any person whom the manufacturer could foresee would be injured by a defect in the goods. If Dr. Allen's complaint describes a situation that falls under that rule of law, the claim is sufficient. Dr. Allen must allege that the equipment was defective, that his injury was caused by the defect, and that as a purchaser of this equipment, it was foreseeable that he would be harmed by a defect in the equipment.

Denials are negative defenses. A defendant may also have affirmative defenses. ABC Dental may claim that Dr. Allen was negligent in the manner in which he had the equipment installed or in the manner in which he used the equipment. Should the court find Dr. Allen to be contributorily negligent, that finding could reduce the amount he could recover or be a bar to any recovery.

Discovery

What discovery tool would be most helpful to the Plaintiff, Dr. Allen? Depositions may be taken from the defendants as well as witnesses. Suppose Dr. Allen knew of another dentist who had similar problems with the same equipment, but was unable to attend the trial as a witness. Dr. Allen's attorney would depose this individual. Lawyers for both parties and a court reporter would be present at a deposition. Dr. Allen will undoubtedly utilize interrogatories to gain more information. He may want to know the names of specific employees or the names of managers of specific departments at ABC Dental. He may want to know some details of the manufacturing process itself. ABC Dental may wish to depose Dr. Allen regarding the manner in which he was operating the equipment. It may wish to depose Dr. Allen's dental assistant regarding care and maintenance of the equipment. It may also include questions in interrogatories to Dr. Allen about who installed the equipment, and then depose the individual who performed the installation.

A motion for summary judgment can be made anytime after the complaint is filed. For instance, there could be a clause in the contract between Mr. Bailey and Dr. Allen that would relieve Mr. Bailey of liability. The judge could conclude that there was no issue of genuine fact and grant Mr. Bailey's motion for summary judgment. Let us assume that the judge grants summary judgment to Mr. Bailey as owner of Fremont Dental.

Trial

Let us assume that ABC Dental, however, demands a jury trial. The first task would be jury selection. During the voir dire examination it is discovered that one potential juror is a dentist. ABC Dental could exercise its preemptory challenge and disqualify the juror. As it turns out, another juror is one of Dr. Allen's patients. That juror would be challenged for cause.

After the attorneys for Dr. Allen and ABC Dental present their opening arguments, each puts forth his case-in-chief. Dr. Allen has the burden of proving the matters asserted in the complaint. Dr. Allen will testify with regard to the incident and his injuries. His physician will testify as to his injuries. Dr. Allen's witnesses may include other individuals having difficulty with the same equipment, Dr. Allen's service and maintenance person, the director of ABC Dental's quality assurance department, and so forth.. Each witness is subject to direct examination and cross-examination by the opposing party. After Dr. Allen's attorney rests, ABC Dental's attorney may continue with his case-in-chief or move for a dismissal if he feels the plaintiff's case is not strong enough. If the motion were denied, ABC Dental's attorney would proceed. His witnesses could include: a medical expert who might allege that Dr. Allen's injuries were not as severe as he claimed, any witness who could demonstrate that Dr. Allen was negligent in his operation of the equipment, or a witness who would show that the equipment was damaged during shipment and was not defective when it left ABC Dental. After ABC Dental pre-

Text continued on p. 28

STATE OF CALIFORNIA
Alameda,   ss.

SUPERIOR COURT
Civil Action
Docket No. 99-178

William Allen,
          Plaintiff   }

    vs.   }   SUMMONS

Jack Bailey
d/b/a Fremont Dental
       &   }
ABC Dental, Inc.,   }
          Defendants }

To the Defendants

The Plaintiff has begun a lawsuit against you in this Court. If you wish to oppose this lawsuit, you or your attorney must prepare and serve a written Answer to the attached Complaint within 20 days from the day this summons was served upon you. You or your attorney must serve your Answer by delivering it in person or by mail to the Plaintiff's attorney, or the Plaintiff, whose name and address appear below. You or your attorney must also file your Answer by mailing it to the office of the Clerk of the Superior Court, 18 Federal Street, Fremont before or within a reasonable time after it is served.

IMPORTANT WARNING: IF YOU FAIL TO SERVE AN ANSWER WITHIN THE TIME STATED ABOVE, OR IF, AFTER YOU ANSWER, YOU FAIL TO APPEAR AT ANY TIME THE COURT NOTIFIES YOU TO DO SO, A JUDGEMENT BY DEFAULT MAY BE ENTERED AGAINST YOU IN YOUR ABSENCE FOR THE MONEY DAMAGES OR OTHER RELIEF DEMANDED IN THE COMPLAINT. IF THIS OCCURS, YOUR EMPLOYER MAY BE ORDERED TO PAY PART OF YOUR WAGES TO THE PLAINTIFF, OR YOUR PERSONAL PROPERTY, INCLUDING BANK ACCOUNTS AND YOUR REAL ESTATE MAY BE TAKEN TO SATISFY THE JUDGMENT. IF YOU INTEND TO OPPOSE THIS LAWSUIT, DO NOT FAIL TO ANSWER WITHIN THE REQUIRED TIME.

If you believe the Plaintiff is not entitled to all or part of the claim set forth in the Complaint, or if you believe you have a claim against the Plaintiff, you should talk to a lawyer, you may ask the Clerk for information as to places where you may seek legal assistance.

Dated: August 4, 1999
Kenneth Emmons, Esq.
Attorney for Plaintiff
108 Main Street
Fremont, CA. 90112
(512) 389-2211

Jenifer Tisdale, Clerk
Superior Court
Served on_____

_____
Deputy Sheriff

FIGURE 2-1
Summons.

STATE OF CALIFORNIA	SUPERIOR COURT
Alameda, ss.	Civil Action
	Docket No. 99-178

William Allen,	}	
Plaintiff	}	
vs.	}	COMPLAINT
	}	
Jack Bailey	}	
d/b/a Fremont Dental	}	
&	}	
ABC Dental, Inc.,	}	
Defendants	}	

NOW COMES Plaintiff, by and through counsel, and states:

1. That on or about May 9, 1999, Plaintiff purchased certain dental equipment from Defendant Jack Bailey d/b/a Fremont Dental, all as listed on Schedule A annexed hereto.

2. Said dental equipment was manufactured by Defendant, ABC Dental, Inc., a corporation doing business and existing under the laws of the Commonwealth of Massachusetts.

3. While operating said equipment, according to the manual, it malfunctioned, causing a fire and damage to Plaintiff's property and injury to Plaintiff.

4. The negligence of Defendants in the manufacture and the sale of said equipment was the proximate cause of Plaintiff's injury and property damage.

WHEREFORE, Plaintiff demands judgment against Defendants in the amount of $55,000.00, sufficient to fairly and reasonably compensate him for all past and future damage plus costs and counsel fees and for such other relief as to the court may seem just.

Dated: August 10, 1999

                                      _____
Kenneth Emmons, Esq.
Attorney for Plaintiff
108 Main Street
Fremont, CA. 90112
(512) 389-2211

FIGURE 2-2
Complaint.

STATE OF CALIFORNIA   SUPERIOR COURT
Alameda,   ss.   Civil Action
                                                  Docket No. 99-178

William Allen,   }
            Plaintiff   }
                                  }
        vs.   }   ANSWER
                                  }
Jack Bailey   }
d/b/a Fremont Dental   }
        &   }
ABC Dental, Inc.,   }
            Defendants   }

NOW COMES Defendant, Jack Bailey, by and through counsel, and admits, denies, and alleges as follows:

1.   This Defendant admits the allegations contained in Paragraphs 1 and 2 of Plaintiff's Complaint.

2.   Answering Paragraph 3 of Plaintiff's Complaint, this Defendant lacks information or knowledge sufficient to form a belief as to the truth or falsity of the allegations contained therein, and therefore, denies the same.

3.   This Defendant denies the allegations contained in Paragraph 4 of Plaintiff's Complaint.

WHEREFORE, having fully answered Plaintiff's Complaint, this Defendant asks the Court to enter judgment in favor of this Defendant and against the Plaintiff and award Defendant his costs.

Dated: August 28, 1999   _____
                                               Joseph Campbell, Esq.
                                               Attorney for Defendant
                                               Jack Bailey
                                               2 Hoover Boulevard
                                               Fremont, CA. 90112
                                               (512) 389-5680

FIGURE 2-3
Answer.

STATE OF CALIFORNIA   SUPERIOR COURT
Alameda,   ss.   Civil Action
                                            Docket No. 99-178

William Allen,   }
                    Plaintiff   }   DEFENDANT JACK BAILEY d/b/a
                                        }   FREMONT DENTAL'S
        vs.   }   INTERROGATORIES PROPOUNDED
                                        }   UPON THE PLAINTIFF
                                        }
Jack Bailey   }
d/b/a Fremont Dental   }
        &   }
ABC Dental, Inc.,   }
                    Defendants   }

Pursuant to rules 80(f) and 33 of the California Rules of Civil Procedure, the Defendant Jack
Bailey hereby requests that the Plaintiff, William Allen, answer under oath and in
accordance with said Rule 33, the Interrogatories below within thirty (30) days of their
service upon said Plaintiff.

Pursuant to Rules 80(f) and 34 of the California Rules of Civil Procedure, the Defendant also
requests that the Plaintiff produce for inspection and copying all of the documents requested
herein and all of the documents identified in the Plaintiff's contemplated answers to these
interrogatories. The Plaintiff or the Plaintiff's attorney may submit copies of all said items
together with the answers to these interrogatories.

1.   What is your full name, home address, business address, date of birth, and social
      security number?

2.   Please state if you purchased certain dental equipment from Defendant. If so, list the
      date, cost, and description of said equipment; and, whether you purchased said
      equipment as new or used?

3.   Please describe how said equipment malfunctioned.

4.   What property was damaged, if any, and the cost of each item damaged and the
      extent of damage to each such item. Please describe the nature of your injuries.

Dated: August 11, 1999   _____
                                            Joseph Campbell, Esq.
                                            Attorney for Jack Bailey
                                            2 Hoover Boulevard
                                            Fremont, CA. 90112
                                            (512) 389-5680

FIGURE 2-4
Interrogatories.

STATE OF CALIFORNIA
Alameda,   ss.

SUPERIOR COURT
Civil Action
Docket No. 99-178

William Allen,
                Plaintiff   }
                                    }
    vs.   }
                                    }
Jack Bailey   }
d/b/a Fremont Dental   }
        &   }
ABC Dental, Inc.,   }
                Defendants   }

PLAINTIFF'S REQUEST FOR
ADMISSION TO DEFENDANT
JACK BAILEY

Pursuant to Rule 18 of the California Rules of Civil Procedure, Plaintiff requests Defendant Jack Bailey to make the following admissions within 30 days. Such admissions are made only for the purpose of this action. If you fail to serve your response within the above time, you will be deemed to have admitted each request.

Request for Admission No. 1.

That Defendant sold certain dental equipment to Plaintiff.

Request for Admission No. 2.

The Defendant knew or should have known that the equipment was used equipment instead of new as alleged and that said equipment was defective.

Request for Admission No. 3.

That collusion existed between Defendant Jack Bailey and Defendant ABC Dental, Inc., as Defendant Bailey is the brother of the President/Treasurer of Defendant ABC Dental, Inc.

Dated: September 15, 1999

_____
Kenneth Emmons, Esq.
Attorney for Plaintiff
108 Main Street
Fremont, CA. 90112
(512) 389-2211

FIGURE 2-5
Request for admission.

sents its defense, both parties present concluding arguments, beginning with the defendant. The judge will then instruct the jury about what the issues are according to law, who has the burden of proof, and what they must find in order to render a decision for one side or the other. The jury then retires, deliberates, and reaches a verdict. The verdict may stipulate the party for whom the jury finds and what damages should be recovered (if in favor of the plaintiff). The verdict must be unanimous or by whatever majority the state law requires. If a jury cannot reach a decision, a new trial may be ordered.

The clerk is called upon to enter judgment. The judge then entertains any posttrial motions. If the judgment were in favor of Dr. Allen, ABC Dental could assert that an error occurred during the trial, such as admission of inadmissible evidence, an error in instructions to the jury, or improper conduct on the part of a jury member.

Appeal

An appeal may be made to a higher court only after final judgment. If ABC Dental appealed the judgment, the basis for the appeal must be an error that affected the outcome of the trial.

Appeals courts do not review a trial court's decision on matters of fact; they review only questions of law. Objections should be raised during the trial for an appellate court to consider. If certain evidence was introduced in court by Dr. Allen's attorney that is not admissible, ABC Dental's attorney could not appeal the final decision on the basis of the inadmissible evidence unless the objection to the evidence had been raised at trial. The parties may make various and numerous other motions throughout the course of a trial. However, this example was constructed to simplify a complicated legal maze for the health care professional.

Figures 2-1 through 2-3 are examples of how a typical summons, a typical complaint, and a typical answer would appear and as they pertain to this case. A summons and a complaint are served upon a defendant by a deputy sheriff or another public official authorized to serve legal process. That person signs the original summons, indicating that he or she made personal service upon the defendant, and returns it to the plaintiff or the plaintiff's attorney ("return of service"). The original summons and complaint are filed in court. Service must take place upon each defendant named in the complaint. Each defendant is required to file an answer to the complaint. Failure to file an answer could result in a default judgment against that defendant. See the warning in the summons.

Figure 2-4 is a representation of interrogatories (a method of discovery). Interrogatories may be served upon any party to the action by any opposing party to the action. Failure to respond to interrogatories could result in not being allowed to prove or dispute at trial the issues that they involve. Interrogatories must be served and responded to prior to trial.

Figure 2-5 is a representation of a request for admission, another method of discovery. Both plaintiff and defendant have the right to serve a request for admission upon the other. Requests for admission must also be completed prior to trial.

SUGGESTED READINGS

Federal Rules of Civil Procedure, Westbury, NY, 1999, The Foundation Press.

Weinstein J, Mansfield J, Abrams N, Berger M: *Evidence*, Westbury, NY, 1987, The Foundation Press.

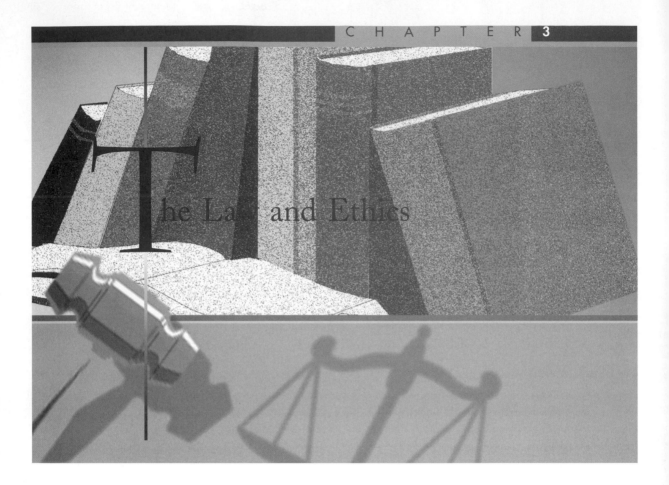

The Law and Ethics

LEARNING OUTCOMES

After reading this chapter, you should be able to:
- Discuss the Code of Ethics of your chosen profession.
- Relate the development of ethics to the development of the law.
- Describe the possible legal consequences for a defendant in a civil lawsuit versus a criminal lawsuit.
- Understand how dental laws regulate a breach of ethics or of law.

KEY WORDS

CIVIL TORT ACTION   TORT
ETHICS   TORTIOUS

ETHICS

Ethics can be defined as the study or realm "of moral action, conduct, motive or character" or concerned with "conforming to professional standards of conduct."[1] The first section of the definition might be viewed as something wholly limited to an individual's personal feelings at a particular moment in time and frustrates a standardization of ethics. On the other hand, if the dental professions are viewed as a single entity, it becomes imperative that ethics, as defined in the second section, be applied as a common goal for everyone in the dental professions. Ethics encompasses common principles, values, conduct, and obligations in interacting with each other. As dental health care professionals, these principles, values, conduct, and obligations are significant in relation to our providing dental services for our patients. Over time, the ethical beliefs of the individual members of the dental professions are molded into standards of professional responsibility. Such commonality is evident in the codes of ethics developed by the American Dental Association, the American Dental Hygienists' Association, the American Dental Assistants' Association, and the National Board for Certification for Dental Technologists. (See Appendixes A to D, pp. 247-266.) Appendix E (p. 267) is a code of ethics for dental technologists, outlined by the American Dental Association and the Federal Trade Commission. These documents were developed to assist members of the dental professions to judge what is ethical in a given situation that may arise. These codes also demonstrate to the public that the professions intend to be accountable, and to hold their members accountable, for the stated ethical principles. What is the relationship between ethical questions and legal questions? A law can be ethical or unethical. However, there are ethical questions with no correlation to the law and ethical questions having legal ramifications. There are very few absolutes and a multitude of conflicting opinions regarding ethics. Legal issues are settled by using statutes and judicial decisions for guidance. Ethical issues are subject to individual interpretations as to the right or wrong of particular situations.

> **ETHICS**
>
> Code or standards of conduct. Each health profession defines professional ethics in written standards of professional behavior.

Ethics Case Example

Mary Dow is a dental hygienist who is presently without a job. Her friend requests that she work for her employer, Dr. Elden, for two weeks while she is on vacation. Ms. Dow quickly agrees to this proposal. During the second day, Ms. Dow notices a definite odor of alcohol on the dentist's breath. Thinking that perhaps the doctor has been having a difficult day, she dismisses the incident. Two days later, Dr. Elden appears to have been drinking when he returns from lunch. Ms. Dow is a bit more distressed over this incident, but is comforted by the fact that her position is only temporary. The following Monday morning, Dr. Elden seems to have been drinking and he is rather irritable; however, he keeps all of his appointments. In the late afternoon, one of Ms. Dow's patients is in a great deal of pain and Dr. Elden is summoned to administer local anesthesia. After Dr. Elden leaves the operatory,

---

[1]*Black's Law Dictionary, Abridged*, ed 5, St Paul, 1979, West Publishing Co.

the patient turns to Ms. Dow and says, "He's been drinking, hasn't he? Does he do this often?"

1. *What, if any, should be the appropriate response from Ms. Dow?*
2. *What ethical issues are involved?*
3. *Should Ms. Dow confront Dr. Elden?*
4. *Should Ms. Dow report these incidents to the friend who works permanently for Dr. Elden?*
5. *Should Ms. Dow report the incidents to the State Board of Dental Examiners?*

The answers exist within each of us as individuals, and we must do what our consciences or ethics tell us to do and always in the best interest of the patient. The American Dental Association and other dental professional associations dictate ethical behavior for their members. Also, ethics is sometimes incorporated into state laws relating to the practice of dentistry, dental hygiene, dental assisting, and dental laboratory technology. In view of these codes of ethics, how would you respond to the following?

1. *Is Dr. Elden bound to those stated ethical standards?*
2. *Does the patient have a right to a truthful answer?*
3. *Is the duty to tell the truth unconditional?*
4. *Do we tell the truth regardless of harmful consequences?*
5. *Or do we cover up the truth regardless of harmful consequences?*
6. *Do health care providers have a legal or ethical obligation to protect patients from harmful care?*

These are some of the questions that Ms. Dow or any of us would need to ask in order to provide dental health care competently. Dr. Elden's conduct may not have been illegal, but it was certainly unethical.

Conduct

Conduct is an essential element of ethics. This fact indicates that there is a correlation between ethics and the law: civil, criminal, and dental. Nevertheless, the scope of professional services does not include all forms of a health professional's conduct simply because he or she is a health professional. The conduct must be within the norm of the standards of professional responsibility attributed to the health profession, whereas conduct that is **tortious** will run contrary to law. Consider the case of *Niedzielski, Doe et al v. St. Paul Fire & Marine Insurance Company.*[2] Mary Doe took her 10-year old daughter, Jane, to the dental office of Eugene Niedzielski, D.D.S., on August 28, 1981, to have Jane's decayed tooth repaired. A dental assistant took Jane to the examination room and then left the office for her lunch break. Once the dental assistant left the office, the dentist entered the examination room where Jane was sitting, shined a light into Jane's eyes, and placed a folded towel over her face so as to obstruct her vision. The dentist sexually assaulted her. Afterward, he took x-rays and placed a filling in Jane's tooth. After

TORTIOUS

Characterized by wrongful conduct that subjects one to liability in tort. The courts are constantly changing the definition of tortious conduct through court decisions.

[2]589 A.2d 130 (N.H. 1991).

leaving the dentist's office, Jane informed her mother of what had happened, and the local police were notified. The Does filed a **civil tort action** against the dentist in September 1984 and won judgment. The dentist's professional liability insurance provider, St. Paul Fire, refused to pay the judgment. The Doe's and Dr. Niedzielski filed suit against St. Paul Fire, arguing that the alleged assault was covered by professional liability insurance because Jane Doe's damages arose as a result of her presence in the dental office for the purpose of receiving professional services. The court ruled that the dentist's professional liability insurance was intended to cover only routine services typically associated with dentistry, not intentional acts such as the sexual assault that occurred. This case clearly illustrates the fact that not every act occurring in a dental office can be characterized as a professional service or as failure to provide a professional service. Clearly, Dr. Niedzielski's actions do not constitute professional services and are not covered under the insurance policy in question. Clearly, the doctor's conduct was both illegal and unethical.

Code of Ethics

The purpose of a professional code of ethics is to achieve high levels of ethical consciousness, decision making, and practice by members of the profession. Specific objectives of the Code of Ethics for Dental Hygienists (see Appendix B) that are applicable to every health professional are as follows:

1. To increase professional and ethical consciousness and the sense of ethical responsibility
2. To lead the members to recognize ethical issues and choices and to guide them in making more informed ethical decisions
3. To establish a standard for professional judgment and conduct
4. To provide a statement of the ethical behavior that the public can expect from the members

CRIMINAL LAW

A crime is a social harm that has been defined and made punishable by law. It is an offense against the people, and the state may institute criminal proceedings in a court of law. Compare this with a **tort,** which is a civil wrong against an individual(s) or entity, and the injured party may seek damages. The victim of a crime does not bring criminal action. Only the state in the person of a prosecutor may initiate formal criminal charges. Criminal law is dealt with separately by the legal system. Various elements must be present to constitute a crime. These elements have specific definitions. The federal government and each state define what constitutes a crime and list the elements of each crime. For instance, murder, rape, and burglary are criminal acts. In a case of burglary, elements necessary to prove against a defendant are that the defendant (1) entered the dwelling of another, (2) did so by breaking into the dwelling, and (3) had the intent to commit a crime. Negligence, medical malpractice, divorce, and contract disputes are civil actions. In a civil lawsuit the basic questions are:

1. *How has the defendant injured the plaintiff?*
2. *What remedies are available to compensate the plaintiff for his or her injury?*

In a criminal action the basic questions are:
1. *How has the defendant injured society?*
2. *What sentence is necessary to punish the defendant for that injury?*

Criminal law seeks to punish the offender, while civil law seeks to compensate the victim.

The Four Purposes of Punishment

Theoretically, there are four purposes of punishment under criminal law:
1. To reform the criminal
2. To incarcerate the criminal while he or she is being reformed
3. To provide retribution for misdeeds (The criminal owes a debt to society, and, hopefully, the punishment will fit the crime.)
4. To provide a deterrence to a crime

Many feel that the last two purposes are inconsistent with reformation of the criminal. The question arises daily as to whether the death penalty serves as a deterrent to crime. Statistics appear to refute that theory.

REMEDIES FOR CIVIL ACTIONS

A traditional legal remedy is an award for damages. The measure of damages varies with the type of case. Generally, the types of damages include the following:
1. *Special damages.* Actual expenses (medical bills or lost income)
2. *General damages.* Damages that are less easy to determine—for example, pain and suffering or decreased future earning capacity
3. *Contract damages.* Damages for breach of contract, which are equal to the difference between the value of the performance promised and the value of the performance received
4. *Punitive damages.* Awarded to punish deliberate wrongful conduct

Large awards in medical malpractice cases are primarily due to general and punitive damages.

DENTAL LAW

State boards of dentistry are created by the state legislatures. A legislature delegates the authority of a board through its licensing statute. The board interprets the statute through rules and regulations for the dental professions. The board also must follow the procedures required by any other applicable statutes. Failure to comply could result in a court's rejection of a board decision.[3,4] The board's primary responsibility is to maintain high-quality health care by disciplining incompetent health care providers before and/or after patients are injured. Should a health care provider be in violation of the rules and regulations of the board, he or she may be reprimanded in some manner or have his or her license revoked. However, this will result in court

---

[3]*Lopez v. New Mexico Board of Medical Examiners*, 754 P.2d 522 (1988).
[4]*Ramirez v. Ahn*, 843 F.2d 864 (5th Cir. 1988).

action only if the violation relates to a criminal matter or a patient decides to pursue court action. Revocation of a license may be appealed to a court of law. A health practitioner may also be found guilty in a criminal or civil matter and remain licensed in his or her profession. A state board of dentistry cannot revoke certification unless that body initially granted the certification. Only the certifying body can revoke certification. A dental health care professional may also perform an act that is a breach of the state's dental rules and regulations as well as a breach of ethics and therefore be subject to sanctions or revocation of his or her license.

In addition to the rules and regulations of state boards of dentistry, criminal statutes and case law, and civil statutes and case law, other entities control the dental professions, such as public health laws and local ordinances. These often vary from state to state, and dental health professionals should be aware of their specific local ordinances and state laws, rules, and regulations. In fact, it is their ethical duty to know what state laws or local ordinances govern the practice of their professions.

SUMMARY OF THE LAW AND ETHICS

A single act or omission by a dental health professional may be:

1. A breach of ethics
2. A cause for revocation of membership in a professional association (or other action)
3. A cause for disciplinary action by a licensing board (including loss of a license)
4. A cause for civil action in a court of law
5. A cause for criminal action resulting in incarceration
6. A combination of any of the above

Having sexual relations with a patient is an example of behavior that might trigger all above actions. However, ethical conduct is not defined in the same way by everyone, as mentioned earlier. For instance, in a survey of physicians regarding sexual contact with patients,[5] the results were as follows:

Ninety-four percent stated that they were opposed to sexual contact with current patients.

Thirty-seven percent were opposed to sexual contact with former patients.

It is possible to put forth an infinite number of ethical questions pertaining to such results. As you read the remainder of this book, examine the differences and similarities between the law and ethics.

SUGGESTED READINGS

Mason JK, McCall RA: *Law and medical ethics*, London, 1983, Butterworths.
Sexual misconduct in the practice of medicine, *JAMA* 266:2741, November 20, 1991.
Weinstein BD: *Dental ethics*, Philadelphia, 1993, Lea & Febiger.

---

[5]Gartrell N et all: Physician-patient sexual contact: prevalence and problems, *Western Journal of Medicine* 157:139, August 1992.

AUTHOR'S CASE STUDY COMMENTS

Reread the Case Study and Study Questions for Section I.
Questions 1 through 10 are examined in the following analysis:

1. Did Ms. Casey exceed her authority? If so, how?

It would appear that Ms. Casey, a registered dental hygienist, had no authority to render this type of treatment for Dr. Albright's patient. State dental practice acts identify what procedures each member of the dental professions may legally perform. In states where it is legal for a dental hygienist to perform local anesthesia, usually he or she may do so within the scope of his or her functions as a dental hygienist. Since states vary in defining the scope of practice for dental hygienists, the Indiana Dental Practice Act would need to be examined.

2. Did Ms. Smythe exceed her authority? If so, how?

Although Ms. Smythe was not certified to perform CPR, she would probably not be held liable unless it was shown that she improperly performed CPR for Mr. Burton, and Mr. Burton suffered harm as a result of her improper administration of CPR. However, Ms. Smythe may have performed an illegal act by completing the restorations for Dr. Albright. Again, we would need to examine the Indiana Dental Practice Act, since this is a legal function for dental assistants and/or hygienists in some states.

3. Did Dr. Halper provide competent dental health care to Mr. Burton?

The facts do not indicate that Dr. Halper acted in an illegal or unethical manner.

4. Is the Ohio Board of Medical Examiners the proper body to receive Mr. Burton's complaint?

The Ohio Board of Medical Examiners is certainly not the appropriate entity to receive Mr. Burton's complaint. Complaints regarding members of the dental profession, acting in that capacity, should be heard by the state board of dentistry or by a similar board organized to hear such complaints. Procedure usually dictates taking complaints regarding dental professionals to the state boards of dentistry prior to initiating any court action. In this particular situation the Indiana Board of Dentistry should be notified, since Dr. Albright's practice and licensure are in Indiana.

5. Is the Ohio Supreme Court the proper court to take Mr. Burton's litigation? If not, name the proper court.

Litigation, in its initiating stages, must proceed in a trial court. A trial cannot be initiated in a court of appellate jurisdiction only. The Ohio Supreme Court is a court of appellate jurisdiction and therefore cannot hear a trial. In this instance, both parties are not residents of the same state; therefore, litigation could be initiated in federal district court. There is also a monetary requirement of $75,000 to file a lawsuit in federal district court. Mr. Burton cannot sue for one million dollars merely on a whim. The dollar figure requested for damages must be realistic in view

AUTHOR'S CASE STUDY COMMENTS—cont'd

of the injury. Should Mr. Burton file his lawsuit in U.S. District Court in Ohio, Dr. Albright can request a change of venue to U.S. District Court in Indiana.

6. What must Mr. Burton's attorney do to secure personal jurisdiction of Dr. Albright?

Personal jurisdiction is obtained by serving a defendant with copies of a summons and a complaint. This is accomplished by a U.S. marshal (or someone authorized to legally serve process) personally serving Dr. Albright with the summons and complaint. The summons and complaint, signed by the U.S. marshal, indicating that he or she served the defendant, must then be filed in federal court.

7. In preparation for trial, is Mr. Burton entitled to copies of his dental records and procedures utilized by Dr. Albright in his treatment of Mr. Burton? If so, what method should be used to obtain them?

Prior to trial, both plaintiff and defendant are entitled to discovery. Serving Interrogatories on the other party is the procedure whereby one party submits a series of questions to the other party, who must answer those questions under oath and within a stipulated period of time. In order to secure copies of real evidence such as documents, a party would submit to the other party a request for production of documents. Here, Mr. Burton is entitled to his dental records. All questions and documents requested must be relevant to the issues in dispute.

8. Is Dr. Albright entitled to a jury trial if Mr. Burton objects to a jury trial?

In most jurisdictions, a jury trial will be allowed at the request of one party. There are no jury trials in state district courts. Trial by jury is a constitutional right in criminal actions in which the defendant may be incarcerated.

9. Could Dr. Albright, Ms. Casey, and Ms. Smythe lose their professional licenses? If so, by whose authority?

The Board of Dental Examiners has the authority to restrict or revoke a dental license. Only Dr. Albright and Ms. Casey are licensed. Ms. Smythe is certified. The Board has no power over certification unless that board issued the certification in question.

10. What ethical considerations does Ms. Casey have regarding the dental receptionist's mishandling of money?

Ms. Casey has an ethical dilemma regarding the receptionist's behavior with Dr. Albright's money. Should she report what she saw to Dr. Albright? Should she remain quiet because it is none of her business? Should she first speak to the receptionist to have her explain her behavior and/or return the money? Is this her responsibility? The Code of Ethics for Dental Hygienists refers to the principle of complementarity, which "assumes the existence of an obligation to justice and basic human rights. It requires us to act toward others in the same way they would act toward us if roles were reversed. In all relationships, it means considering the values and perspective of others before making decisions or taking actions affecting them."

AUTHOR'S CASE STUDY COMMENTS—cont'd

Does this mean that Ms. Casey is ethically bound to discuss the situation with the receptionist? The Code of Ethics also states that the dental hygienist should "document and report inappropriate, inadequate or substandard care and/or illegal activities by a health care provider, to the responsible authorities." Is the receptionist considered a health care provider? If in fact the receptionist is stealing, her behavior is a crime and she would be prosecuted under criminal law. If Ms. Casey says nothing, is she aiding and abetting a crime? Is it possible that the receptionist is acting at the request of Dr. Albright? The ultimate decision must be made by Ms. Casey, keeping in mind the ethical standards of her profession.

LEGAL RIGHTS THAT DEFINE RELATIONSHIPS BETWEEN INDIVIDUALS

CASE STUDY 1

Dr. Kenneth Hastings and Ms. Sara Andrews, his dental assistant, attended a continuing education program that provided information regarding a new nonsurgical procedure for the treatment for periodontal disease. Research relating to this procedure looked very promising, and both Dr. Hastings and Ms. Andrews were anxious to implement it. The following Monday morning Mr. Wayne Arnold, a well-known state politician, was Dr. Hastings' first patient. Mr. Arnold's appointment was a restorative visit for two occlusal restorations, on teeth #19 and #20. After an examination of Mr. Arnold's teeth and gingiva, Dr. Hastings concluded that Mr. Arnold was a perfect candidate for the new periodontal procedure.

After restorations were placed on teeth #19 and #20, Dr. Hastings completed the new procedure on teeth #13, #14, and #15. The treatment went smoothly. Then Dr. Hastings told Mr. Arnold that a periodontal procedure utilizing a new technology had been successfully performed on three of his teeth in the maxillary left quadrant. Mr. Arnold was obviously upset upon finding that three additional procedures had been performed in his mouth. However, he seemed to be more agreeable when Dr. Hastings offered to charge only half of the fee for this particular procedure.

Mr. Arnold had brought Danny, his 5-year-old son, with him to this appointment. Anxious to get his son home, Mr. Arnold decided to discuss the matter with Dr. Hastings at a later time. Just as Dr. Hastings was completing treatment for Mr. Arnold,

his son injured himself on a broken toy while playing in the reception area. Another child had broken the toy earlier, but no one had taken time to fix or replace it. Danny's face was badly lacerated by a piece of metal that was partially attached to the toy. Ms. Andrews helped Danny up and bandaged the wound so that Mr. Arnold could take him to the family doctor.

Two days later, Mr. Arnold called Dr. Hastings' office for an appointment, as he was in pain in the maxillary left quadrant of his mouth. Dr. Hastings examined the patient and gave him a prescription for an antibiotic. After Mr. Arnold left the premises, Ms. Andrews commented to Dr. Hastings that she had remembered several contraindications regarding the new periodontal procedure. Dr. Hastings then carefully read the directions that came with the treatment solutions. The literature clearly stated that this particular procedure should not be utilized in treating patients who were iodine sensitive. Mr. Arnold's medical history clearly indicated that he was allergic to iodine. Three days later, Mr. Arnold again called Dr. Hastings' office, as the pain had not subsided and in fact had become more severe. Dr. Hastings told Mr. Arnold that he could do no more for his medical problem and referred him to his family physician for treatment. Mr. Arnold sought the services of another dentist, Dr. Michael Jones, who refused to treat him. He was finally able to acquire the services of an oral surgeon, Dr. Robert Roberts.

After all treatment was completed, Mr. Arnold unfortunately lost three teeth, #13, #14, and #15. Dr.

Roberts had never seen a similar condition quite as severe and asked permission to take pictures of Mr. Arnold's mouth prior to treatment. Later, Dr. Roberts was able to utilize these pictures in a continuing education program he was presenting during a statewide dental meeting. He also published the pictures in a pathology textbook he authored.

Dr. Hastings openly blamed Ms. Andrews for the mistake in treatment of Mr. Arnold, and she became very unhappy with her employment. A friend informed her of Dr. Roberts' search for a dental assistant. Ms. Andrews sent a resume to Dr. Roberts and during an interview found that this new position would pay $30 more per week than her present salary. Dr. Roberts contacted Dr. Hastings for a recommendation regarding her qualifications. Not wanting to lose her as an employee, Dr. Hastings reported falsely that Ms. Andrews was incompetent and often late for work. As a result, the position was offered to another applicant.

RESPONSE TO CASE STUDY   Frederick D. Williams, Esq.

Immediately evident from the case study is the fact that the new nonsurgical procedure for the treatment of periodontal disease "looked very promising." From this, I can only assume that this procedure has not been approved by the Federal Drug Administration. Assuming that it was, Mr. Arnold was not asked whether he wanted the treatment. Therefore, lack of informed consent is Dr. Hastings' first tort. This tort is compounded by the fact that Dr. Hastings failed to thoroughly read and adhere to the instructions pertaining to the application of this new procedure. More specifically, the procedure is not to be used on patients who are iodine sensitive. Mr. Arnold's records indicated that he was allergic to iodine. Clearly, Dr. Hastings breached the standard of care demanded of him. We are then presented with an essential question. Was it foreseeable that the possibility of injury or harm to Mr. Arnold would be imminent if the procedure's warning were not adhered to completely? I submit that it was forseeable and that, as a consequence, Dr. Hastings was negligent and is liable in tort to Mr. Arnold for the subsequent loss of teeth #13, #14, and #15.

Dr. Michael Jones refused to treat Mr. Arnold. It is my opinion that he had a perfect right not to accept Mr. Arnold as a patient, particularly since there was no prior relationship (doctor-patient) between them.

Dr. Roberts secured Mr Arnold's permission to take photographs of his mouth prior to treatment. However, Dr. Roberts did not secure Mr. Arnold's permission to use the photos in an educational program or to publish said photos. Such unauthorized use by Dr. Roberts constitutes an invasion of Mr. Arnold's privacy.

Mr. Arnold's son, Danny, is injured in Dr. Hastings' office while playing with a broken toy in the reception area. Both are in Dr. Hastings' office as business invitees. As such, they are owed a duty of care against hidden harmful devices or harmful instruments (in this case a broken toy). The facts are clear that the toy has been broken for some time and that all dental personnel in the office are aware of this fact. We are again presented with the same issue. Is it foreseeable that a child could injure himself on a broken toy exposed in an open area of an office? The preponderance of cases indicates the affirmative. There is no doubt that Dr. Hastings is liable in tort for injury to Danny, particularly since he knew or should have known of the existence of a dangerous condition in his office. Ms. Andrews applied first aid to the child, and it does not appear that she acted in a negligent manner.

Dr. Hastings' attempt to blame Ms. Andrews for the mistreatment of Mr. Arnold is an exercise in futility, as she was operating under his direct supervision. The doctrine of respondeat superior

RESPONSE TO CASE STUDY—cont'd

is applicable in this instance. Under this doctrine an employer is responsible for all acts of an employee when the employee is acting within the scope of his or her employment.

Not content with all of his accumulated liability as discussed herein, Dr. Hastings now adds a final tort. When he reported to Dr. Roberts, a third party, that Ms. Andrews was incompetent and often late for work, he misrepresented the truth and committed the tort of defamation.

RESPONSE TO CASE STUDY
Christina Corbin-Price, R.D.H., B.S.

An intentional tort arises from an act that the defendant consciously desired to perform, either in order to harm another or knowing with substantial certainty that injury to another could result. When a person consents to the act that harms him, there is no liability for the damage done. However, in this case Dr. Hastings did not get consent from Mr. Arnold for performing the new periodontal procedure. Therefore, Mr. Arnold was not informed of the periodontal problem, the new procedure, and the risk involved in the new procedure. Because of the development of pain where the new procedure had been performed, Dr. Hastings saw Mr. Arnold on an emergency visit. He then prescribed an antibiotic for this pain. Before prescribing an antibiotic, Dr. Hastings failed to review Mr. Arnold's medical history. The medical history listed Mr. Arnold's sensitivity to iodine. Has Dr. Hastings committed negligence (an unintentional tort)? Negligence has been committed when someone has suffered injury caused by the failure of another to live up to a required duty of care. Generally, the tort of negligence requires the presence of the following four elements:

1. The defendant owed a duty of care to the plaintiff.
2. The defendant breached that duty.
3. The plaintiff suffered a legally recognizable injury.
4. The defendant's breach of the duty of care caused the plaintiff's injury.

Clearly, Dr. Hastings is negligent, especially since Mr. Arnold lost three teeth as a result.

In the case of Danny's injuries sustained in Dr. Hastings' office, Dr. Hastings is once again guilty of negligence. The fact that the broken toy was not removed or fixed by Dr. Hastings or an employee puts the child at risk. Therefore, he is liable for damages for injuries sustained. Dr. Robert Roberts is guilty of invasion of the right to privacy. A person's right to solitude and freedom from prying eyes is the interest protected by the tort of invasion of privacy. Obtaining consent to take the photographs of Mr. Arnold was the right thing to do; however, failure to get consent for use of the pictures in any way and using them in the way he did constitute an invasion of privacy.

The last situation involving Ms. Andrews is clearly a case of an intentional tort. Dr. Hastings, her employer, committed slander. The law has imposed a general duty on all persons to refrain from making false, defamatory statements about others. Breaching this duty orally involves the tort of slander. In regard to Dr. Hastings openly blaming Ms. Andrews for Mr. Arnold's treatment, the principal-employer is liable for harm caused by an agent-employee in the scope of employment. This theory of liability involves the doctrine of respondeat superior. This doctrine imposes vicarious, indirect liability on the employer, without regard to the personal fault of the employer, for torts committed by an employee in the course or scope of employment.

CASE STUDY QUESTIONS

1. Does Mr. Arnold have a legal claim against Dr. Hastings?
2. Did Dr. Hastings owe a duty to Mr. Arnold?
3. Did the treatment Dr. Hastings provided for Mr. Arnold fall below the required standard of care?
4. What must Mr. Arnold legally prove to recover damages against Dr. Hastings?
5. Is Dr. Hastings in any way liable to Danny?
6. Is Dr. Jones liable to Mr. Arnold for refusing to treat him on an emergency basis?
7. Does Ms. Andrews have a legal claim against Dr. Hastings?
8. Does Mr. Arnold have a legal claim against Dr. Roberts?
9. Did Dr. Hastings commit assault and battery?
10. Were the elements of informed consent or informed refusal met in regard to the procedure Dr. Hastings completed for Mr. Arnold?
11. As a consultant for Dr. Hastings' office, what suggestions would you have for other members of his office staff in regard to strategies to reduce the risks of legal liability?

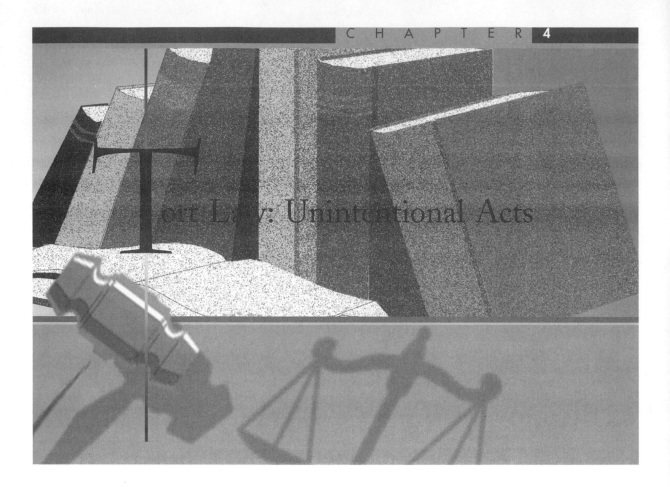

Tort Law: Unintentional Acts

LEARNING OUTCOMES

After reading this chapter, you should be able to:
- Explain the concept of liability.
- Name four elements a plaintiff must prove in court to recover damages from a defendant who has allegedly committed negligent malpractice.
- Describe how expert testimony is utilized in a court of law.

KEY WORDS

CONTRIBUTORY NEGLIGENCE
DUTY
EXPERT TESTIMONY
LIABILITY
MALPRACTICE
MEASURE OF DAMAGES

NEGLIGENCE
PUNITIVE DAMAGES
RES IPSA LOQUITUR
RESPONDEAT SUPERIOR
STANDARD OF CARE

A tort is a legal or civil wrong committed by one person against the person or property of another. The law permits the harmed individual to bring a civil action against the wrongdoer to recover damages (a sum of money) as compensation for the injuries suffered.

Tort law is divided into three categories:

1. Intentional torts: there must be an intent to cause physical or mental harm to another individual or harm to the property of another individual.
2. Unintentional torts (negligence): committed with no intent to harm others; the defendant's conduct represents an unreasonable risk to others.
3. Strict liability: the defendant's behavior is not intentional or negligent; the basis of liability is the nature of the activity. For example, the manufacturer of a defective product would be liable for damages to an individual who is injured as a result of that defect.

This chapter will examine unintentional torts. Chapter 5 will examine intentional torts. Strict liability is rarely applicable in cases relating to dental professionals.

MALPRACTICE LIABILITY

Malpractice includes negligent conduct of all professional individuals. Medical malpractice is negligence in providing medical care. The majority of medical malpractice claims are asserted against physicians, as they are primarily responsible for patient care. However, the legal principles applicable to the conduct of physicians are equally applicable to the conduct of other health care professionals, including all dental health care providers.

One person is **"liable"** to another when he or she is legally obligated to pay for the injury or injuries that he or she causes another individual. In medical malpractice the injury to another is generally caused by a health care professional's failure to adequately perform a legal duty owed to a patient or by a violation of the patient's rights. Compensation for an injury can include not only the cost of medical or dental fees but also amounts for loss of wages, pain and suffering, and other related costs.

A lawsuit for medical malpractice utilizes rules from both tort law and contract law. Contract law is more fully discussed in Chapter 8. Whether one uses tort law or contract law to bring an action against a health care provider depends on the act that the plaintiff alleges to have occurred. The statute of limitations and the amount of damages available are other considerations that affect the choice of law.

Statute of Limitations

The statute of limitations specifies the legal time during which a civil suit for an alleged wrong must be filed with the proper court. The statute of limitations for a tort differs in length from the statute of limitations for an action in contract. The statute of limitations also may vary from state to state. Tort actions must be initiated within one to ten years (depending on the jurisdiction) from the time the wrong was committed or within a given number of years from the time the plaintiff/patient "knew" or "should have known" of the injury.

Generally, breach of contract suits have limitations of from one to ten years, de-

MALPRACTICE

Failure by a professional to exercise reasonable care or to meet a standard of care, which results in harm to another. Professional negligence.

LIABILITY

Responsibility for a breach of duty.

pending on the jurisdiction. Therefore, a particular jurisdiction may have a limitation of two years for tort actions and a limitation of six years for contract actions. If three years have passed since the plaintiff's injury, an action could still be filed on the basis of breach of contract. But a claim could no longer be brought on the basis of tort law unless the plaintiff could show that he did not know of the injury until a time that is less than two years prior to the filing of the lawsuit.

Measure of Damages

Similarly, the **measure** (type and amount) **of damages** varies from jurisdiction to jurisdiction. Choices of tort or contract law are often based upon the type of wrong committed and that law which would allow for the greatest recovery. For instance, most jurisdictions do not allow **punitive damages** for breach of contract suits. Punitive damages are awarded by the court when some particularly outrageous act has been committed. If the plaintiff had six sound teeth extracted by mistake because the radiographs were mounted backward and contract law does not allow for punitive damages, tort law would become the basis of the lawsuit, unless the statute of limitations had run for a tort action.

NEGLIGENCE

Most liability of health care providers involves principles of **negligence.** To recover for negligent malpractice, a plaintiff must prove four elements in a court of law:

1. A duty of care was owed to the plaintiff/patient by the defendant/health care provider.
2. The defendant/health care provider breached the duty by violating an applicable standard of care.
3. The plaintiff/patient suffered injury.
4. The plaintiff/patient's injury was caused by the substandard care resulting from the violation of the standard of care by the defendant/health care provider.

All four elements must be present, or no recovery for damages will be allowed. There must be a causal connection between the patient's injury and the defendant's negligence or breach of duty. The plaintiff must also establish the standard of care and show how the defendant failed to meet that standard. This is usually accomplished through an expert witness. If the requirements of all four elements are met, the plaintiff has a legal right to take the lawsuit to court. The jury decides all questions of fact on the basis of the evidence. The judge takes the jury's findings and applies the law of the jurisdiction of the court.

DUTY

There is no actionable negligence unless the actor has violated a **duty** he or she owed the victim of his or her act or omission. Actionable negligence must arise from violation of a duty imposed upon the actor by common law, statute, or contract. Common law or case law is judge-made law. Judicial decisions interpret legal issues raised in a court of law. Statutes are laws passed by Congress or state legis-

MEASURE OF DAMAGES

Determination of the remuneration that the injured party to a lawsuit will receive.

PUNITIVE DAMAGES

Remuneration awarded to a plaintiff that is greater than actual damages suffered. Punitive damages are designed to punish the defendant for egregious behavior.

NEGLIGENCE

Failure to exercise the degree of care that a reasonable and careful person would exercise under similar circumstances.

DUTY

An obligation, in law, that one owes to another person or a business.

lative bodies. Contract law refers to agreements that the law will enforce in some way. In any discussion of negligence, common law will be the major source of law.

When one affirmatively acts in a way that creates a relationship with another individual, a duty of care is created. In a dental setting the duty can be created in several ways. When a dental health care provider begins treatment with the consent of a patient, the courts will infer a voluntary relationship that gives rise to a duty.[1] Even making an appointment with a new patient to treat a specific condition may create a professional relationship and a corresponding duty of care.[2]

STANDARD OF CARE

In tort law, liability for medical or dental malpractice depends on whether the defendant/health care provider's conduct fell below a certain **standard of care.** The "reasonable prudent person" standard requires that an individual perform a function as any reasonable person of ordinary prudence with comparable education, skill, and training, under similar circumstances, would perform that same function. The standard for health care professionals is higher, as they have skills and knowledge beyond ordinary individuals. Their conduct is evaluated by being compared to what a reasonably competent member of the profession practicing in the same specialty as the defendant would do to conform to acceptable professional practice. Should a practitioner from one profession practice beyond the scope of that profession, he or she may be held to the level of care of the profession whose members would have been qualified to handle the condition.[3] A dentist who did not utilize a rubber dam and undertook endodontics was held to the standard of a specialist (endodontist).[4] A dentist performing an occlusal equilibration procedure was held to the standard of a specialist even though there is no such specialty in dentistry. If a dental hygienist or assistant performs a procedure that is designated by law to be performed by a dentist in the particular state where he or she practices and the patient sues for negligence, the hygienist or assistant could be held to the standard of care for a dentist in a court of law, thus increasing the likelihood of liability.

> **STANDARD OF CARE**
>
> The degree of care that a reasonably prudent professional should exercise.

The courts evaluate the standard of practice of a health care professional on the basis of the local community or a similar community. As the education and practice of health care providers have become more uniform, courts have been leaning toward a national standard.[5] The standards for evaluating medical and dental care are not decided by a judge or a jury. They are not generally developed by government agencies or state licensing boards. They are developed by members of the profession. The standards are established and reported in professional journals and meetings, as well as in educational settings. Rules and regulations relating to medical and dental services are adopted by professional organizations and institutions, such as hospitals and professional societies. These rules and guidelines may be used to establish a standard of care in malpractice litigation. Access to the computer

---

[1]*Davis v. Weiskoff,* 439 N.E.2d 836 (1982).
[2]*Lyons v. Weiskoff,* 239 N.E.2d 103 (1977).
[3]*Simpson v. Davis,* 549 P.2d 950 (1976).
[4]*Short v. Kenkade,* 685 P.2d 210 (Colo. App. 1983).
[5]*Blair v. Eblen,* 461 S.W.2d 370 (Ky. 1970).

plays an increasingly critical role in establishing such standards. In medicine, MEDLINE has the largest database, containing several million references and articles from thousands of journals.[6] Any health care provider using inappropriate procedures can be challenged in court by the use of computer research. Today, computer skills are extremely valuable in retrieving information relating to specific modes of treatment. Gathering information prior to treatment decisions enables the health care provider to practice within a generally accepted standard of care and protects him or her from legal liability. If named as a defendant in a malpractice lawsuit, a provider can use such guidelines as an affirmative defense by showing compliance with a specific standard of care. MEDLINE is an online database, indexed by the National Library of Medicine. Therefore, the available information represents the latest patient treatment information for the medical or dental professional. This service is available twenty-four hours a day. Members of each profession (whether or not they are members of the professional organization representing their profession) one day may be held to such standards in a court of law. Knowing of the existence and content of these standards set primarily by professional organizations is essential to protecting both practitioner and patient. It is also essential that the members of professions help their organizations to keep standards current with practice and technology. One would not want to be held to an outdated standard in a court of law.

Dental offices utilize various materials and equipment for diagnosis and treatment. Each material or piece of equipment is sold with the manufacturer's explicit instructions regarding use. The standard of care may be shown in court by introducing these documents to prove negligence.[7] These documents are utilized to show what the defendant should have known or what he or she should have done.[8] A manual may reveal substandard care.[9] In one case, a defendant's defense for not using a rubber dam was possible damage to the teeth; however, a portion of a textbook on endodontics was introduced to provide evidence of the standard of care.

EXPERT TESTIMONY

EXPERT TESTIMONY

Testimony offered by a specialist in a particular field. For example, a radiologist's testimony about interpretation of radiographs.

Expert testimony is usually required in order to show professional negligence. An expert must establish the standard of care, show how the defendant's conduct deviated from the standard of care, and show the causal relationship between the injury and the defendant's negligence. Courts differ on the qualifications of an expert witness. The Federal Rules of Evidence state that an expert may be qualified by "knowledge, skill, experience, training and education."[10] Therefore, an expert is not always an individual with the greatest amount of formal

---

[6]Gould K, Lang P: MEDLINE: an information resource for dental hygienists, *Journal of Dental Hygiene* 70(5):206-210, September-October 1996.
[7]*Winkjer v. Herr,* 277 N.W.2d 579 (N.D. 1979).
[8]*Holloway v. Hauver,* 322 A.2d 890 (1974).
[9]*Sprowl v. Ward,* 441 S.2d 898 (Ala. 1983).
[10]Federal Rules of Evidence, Rule 702, Washington, DC, 1983, US Government Printing Office.

education. He or she is often one who has the requisite knowledge, skill, or experience. Most malpractice suits require experts with many years of education in the medical or dental professions. In most state courts, during medical or dental litigation, expert testimony must be based upon "a reasonable degree of medical and scientific certainty."

Documents, such as professional journals, textbooks, and research results, may be admitted to support or refute an expert's testimony. A document may be admitted into evidence, and the expert may testify regarding his or her own conclusions and conclusions from the literature.[11] In one case, portions of the *Physician's Desk Reference* (PDR) were admitted to assist in determining if a physician's conduct fell below the standard of care.[12]

A party intending to use an expert witness must:

1. Qualify the witness as an expert (establish his or her knowledge, skill, experience, training, or education).
2. Convince the court that the proposed expert's testimony will assist in deciding a factual issue or understanding the evidence presented.
3. Provide a correlation between the proposed expert's opinion and the facts that support that opinion.

It is the judge's decision as to whether a proposed expert witness qualifies.

RES IPSA LOQUITUR

As previously discussed, to prove negligence the plaintiff must prove that the defendant failed to meet a professional standard of care and that the plaintiff was injured as a result. Usually, the plaintiff introduces direct evidence to establish negligent malpractice. The plaintiff can also prove negligence indirectly by circumstantial evidence. The doctrine of **res ipsa loquitur** ("the thing speaks for itself") is utilized to establish negligence by circumstantial evidence. This doctrine eliminates proving fault (substandard care); however, causation must still be established. Therefore, when utilizing this doctrine, the plaintiff is not required to have an expert witness to testify regarding the standard of care in order to prove negligence.[13] The plaintiff must show the existence of three conditions in order to utilize the doctrine. The injury must:

1. Be of a type that does not normally occur unless there has been negligence.
2. Be caused by an agency or instrumentality under the exclusive control of the defendant.
3. Not be due to the plaintiff's contributing to his or her own injury in any way.[14,15]

RES IPSA LOQUITUR
"The thing speaks for itself." That is, the instrument that caused the damage was under the defendant's exclusive control.

---

[11]*Young v. Horton*, 855 P.2d 502 (Mont. 1993).
[12]*Bowman v. Songer*, 820 P.2d 1110 (Colo. 1991).
[13]*Van Zee v. Sioux Valley Hospital*, 315 N.W.2d 489 (S.D. 1982).
[14]*Anderson v. Somberg*, 338 A.2d 1 (N.J. 1975).
[15]*Loizzo v. St. Francis Hospital*, 459 N.E.2d 314 (Ill. App. 1984).

When the three conditions are present, the court may decide that the doctrine is applicable. The plaintiff does not automatically prevail. The court rules the doctrine applicable. The defendant may introduce evidence to the contrary to prove that he or she is not responsible for the injury. For instance, the doctrine is not applicable if evidence or testimony is presented that there was more than one cause for the injury.[16]

Just as a criminal defendant is brought to court with a presumption of innocence until proven guilty of the charged criminal behavior "beyond a reasonable doubt," a health care provider is entitled to a presumption that he or she has practiced within the standard of care. It is up to the plaintiff to prove the defendant's negligence by a "preponderance of the evidence." However, if the plaintiff is allowed by the court to utilize the res ipsa loquitur doctrine, the presumption would then be that the defendant was negligent, and the burden of proof shifts to the defendant, who must prove that his or her acts were not negligent.

Res Ipsa Loquitur in Dentistry and Medicine

Examples of when res ipsa may be utilized in medical or dental cases include the following:
1. When an instrument or a foreign object is left in a patient's body after an operation
2. When dental treatment has been performed on the wrong tooth
3. When a patient is injured while he or she is unconscious

The purpose of the doctrine is to assist a plaintiff in proving his or her case when there has clearly been an injury but circumstances make it difficult to demonstrate fault. Some states do not permit the use of the doctrine, as they deem it unfair to health care providers.

RESPONDEAT SUPERIOR

If an employee commits a tort during the "scope of his or her employment," the employer will be jointly liable with the employee. This doctrine applies to all torts, but this tort must have occurred while the employee was acting on behalf of the employer. Business trips and other short trips for business purposes are considered within the scope of employment. However, traveling from home to work is not considered acting within the scope of employment. Under this doctrine, known as **respondeat superior** ("let the master answer"), the dentist is the principal (or employer) and the dental assistant, the dental hygienist, and others employed by the dentist are his agents (or employees). The dentist is legally responsible for wrongs committed by employees in the scope of their employment. Although this does not absolve the employee from blame, it may give the patient another party to sue. If an employer is otherwise blameless for the negligent act of an employee, the employer will still be obligated to pay damages to an injured party under respondeat

RESPONDEAT SUPERIOR

The principle that, generally, an employer is liable for the wrongful acts of an employee if the employee was acting within the scope of his or her employment.

---

[16]*Storniolo v. Bauer,* 574 N.Y.S.2d 731 (N.Y. App. Div. 1991).

superior. However, the employer may recover the amount of damages (in part or in whole) from the employee in a separate court action.

CONTRIBUTORY NEGLIGENCE

Contributory negligence is an affirmative defense and can be a complete bar against a plaintiff's recovery in states where it is recognized. The defendant must establish evidence that the plaintiff was guilty of contributory negligence. Actions of each party are held to the standard of how the reasonably prudent person would act under like circumstances. If a patient does not take reasonable care to protect his or her own safety and fails to act according to this standard, his or her actions are considered to have contributed to his or her injury, and constitute a bar to receiving any recovery from a health care provider. In some states this is a complete defense against recovery of damages. Other states use a comparative negligence theory, which attempts to proportion liability between the plaintiff and the defendant on the basis of their relative degrees of fault. In such a case, the plaintiff is not barred completely from recovering damages because of his or her contributory negligence. The recovery is reduced by a proportion equal to the ratio between the plaintiff's own negligence and the total negligence involved in the accident. A few states follow a pure comparative negligence system. Under this system a plaintiff is allowed partial recovery only if his or her negligence is either less than or no greater than the defendant's. If the plaintiff's negligence is more than the defendant's, the plaintiff can recover nothing. This can be an important legal defense for a dental health care provider. For instance, a patient's noncompliance with a provider's recommendations is certainly a form of contributory negligence.

> **CONTRIBUTORY NEGLIGENCE**
>
> A situation in which the plaintiff's negligent actions or omissions have contributed to his or her own injury.

SUGGESTED READINGS

Ahlowalia K, Lang W: Accessing MEDLINE from the dental office, *Journal of the American Dental Association* 127:510-516, 1996.

Vick V: The Internet in dentistry, *Dental Hygiene News* 11(1):10-13, 1998.

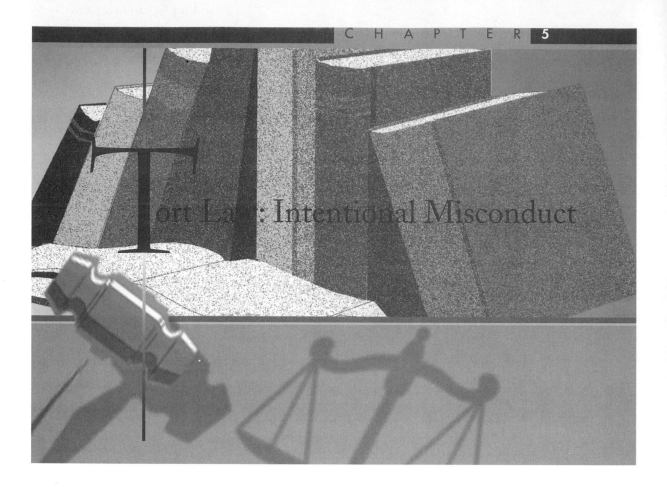

Tort Law: Intentional Misconduct

LEARNING OUTCOMES

After reading this chapter, you should be able to:

- Discuss the difference between intentional and unintentional torts, giving examples of each.
- Recognize what types of court actions may be taken against an individual who invades another person's privacy.
- Differentiate between intentional infliction of mental distress and negligent infliction of mental distress.
- Discuss an example of a situation in which a defendant is found guilty of fraud, or intentional misrepresentation, listing all elements that the plaintiff must prove in a court of law.
- Describe a situation in which an individual may recover damages in a court of law for interference with advantageous relations.

KEY WORDS

APPROPRIATION
ASSAULT
BATTERY
BUSINESS TORT
DEFAMATION
FALSE LIGHT
FRAUD

INJURIOUS FALSEHOOD
INTENTIONAL TORT
INTRUSION UPON SECLUSION
PUBLICITY OF PRIVATE LIFE
SLANDER PER SE
WRONGFUL DISCHARGE

INTENTIONAL AND MISCELLANEOUS TORTS

Intentional torts are more serious than negligent acts and are subject to a greater burden of proof. The plaintiff must prove that the defendant actually intended to commit the alleged act. The plaintiff must show that the defendant acted for the purpose of achieving a result that harmed the plaintiff's interest or that the defendant realized that such a result was substantially certain to follow from his or her action. The action need not be hostile, just intentional.

Certain disadvantages exist for a defendant, as well as advantages for a plaintiff, in a lawsuit claiming damages for an intentional rather than an unintentional (negligent) act. A few are as follows:

1. No expert witness is necessary in order to establish the standard of care on behalf of the plaintiff.
2. A plaintiff may recover damages even though there has been no physical harm.
3. Intentional torts are not always covered by liability insurance, leaving the defendant totally and personally liable.[1]
4. Punitive damages, as well as actual damages, are likely to be awarded in cases of intentional misconduct.

In this chapter the torts of assault, battery, defamation, invasion of privacy, infliction of mental distress, fraud or intentional misrepresentation, interference with advantageous relations, and wrongful discharge are discussed.

INTENTIONAL TORT

A tort that is committed with intent to cause physical or mental harm to another individual or the property of another.

ASSAULT AND BATTERY

Assault is any action that produces an apprehension or fear of bodily harm. **Battery** is the intentional infliction of harmful or offensive bodily contact[2] or nonconsensual contact with another that is harmful or offensive. Offensive contact includes any contact that is damaging to a "reasonable sense of dignity." A health care provider often performs procedures that are painful to the patient. These are not usually considered battery, as in most cases the patient has consented to the procedure.

However, the law protects a patient from unauthorized contact to his or her person. For an assault to occur, the patient/plaintiff must be aware of the threat. For a battery to occur, there must be lack of consent to physical contact or actual bodily harm. For instance, if a dental patient refuses local anesthesia for a dental procedure and the dental hygienist or dentist attempts to administer an injection (and the patient is aware of the attempt), an assault has been committed. However, if the injection is actually administered, battery has occurred. In each case the patient would have grounds for a lawsuit.

ASSAULT

Threatening to do bodily harm to another individual. Assault can be a civil or a criminal offense.

BATTERY

Committing bodily harm. Battery can be a civil or a criminal offense.

DEFAMATION

Defamation is the communication, to a third person, of an untrue statement about another person, exposing that person to contempt or damaging his or her reputation. Written defamation is libel, and oral defamation is slander. A statement is not

DEFAMATION

Publishing written or printed matter (libel) or making oral statements (slander) that damage the reputation of another person.

[1]*Niedzielski, Doe et al v. St. Paul Fire & Marine Insurance Co.*, 589 A.2d 130 (N.H. 1991).
[2]*Restatement of the law of torts, second*, St Paul, 1999, The American Law Institute, §§ 13, 18.

defamatory if it is true. If the plaintiff is a private individual, he or she must prove that the defendant was negligent in believing the truth of the statement. If the plaintiff is a public official or a public figure (e.g., politician or entertainer), the plaintiff must prove that the defendant had knowledge of the falsity of the statement or reckless disregard for whether the statement was true or false.[3,4] Certain types of statements are covered by a qualified privilege and are not subject to allegations of defamation. Employment recommendations and evaluations are in this category and cannot be considered defamatory, unless made with malice.

Slander Per Se

Generally, a plaintiff alleging slander is required under the law to prove special damages (financial losses). There are four exceptions to this requirement, which are classified as **slander per se.**

1. Statements that charge the plaintiff with engaging in criminal conduct. The criminal conduct must be a major crime punishable by imprisonment or involving moral turpitude.
2. Statements alleging that the plaintiff is unfit to conduct his or her business, profession, trade, or office
3. Statements alleging that the plaintiff has a venereal or other loathsome and communicable disease
4. Statements charging that the plaintiff has engaged in serious sexual misconduct

INVASION OF PRIVACY

Four categories of invasion of privacy involve various aspects of an individual's right to privacy:

1. **Intrusion upon seclusion.** Intrusion upon seclusion is an intrusion into one's solitude that would be "highly offensive to a reasonable person."[5] It occurs only when a private place is invaded, such as one's yard, home, or automobile. The taking of a photograph of someone in public is excluded, unless the photograph was of a private part of the individual's anatomy.
2. **Appropriation.** Appropriation is the use of any person's name or likeness for advertising purposes or other financial benefit without that person's consent. Appropriation can occur in dentistry when pictures of patients are displayed for the purpose of advertising certain procedures. Photographs for textbooks, brochures, and so forth, should never be used without the consent of the persons in the photographs.
3. **Publicity of private life.** Publicity of private life is the publicizing of details of a person's private life, which may be an invasion of his or her privacy. As with intrusion upon seclusion, the effect must be "highly offensive to a reasonable person."[6] The information publicized must be strictly private and

SLANDER PER SE

To prevail in a lawsuit based upon slander, the plaintiff must prove that he or she sustained some special monetary harm. However, there are four types of slander, called slander per se, in which such proof is not necessary: statements that the plaintiff (1) engaged in criminal behavior, (2) suffers from a loathsome disease, (3) is unfit to conduct his or her business, or (4) engaged in serious sexual misconduct.

INTRUSION UPON SECLUSION

An "invasion of privacy" tort. A person may sue if his or her solitude is intruded upon. The intrusion must be highly offensive to a reasonable person.

APPROPRIATION

The wrongful use or reproduction of a person's name or likeness for financial gain.

PUBLICITY OF PRIVATE LIFE

An "invasion of privacy" tort. Publicizing details of a person's private life. The invasion must be highly offensive to a reasonable person.

---

[3]*Dun & Bradstreet v. Greenmoss Builders*, 105 S.Ct. 2939 (1985).
[4]*Gertz v. Welch*, 418 U.S. 323 (1974).
[5]*Restatement of torts, second*, § 652B.
[6]*Restatement of torts, second*, § 652D.

must not be in a public record. Information publicized must not be of legitimate public concern.[7] Private lives of public officials are often considered of legitimate public concern, and release of information of public concern is not an invasion of privacy. The private details must be publicized and not simply released to a few people, unlike the situation in defamation, in which case publication may involve transmitting the false information to only one other individual. Therefore, publicity of private life includes the transmission of truthful information that if divulged to others would be highly offensive to a reasonable person and is not of legitimate concern to the public.

4. **False light.** One can bring an action for false light if by the actions of another person, one is placed before the public eye in a false light and the false light would be highly offensive to a reasonable person.[8] In cases of false light the defendant must have known that he was portraying the plaintiff in a false light or have acted with reckless disregard for the truth or falsity of the information released to the public.

FALSE LIGHT

An "invasion of privacy" tort. A person may sue if he or she is placed in a false light before the public. The false light must be highly offensive to a reasonable person.

INFLICTION OF MENTAL DISTRESS

In most situations involving claims for mental distress, it is initial physical injuries that produce the mental distress. In such cases, liability is usually based on traditional negligence or intentional tort theories. The elements of mental distress are usually compensable as part of the damages recoverable in tort action. The initial injury may be solely emotional and not covered by another tort theory.

Two categories for liability for infliction of mental distress are as follows:

1. Intentional "outrageous conduct," by which the defendant intentionally or recklessly inflicts severe emotional distress on the victim.[9]
2. Negligent conduct or intentional conduct that would not be considered "outrageous"

The most significant difference between the two is that most courts do not require that the mental distress has produced physical consequences when the conduct is outrageous. However, physical symptoms must have occurred to be actionable when a case is based upon behavior that is less than "outrageous."

FRAUD OR INTENTIONAL MISREPRESENTATION

Fraud is the intentional perversion of truth for the purpose of inducing another person to rely on it and part with something of value or surrender a legal right. The elements of fraud, or intentional misrepresentation, that a plaintiff must prove in a court of law are as follows:

1. The defendant's action to induce the plaintiff was intentional, not negligent.
2. The misrepresentation was material (substantial and important to the plaintiff's decision).
3. The misrepresentation was known to be untrue by the person asserting it.
4. The misrepresentation caused loss or harm to the victim.

FRAUD

Telling an intentional untruth for the purpose of inducing another person to rely on the falsehood and to surrender something of value.

---

[7]*Restatement of torts, second*, § 652D(6).
[8]*Restatement of torts, second*, § 652E.
[9]*Restatement of the law of torts*, St Paul, 1947, The American Law Institute.

5. The plaintiff relied on the misrepresentation, and it was justifiable that he do so (justifiable reliance by the plaintiff/victim).

For example, if a health care professional provided unnecessary services for a patient by mistake, the wrong would likely be considered negligence. If services provided were concealed from the patient, the wrong becomes fraud or intentional misrepresentation. If the professional took steps, such as destroying or altering patient records, to conceal the source of the patient's injury, the party would be guilty of express misrepresentation and could be liable for all injuries (including nonphysical injuries) resulting from the misrepresentation.

INTERFERENCE WITH ADVANTAGEOUS RELATIONS

Listed below are the three **business torts** that protect certain business interests:

1. Injurious falsehood
2. Interference with contract
3. Interference with prospective advantage

The tort of **injurious falsehood** protects one against false statements made against one's business, product, or property. The plaintiff must prove that a statement is false, that the statement was published (communicated to at least one other individual), and that the defendant acted out of ill will or spite for the plaintiff, and there must be monetary harm.

The tort of interference with contract protects one's interest in having existing contracts performed by the other party to the contract. The tort claim is against a party who induces another party to breach a contract with the plaintiff. The defendant's actions must be intentional.

The tort of interference with prospective advantage protects one from loss of the benefits of prospective or potential contracts or relationships with others. Names and definitions of this tort vary from state to state. Generally, the possibility of tort actions for interference with contractual relations prevents a wrongdoer from interfering with the gainful employment of another person.

WRONGFUL DISCHARGE

An employee who has been illegally terminated may sue the former employer for **wrongful discharge.** If the lawsuit is successful, a plaintiff may be able to claim compensation for all injuries suffered, including lost wages and mental distress. Absent a contract to the contrary, most employees are considered employees at will and can be fired for any reason that is not illegal (see Chapter 16). There are several possible exceptions to an employer's freedom to terminate an employee. The first exception is if the court finds that the firing violates public policy. This may be the case in sexual harassment cases or in whistleblower cases, in which a particular violation is reported to the authorities. The second exception relies on the terms in employee manuals. These manuals can be construed as terms of an employment contract. If safeguards in the employee manual are violated and apply to the specific situation, an employer may be held liable for wrongful discharge. Third, the law implies that all contracts include the covenant of good faith and fair dealing. Thus, employers must give a good reason and provide a fair process when terminating an employee.

BUSINESS TORT

A wrongful act committed in the course of business.

INJURIOUS FALSEHOOD

Defamation that causes actual damages.

WRONGFUL DISCHARGE

The termination of an employee from his or her job on the basis of reasons that violate the law, such as race, age, or religion.

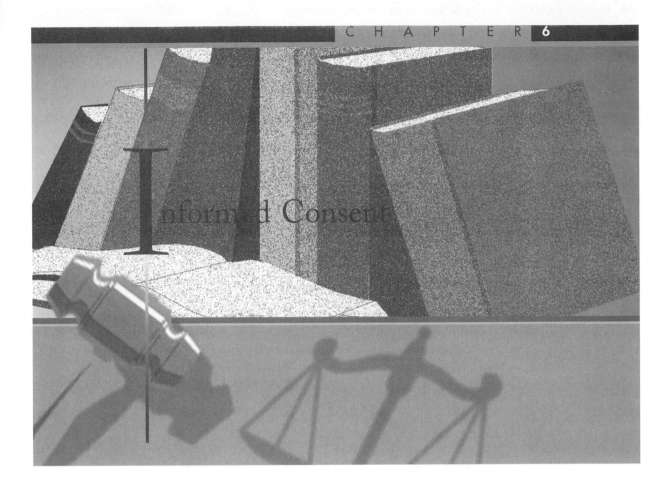

CHAPTER 6

Informed Consent

LEARNING OUTCOMES

After reading this chapter, you should be able to:
- Differentiate between implied consent and express consent.
- Describe situations in which consent may be considered incompetent.
- Explain which information a patient must understand in order for his or her consent to be considered informed.
- Design an informed consent form for a dental procedure.

KEY WORDS

CAUSATION
CONSENT
EXPRESS CONSENT
IMPLIED CONSENT
INFORMED CONSENT

INVALID CONSENT
MISREPRESENTATION
NONDISCLOSURE
OVERBROAD LANGUAGE

A patient's consent to medical or dental treatment that is given after the patient understands the nature of his or her condition, the treatment options, the risks involved in treatment, and the risks if no treatment is sought.

The right of **informed consent** is the patient's right to information and self-determination (freedom to make personal choices). Put simply, it is the patient's right to know and participate in decisions regarding his or her own health care.

Three questions are critical in regard to the patient's right of informed consent:
1. Whether the patient actually consented to a medical procedure
2. Whether the patient's consent was actually informed
3. Whether misrepresentation or nondisclosure of material information negated informed consent

The patient's right of informed consent sets requirements for the relationship between health care provider and patient. As a result of these requirements, patients are requested to sign consent forms indicating that they understand all aspects of treatment. These forms are required to be signed prior to certain medical or dental treatment. As discussed in Chapter 5, treatment provided with no valid informed consent could be considered battery. In a lawsuit for battery, a plaintiff/patient must establish that he or she was not informed of the medical or dental procedure performed and that a touching without consent therefore occurred. A plaintiff/patient may recover in a lawsuit for battery even if there has been no physical harm to the plaintiff. The plaintiff is also not required to show that consent would not have been given if he or she had been asked. If consent is given but the patient was not sufficiently informed, a health care provider may be liable for negligence.[1]

In *Salgo v. Leland Stanford Jr. University Board of Trustees*,[2] the court held that even a written consent is ineffective if the patient failed to understand material information about the procedure to be performed. Information must include the nature of the procedure and its risks.

REQUIREMENTS OF CONSENT

In a lawsuit in which informed consent is questioned, the defendant must establish the patient's consent to undergo treatment. There are two types of **consent:**

CONSENT

Approval or permission.

IMPLIED CONSENT

Permission that is inferred from the behavior of the parties rather than written or spoken.

EXPRESS CONSENT

Permission given specifically by words, written or oral.

1. **Implied consent.** Based on conduct. Consent is presumed from certain actions of the patient. Implied consent is given when the patient comes to the dental office and sits in the dental chair. However, implied consent would apply only to examination, diagnosis, and consultation. From that point on, the dentist may not assume the patient's consent, even if treatment is needed. The health care provider's understanding that particular conduct by the patient indicated consent must be reasonable. Implied consent is usually considered valid when an emergency situation exists.
2. **Express consent.** An affirmative statement that is communicated either verbally or in writing. Both verbal consent and written consent are binding. There are situations in which it is desirable to have the patient's consent in writing, to prove at a later time exactly what consent was given—for example, when a patient's photograph, in which he or she is identifiable, is to be shown to others. This is why textbook photographs often show a portion of the pa-

[1]*Chouinard v. Marjani*, 575 A.2d 238 (Conn. App. 1990).
[2]317 P.2d 170 (Cal. App. 1957).

tient's face blocked from view, so that his or her identity is unknown. Written consent for a particular treatment is required by law. A patient's express consent must be in writing for treatment that will require more than one year to complete.

Regardless of the reasonableness of the treatment, a health care provider may not act beyond the patient's authorization, except when the patient's life or health is seriously threatened.

If a patient has previously refused consent to a particular procedure, a court will more closely scrutinize the issue of consent. Obviously, it would be preferable to have written consent. A written consent form is an important piece of evidence should the patient make the claim that informed consent was not given. A signed consent form will generally create a presumption that informed consent to a particular treatment was given. The burden of proving that consent was not given would then shift to the patient.

COMPETENCY OF CONSENT

A patient giving consent must be mentally competent and able to comprehend the material facts. Consent must be voluntary and based on sufficient knowledge to make an intelligent choice. Absent an emergency requiring immediate treatment to save the patient's life or to prevent serious bodily harm, consent by a parent or guardian should be obtained for minors or for mentally incompetent individuals who are not legally able to give consent for themselves prior to treatment.[3] A dentist or a dental hygienist should not proceed with dental treatment for a child without parental consent, either orally (by telephone or in person) or in writing. For the consent to be legal, a patient must be in the legal custody of the person giving the consent. Consent by a minor has been found valid by the court when the minor was found to be mature enough to understand the nature and consequences of the treatment and to knowingly consent.[4] Many states have enacted legislation legalizing a minor's consent for certain procedures. Check your state's statute to see how applicable it is to various dental procedures.

Consent is implied in emergencies in which immediate treatment is necessary but the patient is unable to give consent. The patient may be unconscious or in a state of shock, or he or she may be a minor or mentally incompetent. Consent may be presumed if the emergency is a true emergency (one in which the patient is in danger of death or serious bodily harm).

Invalid Consent

Unless an emergency exists, a patient's consent will be invalid if gained by fraud, under duress, or by misrepresentation. Thus, consent is invalid if a health care provider is aware that the patient is acting with belief in an untrue statement of fact, or when the patient is a minor, incompetent, or not in a lucid state (disoriented as a result of trauma or medication). Consent may be found invalid because of duress

INVALID CONSENT
Permission given with no force of law. For instance, a person may sign an informed consent form that appears legal. However, if he or she is under the age of majority or is mentally incompetent, the consent is invalid.

[3]*Zoski v. Gaines*, 260 N.W. 99 (1935).
[4]*Melcher v. Charleston Area Medical Center*, 422 S.E.2d 827 (W.Va. 1992).

if it was signed while the patient was in severe pain. Also, for consent to be valid, it must be for a procedure that is legal. A patient could not legally consent to a treatment for cancer that is illegal to perform in the United States. When a patient cannot provide valid consent, because of minority or incapacity, and substitute consent is required, state statutes often identify specific persons, such as parents, guardians, or spouses, to provide the required consent. In some cases, court approval is required. Courts utilize child neglect statutes to appoint a guardian to consent for a child or give the court authority to approve treatment. Usually, treatment involves procedures to prevent death or serious injury. Courts look to the best interest of the child in deciding whether to appoint a guardian to ensure appropriate medical care for the child.[5] Abuse and neglect statutes have been utilized by public agencies to require parents to obtain dental care for their children.

Without clear consent of the patient, a health care professional must act with caution, and must consider factors such as age, mental capacity, existence of an emergency, and the relationship to another person who is giving substitute consent. State laws are unclear and differ from jurisdiction to jurisdiction (state to state).

CONTENT OF THE INFORMED CONSENT

A patient's consent must be informed. Prior to many medical or dental treatments, the patient must receive specific information. The health care provider must disclose several factors prior to treatment to satisfy the requirements of informed consent. The question of who must disclose is addressed in *Nevauex v. Park Place Hospital*.[6] The duty rests with the health care provider performing the medical procedure in question, regardless of who ordered the treatment. Each state has its own standard of disclosure to meet the requirements of informed consent. The following is an overview of criteria, based on cases found throughout our court system.

Diagnosis

The patient must be informed of a diagnosis and also must be given a description of tests, and alternatives to them, that support the diagnosis. In the patient-professional relationship, a health care provider has the duty to disclose the diagnosis.

Nature and Purpose of Treatment

The mode of treatment should be described to the patient and should include expected outcomes. The probabilities of success and failure should also be disclosed.

Risks and Outcomes

For disclosure of risks to be required, the risks must be material to the patient's decision making.[7] Remote risks or those commonly known to patients need not be disclosed.[8] For instance, the risk of infection should be known to every patient.[9]

---

[5]*Custody of a Minor*, 393 N.E.2d 836 (Mass. 1979).
[6]656 S.W.2d 923 (Tex. Ct. App. 1983).
[7]*Harbeson v. Parke Davis*, 746 F.2d 517 (9th Cir. 1984).
[8]*Shinn v. St. James Mercy Hosp.*, 675 F.Supp. 94 (N.Y. 1987).
[9]*Kissinger v. Lofgren*, 836 F.2d 678 (1st Cir. 1988).

Courts have held that if a risk is small, disclosure is not needed, unless the small risk is death.[10] If a patient asks a specific question regarding a particular risk, the duty to disclose may include the information necessary to explain that particular risk.[11] If a patient specifically inquires about a risk, he or she has a right to know, even if disclosure would not otherwise be required.[12]

Alternatives

Patients should be provided information on alternative methods of diagnosis and treatment, their risks and consequences, and their probability of success.[13]

Prognosis If Treatment Is Refused

A health care provider has a duty to inform the patient of the likely prognosis if he or she refuses a treatment or test viewed as valuable by the professional. Every patient has a right to "informed refusal." Patients refusing dental radiographs need to know the possible consequences of their refusal. If a patient wishes to refuse a procedure or test, the health care provider has a duty to advise the patient of all material risks that a reasonable person would want know about, before the patient decides not to undergo the procedure or test. It is always good practice to document a patient's refusal. One should have the patient write his or her refusal or have a witness sign the documented refusal. Remember that absent a compelling state interest, a competent adult has a constitutionally protected right to refuse treatment, including lifesaving treatment.[14] In some situations, a compelling state interest exists for the protection of both the individual and society. An example of such an interest is the prevention of the transmission of disease, which is accomplished by means of a state statute requiring vaccinations.

Prognosis With Treatment

A patient cannot make an informed choice without information regarding prognosis. There are cases in which physicians have argued "therapeutic privilege"; for example, if life expectancy is in question, a physician may choose to withhold information so that a patient will not give up hope of recovery. Some courts, however, have required disclosure of all material risks,[15] and others have indicated that the duty to disclose encompasses diagnosis, general nature of the procedure, and probability of success.

CAUSATION, MISREPRESENTATION, AND NONDISCLOSURE

If a plaintiff/patient proves a violation of a duty to disclose, he or she is not entitled to recover damages without proving that it was the cause of injury; the **nondisclosure** of information must have affected the plaintiff/patient's decision to proceed with or refuse treatment. Courts utilize either of two tests of **causation**—the ob-

NONDISCLOSURE

Failure to divulge facts. Nondisclosure need not be associated with deception.

CAUSATION

Derivation, basis, or origin of some specific condition or event.

---

[10]*Cobbs v. Grant*, 502 P.2d 1 (Calif. 1972).
[11]*Korman v. Mallin*, 858 P.2d 1145 (Alaska 1993).
[12]*Harbeson*, supra.
[13]*Moore v. Baker*, 989 F.2d 1129 (11th Cir. 1993).
[14]*Lane v. Candura*, 376 N.E.2d 1232 (Mass. 1976).
[15]*Canterbury v. Spence*, 464 F.2d 772 (D.C. Cir. 1972).

jective reasonable person test (what a reasonable patient would have done) or the subjective test (what this particular patient would have done). Some courts require both tests to show causation.[16]

Should a health care professional make fraudulent or negligent **misrepresentations** to a patient that result in harm to that patient's health, the professional is liable for the injury caused by the patient's justifiable reliance on the misrepresentation. Note that the patient's reliance on the misinformation must be justifiable. The reliance must be warranted; that is, it must be consistent with ordinary caution and prudence on the part of the patient.

Health care providers may be liable for both their own nondisclosure and nondisclosure by others. For instance, should a health provider discover a condition that is a risk to a patient's health, regardless of who caused the injury, the condition must be disclosed, or the health care provider risks liability for negligence. A health professional attempting to protect another could risk a lawsuit based on negligence. Should an injury to a patient occur, all participants in the treatment have the duty to disclose or risk liability for nondisclosure. A patient/plaintiff who proves a violation of the duty to disclose can recover all proximately caused damages, including nonphysical damages and physical damages.

Depending on the jurisdiction, the running of the statute of limitations could be suspended if nondisclosure of information were established later. This would have the overall effect of increasing liability, as the statute would not begin to run until the patient discovered the injury. For example, a state's statute might provide that a medical malpractice suit must be filed within two years. If the patient/ plaintiff did not discover the injury for five years, the patient would be allowed to bring the action to court unless he or she should have known of the injury sooner. (See Chapter 4 for discussion of statute of limitations.)

OVERBROAD CONSENT FORMS

The language in consent forms is often overbroad. **Overbroad language** includes authorization of any treatment for the patient's condition or a statement that all risks have been explained to the patient. Under such circumstances, a patient could claim that the oral disclosure that a health care provider made was deficient.[17] It could also be claimed that the patient's consent to treatment was not specific.[18] The language in a preprinted, boilerplate form often bears little relationship to the actual treatment and may not be useful in a court of law.

Ideally, patient consent should be documented in the progress notes as well as on a separate form in the record. This is especially true of procedures involving endodontics, oral surgery, orthodontics, periodontal surgery, implants, esthetics, or other higher-risk treatment.

All informed consent forms are to be signed and dated by the patient and the provider. The signed form should document the discussion between the patient and

---

[16]*Harnish v. Children's Hospital,*, 439 N.E.2d 240 (Mass. 1982).
[17]*Bourgeois v. McDonald,* 622 So.2d 684 (La. App. 1993).
[18]*Cross v. Trapp,* 294 S.E.2d 446 (W.Va. 1982).

the provider, and the patient's treatment decision should be based on information given to the patient during the discussion.

SUMMARY

For valid consent to occur, the individual consenting must be legally competent, the consent must be for a specific procedure, and the treatment consented to must be legal. Consent cannot be obtained by fraud, under duress, or by misrepresentation, and it must be informed. The requirements of informed consent are time consuming for those involved in the delivery of health care. However, they provide patients with the power to make decisions regarding their health.

If treatment proceeds with no informed consent, a patient can prevail in a court of law with no expert testimony. This means that the patient/plaintiff need not allege or prove a violation in the standard of care. This also means that no error of treatment or diagnosis need be alleged or proven.[19] Therefore, providing informed consent is a safe practice for health care providers and allows patients the dignity of making choices regarding their medical and dental care.

SUGGESTED READINGS

Kirby MD: Informed consent: what does it mean? *Journal of Medical Ethics* 9:69-75, 1983.
Tromblt RM: Taming the paper tiger, *Dental Teamwork* 9(4):18, July-August 1996.

---

[19]*Harnish*, supra.

AUTHOR'S COMMENTS FOR CASE STUDY 1

Reread Case Study 1 and the Study Questions at the Beginning of Section II.
Questions 1 through 4 are examined together in the following analysis:

1. Does Mr. Arnold have a legal claim against Dr. Hastings?
2. Did Dr. Hastings owe a duty to Mr. Arnold?
3. Did the treatment Dr. Hastings provided for Mr. Arnold fall below the required standard of care?
4. What must Mr. Arnold legally prove to recover damages against Dr. Hastings?

In the case study it appears that Mr. Arnold does have a legal claim of negligence against Dr. Hastings.

The four elements that Mr. Arnold must establish in court to show negligence are as follows:

1. A duty was owed to the plaintiff (Mr. Arnold) by the defendant (Dr Hastings).
2. There was a breach of that duty.
3. An injury was suffered by the plaintiff.
4. The injury was caused by the breach of duty.

Duty. Mr. Arnold was Dr. Hastings' patient, and treatment was provided. Therefore, the relationship between the two indicated that a clear obligation of due care (reasonable care under the circumstances) was owed to Mr. Arnold by Dr. Hastings. Also, Dr. Hastings owed Mr. Arnold a duty to inform him of the dental procedure he was about to perform and to obtain Mr. Arnold's informed consent prior to treatment.

Breach. Dr. Hastings breached his duty of care. Proving this breach consists in demonstrating that the dentist did not provide treatment with the skills and knowledge comparable to those possessed by members of the dental profession in good standing. First, Dr. Hastings' competence should be called into question in relation to a procedure he performed for Mr. Arnold with very little training and no previous experience. Second, the standard of care has clearly been breached by Dr. Hastings' omission in not thoroughly reading all of the instructions accompanying the materials for the periodontal procedure. Written instructions such as these may be introduced into evidence in a court of law. In addition, Dr. Hastings did not adequately review Mr. Arnold's medical history prior to treating him. Remember that an expert witness would have to testify in court that Dr. Hastings' care fell below the standard of care.

Injury. Mr. Arnold's loss of three teeth is an obvious injury. He may also establish damages such as lost wages, pain and suffering, and other related expenses.

Causation. It is not clear from the information provided in the case study, but it is likely that Mr. Arnold's loss was caused by Dr. Hastings' negligent treatment of those particular teeth. Causation would be established by a witness who may be deemed an expert in dentistry by the court. One of the dentist's duties to the patient is not to abandon the patient once treatment has started. Mr. Arnold also has a claim of abandonment against Dr. Hastings. Abandonment is discussed in Chapter 8.

AUTHOR'S COMMENTS FOR CASE STUDY 1—cont'd

5. Is Dr. Hastings in any way liable to Danny?
This question addresses the issue of whether Danny has a claim against Dr. Hastings. A business invitee is one who is invited by the owner onto the premises to do business with him. Here, Mr. Arnold and Danny would be considered business invitees. Dr. Hastings has a duty to keep his property in safe condition and to warn patients and anyone else entering the office as a business invitee of any hazards that might exist. This duty applies to furniture, fixtures, toys, and dental equipment and dental instruments, as well as conditions outside of the office, such as broken steps or icy sidewalks. Dr. Hastings breached his duty to see that the premises were safe. The breach was evident, as the toy had been broken for some time. It seems that no one saw Danny's accident. In this particular situation Danny's attorney may want to utilize the doctrine of res ipsa loquitur. It would then be unnecessary to prove Dr. Hastings' substandard care through an expert witness. The elements of res ipsa are arguably met. A 5-year-old child is not normally injured to that extent without negligence on someone's part. The instrumentality, or in this situation the toy, was under the exclusive control of Dr. Hastings. Finally, we have no information indicating that Danny in any way negligently contributed to his injury. In conclusion, Danny would have a negligence action in which Dr. Hastings would be the defendant.

6. Is Dr. Jones liable to Mr. Arnold for refusing to treat him on an emergency basis?
Mr. Arnold has no claim against Dr. Jones for not providing emergency treatment. Mr. Arnold was not a patient of record in Dr. Jones' office, and Dr. Jones did not begin any treatment. Therefore, Dr. Jones owed no duty to Mr. Arnold and could not be liable for his injury.

7. Does Ms. Andrews have a legal claim against Dr. Hastings?
Yes, Ms. Andrews does have a claim. Although employment recommendations are protected against allegations of defamation, there is no protection if statements about an employee are made with malice. Here, Dr. Hastings deliberately lied regarding Ms. Andrews' performance in order to keep her as an employee. Ms. Andrews has a claim of interference with advantageous relations as well as defamation.

8. Does Mr. Arnold have a legal claim against Dr. Roberts?
Although Dr. Roberts asked permission to take the photographs, he did not get permission (preferably written) to use the photographs in a public display. Dr. Roberts will have committed an invasion of Mr. Arnold's privacy should he use recognizable photographs of Mr. Arnold. Dr. Roberts' textbook was written for financial gain, and Mr. Arnold is a well-known politician throughout the state. Depending how Dr. Roberts uses the photographs, it may also be alleged that he is guilty of appropriation.

AUTHOR'S COMMENTS FOR CASE STUDY 1—cont'd

9. Did Dr. Hastings commit assault and battery?

10. Were the elements of informed consent or informed refusal met regarding the procedure Dr. Hastings completed for Mr. Arnold?

Negligence actions can result when a patient gives consent for a particular procedure but the consent was uninformed. In this situation not only did Mr. Arnold not have an opportunity to give informed consent, but he had no opportunity to give any consent. The procedure was completed prior to his having any knowledge of it. This is an obvious violation of informed consent. Since treatment was performed with no consent, Mr. Arnold's allegation would be battery (an unconsented touching). Mr. Arnold would have no claim for assault, as he was not in fear of being touched (or receiving treatment) because he was totally unaware of the procedure during treatment.

11. As a consultant for Dr. Hastings' office, what suggestions would you have for other members of his office staff in regard to strategies to reduce the risks of legal liability?

All literature relating to medicaments, instruments, and equipment should be placed in one location. This literature should be available to all members of the dental health team. All employees could then refresh their memories whenever necessary. This would ensure that all medicaments, instruments, and equipment are utilized according to manufacturer's directions, thus providing for the safety of the patient.

In addition, one individual within the office should be designated to oversee all patient consents for dental treatment. That individual needs to monitor information dispensed to patients regarding their treatment. Any necessary written informed consent documents need to be signed. Should a consent be verbal, such consent must be documented in the progress notes of the patient's file.

With children's safety in mind, all members of the dental health team should develop a policy regarding children visiting the office as patients or nonpatients. This policy is to be shared with the patients.

Immediately after seating a patient in the dental operatory and prior to treatment, the dental assistant or hygienist should review the medical history with the patient. It is necessary to establish whether there are new additions to the information. Any positive responses that may be important should be flagged for the dentist to review.

It is the responsibility of all members of the dental health team to see that the office is a safe environment. All areas should be checked on a daily basis, and any necessary changes should be made immediately. If repairs are beyond an employee's ability to address, they should be called to the attention of the dentist.

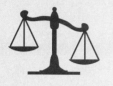

CASE STUDY 2

Mr. Mark Cook is a single, 35-year-old accountant. Although Mr. Cook was a patient of record in Dr. Hastings' dental practice, he had not been to the dental office for three years. Mr. Cook made an appointment with Dr. Hastings after injuring his maxillary right central incisor while playing basketball. During this appointment Dr. Hastings found that the tooth was severely fractured and required endodontic therapy and a crown. Dr. Hastings told Mr. Cook that complete treatment of the tooth would cost $1,000. Mr. Cook agreed to the treatment and the costs. Immediately, Dr. Hastings proceeded with the endodontic therapy during Mr. Cook's emergency visit. Noticing that Mr. Cook's gingiva was inflamed and that there were large calcareous deposits on his teeth, Dr. Hastings recommended that Mr. Cook make an appointment with the dental hygienist, Ms. Elaine Gale. The following day Mr. Cook reported for his appointment with Ms. Gale. After completing a medical history form, Ms. Gale discovered that Mr. Cook had a heart defect. He described this condition as minor and stated that no one had ever required him to have antibiotic therapy prior to dental treatment. Ms. Gale phoned Mr. Cook's cardiologist, who reported Mr. Cook's condition to be hypertrophic cardiomyopathy. Ms. Gale explained to Mr. Cook why the protection of an antibiotic was required for his particular condition. However, Mr. Cook refused to take an antibiotic or to postpone his appointment until a later time; he insisted on having his teeth cleaned immediately. It was currently tax

season, and the demands of Mr. Cook's job permitted no additional free time. Mr. Cook agreed to sign a waiver stating that he assumed the risk of not complying with antibiotic therapy. Ms. Gale performed a gross debridement with the ultrasonic scaler. Because of the profuse bleeding of Mr. Cook's gingival tissue, Ms. Gale requested that he make an appointment for a follow-up prophylaxis in three weeks. Mr. Cook did not keep his appointment. In fact, he did not return to Dr. Hastings' office for nine months. Again Mr. Cook called for an emergency appointment, since he was again in pain. Mr. Cook told the receptionist that the reason he had not returned for his treatment to be completed was that he had been in the hospital for several months. An examination of Mr. Cook's teeth revealed an abscess on tooth #18. No payment was ever made by Mr. Cook for any of the services received in Dr. Hastings' office. As a result, Dr. Hastings refused to treat Mr. Cook. Mr. Cook left and went to the dental office of Dr. Warner. When asked about his medical history in Dr. Warner's office, he did not include information regarding his heart condition. Mr. Cook complained to Dr. Warner about Dr. Hastings, stating that it had been unethical for Dr. Hastings not to have treated him on an emergency basis. Dr. Warner suggested that Mr. Cook report Dr. Hastings to the state board of dental examiners.

The following day Ms. Sarah Charles, the receptionist for Dr. Hastings' office, had lunch with Ms. Ellen Lane, who is employed in Dr. Warner's office as a dental assistant. In their conversation Ms. Lane told Ms. Charles about Mr. Cook's visit to their office and how upset he had been with Dr. Hastings. In an effort to protect her employer, Ms. Charles told Ms. Lane that Mr. Cook was nothing but a deadbeat. She explained that he did not pay his bills and that he had an awful temper. She also explained that Ms. Gale had told her how diseased and dirty his mouth was. Ms. Lane said that Mr. Cook had listed a disease on his medical history that sounded rather serious; she was not sure what it was, but thought it might be related to his having AIDS, and that Dr. Warner had better think twice before treating this patient. Ms. Lane and Ms. Charles were so busy with their conversation that they were not aware that several people in the restaurant could hear every word spoken. One of these people was Mr. Cook's sister, who called him immediately after lunch and repeated every word she had heard.

Ms Clara Jenret is also a dental assistant for Dr. Hastings. She has been with him for eighteen years and just celebrated her sixty-first birthday. Although Dr. Hastings appreciated her years of service, he was anxious to get some new ideas into the office and told Ms. Jenret that he could no longer afford to keep both assistants. He stated that he was very sorry, but her job was being eliminated and he would naturally provide her with two weeks' severance pay. One month later Dr. Hastings placed an advertisement in the local newspaper, requesting applications for a dental assistant's position in his office. He received four applications. One applicant was a 23-year-old man with five years of dental assisting experience in the United States military. Another applicant was a 32-year-old black woman with seven years of dental assisting experience. Another applicant was a 52-year-old white woman with twenty-five years of dental assisting experience. The last applicant was a 24-year-old white woman who had one year of experience selling cellular phones, two years of experience in a hospital setting processing forms for the admissions department, and two years of experience in a local modeling school. Dr. Hastings hired the last applicant because of her diversified experience.

RESPONSE TO CASE STUDY — Laurence P. Minott, Jr., Esq.

Initially, it looks as though there is an enforceable contract between the good doctor and Mr. Cook (i.e., an agreement as to treatment and costs). There may be issues regarding the statute of frauds and the writing requirement, but a lot of that would depend on what may have appeared in the medical intake that was subsequently done prior to the prophylaxis the next day (Mr. Cook signed the release, so I assume that he also signed the medical intake form). There is also the quantum meruit argument in relation to the work accomplished on behalf of and with the express agreement of Mr. Cook.

I question whether the "waiver" is sufficient to fully protect Dr. Hastings and would have to see it in order to be comfortable with the procedure involved. I also wonder where Dr. Hastings' input is in the procedure. Did Ms. Gale undertake this responsibility on her own, or did she confer with the good doctor, who ordered her to do it in the manner that it was accomplished? I also believe that since Dr. Hastings started an endodontic treatment, he should have been concerned when his patient did not return for the ongoing treatments as well as for the sealing of the tooth and crown placement. I believe that in order for him to protect himself, Dr. Hastings should have tried to get Mr. Cook back in for the continuing treatment (regardless of the payment issues) until the treatment and crown were complete. I also think that Dr. Hastings' later refusal to treat Mr. Cook because of his failure to pay is faulty for that same reason (i.e., the incomplete endodontic treatment). I think that it would have been better for Dr. Hastings to have seen him, if for no other reason than to ascertain the status of the endodontic treatment; if that had been completed by another dentist, then Dr. Hastings could refuse further treatment, if Mr. Cook did not pay his bill.

Regarding the issue of not treating Mr. Cook during an emergency (say pain), I am not aware of any requirement that a dentist must see anyone who calls up and says that he is in pain. Without more, the dentist is free to accept or reject clients on a nondiscriminatory basis. For instance, refusal could not violate the Americans with Disabilities Act. Refusing to treat because of prior nonpayment should be acceptable; the problem that I have is with the unresolved matter of the endodontic treatment and crown.

My reaction to the possibility of reporting Dr. Hastings to the board of dental examiners is that should Mr. Cook, who has done a number of things wrong himself, bother to call the board, after a thorough investigation the board would not find actionable fault with Dr. Hastings' actions (other than perhaps for not following up on the endodontic treatment).

In regard to the office help openly discussing patient business in public, that is the obvious wrongdoing in the second part of the scenario; patient confidentiality should not be breached. In addition to that is the matter of information and opinions being passed from the assistants to the rest of the restaurant. Mr. Cook appears to have very good grounds for a slander and invasion of privacy suit against the doctors and their assistants. (If I were Mr. Cook's attorney, I would sue both doctors. I think that of the two matters in the case study, this one is by far the most serious.)

Finally, in regard to the termination of Ms. Jenret, she may have grounds for an age dis-crimination suit. I think that, depending on how the doctor covered his tracks (i.e., financial study regarding the practice; rewriting office manual to downsize staff, etc.), he may be able to defend himself against that allegation, but most likely he will not have done that and then will have really left himself wide open to the allegation. Further evaluation than that would require an extensive examination of labor laws.

Regarding Dr. Hastings' hiring of the model—so what's the problem? It can always be explained that he wants to train her in his own methods rather than having to break old habits of the more experienced assistant and then re-train her. Also, as a private individual, he is not necessarily held to minority hiring practices, and is under no compunction to hire any minority applicant unless he wants to. Although he most probably would lose a lot of respect (assuming that he had any to begin with in relation to his employees), he can hire the applicant with "diversified experience." The applicants probably would not be aware of each other and probably would not have standing to do anything but grouse about not getting the position—remember that they are just applicants, and given the proximity between dentists and assistants in the work setting, a dentist can turn down an application for an assistant's position on grounds that he or she just does not want to work, on a daily basis, in such close quarters with the applicant. Again, although Ms. Jenret may have some grounds, I do not believe that any of the applicants do. We may not *personally* like what Dr. Hastings did, but I do not find it actionable.

Statute of frauds. Many contracts are valid even though they are oral. However, a statute of frauds makes some types of contracts unenforceable unless they are in writing. All states, except Louisiana, have adopted rules relating to some form of a statute of frauds to prevent fraudulent claims.

RESPONSE TO CASE STUDY—cont'd

Quantum meruit. In the event that a breach of contract occurs after a portion of the services have been performed, a party may sue for the reasonable value of the services performed or the benefits actually conferred on the other party to the contract. Therefore, a party may be able to recover on quantum meruit ("as much as he or she deserves") the reasonable value of his or her services.

Standing. A plaintiff must have standing to assert a claim in a court of law. To have standing, one must have an interest or stake in the outcome of the litigation.

RESPONSE TO CASE STUDY — Joan Leland, Dental Office Manager

All of the "mistakes" listed in this case study are more common than one might believe. In reality these things do happen every day in many offices. There are doctors who get so caught up in the multiple stresses of running a practice that they become lax, and neglect some of the things that are most important. These are professionals who have studied the laws regarding taking medical histories prior to treatment, abandonment, medical ethics, patient confidentiality, and discrimination. These dentists know the importance of training each and every staff member in all of these areas. It should not be forgotten that these are laws, not individual preferences or office policies.

It can become easy enough for anyone to neglect his or her responsibilities in regard to confidentiality, ethics, and record keeping. Staff members have two overall concerns that they must never lose sight of: their obligations to the patient and their obligations to the doctor. It is important that the doctor and his office manager have a well-informed, trusted, and professional staff. When an employee breaks this trust, something must be done immediately to correct and end the problem. This may include additional training, a reprimand, or possibly termination to protect the doctor and his patients.

Dr. Hastings' receptionist not only forgot about her legal and ethical duty to her boss and to the patient, but ignorantly exaggerated the inaccurate information. To misconstrue information and actually imply that Mr. Cook may have AIDS or be HIV positive was a very serious allegation. The receptionist placed her employer at risk of a lawsuit, and just imagine how Mr. Cook felt after finding out that this false information had been spread to his new dentist, dental staff, and his family.

Dr. Hastings' problems go further than his receptionist. He abandoned treatment of a patient after being negligent in the first place. Updating a medical history for a patient who had not visited the office for the past three years should have been his top priority when he met with Mr. Cook. These two men had a contract between them from the time that Mr. Cook agreed to the recommended treatment plan. Dr. Hastings could have properly terminated their relationship in writing because of nonpayment long before Mr. Cook had the opportunity to show up for an emergency visit.

Dr. Hastings continued to show negligence with his illegal and unfair treatment of a long-time assistant, who may have been graying at the temples but, it would appear, may have been the only trustworthy staff member in the practice. Following discrimination laws and keeping accurate employee records is also a big key to staying out of the courtroom. Ms. Jenret has the best

RESPONSE TO CASE STUDY—cont'd

reasons to file a suit against her employer of eighteen years. Age discrimination was just the beginning for Dr. Hastings when he began interviewing new applicants for the dental assisting position. He obviously was not in search of the most qualified individual. He then showed discrimination regarding sex and race as well. These applicants, too, would have good claims against the doctor.

Ms. Gale, Dr. Hastings' hygienist, had the good sense to update Mr. Cook's medical history and continued to follow through with a call to his cardiologist. After the cardiologist informed her that premedication prior to dental treatment was required for Mr. Cook, she should have followed through by insisting that he take the antibiotic. She felt that having the patient sign a waiver was sufficient to go ahead with treatment that day. This is a common misconception in many practices. The waiver would not be useful in court as evidence against malpractice. Although Mr. Cook had the right to refuse the antibiotic, Ms. Gale should have protected herself and the practice by rescheduling Mr. Cook for a time when he would be properly premedicated.

Mr. Cook, being a professional accountant, should understand how withholding critical information from someone who is trying to help him could hurt everyone involved. If he had fully disclosed all of his medical history to his new dentist, he not only would have helped the new dentist treat him properly, but may have, in the right situation, saved his own life. This case study never provides the reason behind Mr. Cook's hospital stay or says whether it may have been related to his recent dental visit in which he refused antibiotics. This patient placed himself in jeopardy again by not telling his new dentist about any of this. Dr. Warner was given consent to treat Mr. Cook and had no liability for any heart-related complications that could have occurred, because he was not informed by the patient. This patient neglected his responsibility.

The importance of following the laws that relate to a practice cannot be stressed enough. Constant reminders to keep the entire dental team "on their toes" should be everywhere, every day. There are so many things to remember—safety, ethics, thorough record keeping, confidentiality—and all are vital to the dental practice.

RESPONSE TO CASE STUDY — Geoffrey W. Wagner, D.D.S.

Dr. Hastings and Mr. Cook

1. The phrase "patient of record" implies a number of things. First to my mind is that I am responsible for providing competent care. I have agreed to this when I accept the patient. I have also told patients at an introductory visit that I was not, nor was my office, going to provide anything but emergency care for this single episode.

2. We are not told if the endodontic fill was completed for Mr. Cook. If the fill was not completed, the dentist is obligated to finish this procedure with or without collecting his fee.

3. From the text it seems that the medical history form revealing the heart defect was not completed until Mr. Cook met with the hygienist, Ms. Gale. This was at Mr. Cook's

---

Opinions are those of the writer, Geoffrey W. Wagner, D.D.S. Comments are based on gleanings from risk management seminars, as well as fairness in clinical practice.

RESPONSE TO CASE STUDY—cont'd

second treatment appointment with this office. At this point, were Mr. Cook to have an untoward event involving his heart, possibly the reason he was in the hospital and missed his next dental appointment, I believe that Dr. Hastings and his insurance company could be held accountable for this omission. The waiver that the hygienist had the patient sign is basically a piece of paper that has no merit. My risk management courses tell me that the patient cannot give up the right to protect and safeguard his health.

4. Dr. Warner suggested that Mr. Cook contact the state board of dental examiners regarding his complaints about how Dr. Hastings and/or Dr. Hastings' office had treated him. In Maine there are three avenues for complaints:
   a. Peer review through the state dental association
   b. The state board of dental examiners
   c. 1-800-ISUE4UU

   In some states both options a and b offer a grievance procedure to help resolve a question regarding refusal to treat a patient.

5. The lunch discussion that took place between two dental staff persons, one from Dr. Hastings and one from Dr. Warner, which was overheard by other people in a public area, constitutes a case of slander. All health care personnel need to be made aware of the responsibility they bear to safeguard the privacy of their patients out of the office as well as in the office.

Dismissal of an employee, Ms. Jenret, after 18 years of service. I do not have much information to share about potential wrongful dismissal. I would suggest that the employer in question would have been well advised to speak with his lawyer prior to making this decision. As for his hiring practices, I believe, again, that he would have been well advised to get some legal advice. As for his desire for "new ideas," continuing dental education is mandatory in most states and is designed to require practitioners to be exposed to "new ideas." I would question the doctor's motives.

RESPONSE TO CASE STUDY — Carolyn A. Hartnett, C.D.A., R.D.H., M.Ed.

This case study cleverly illustrates several important ethical and legal aspects of health care practice, involving contractual agreements between patient and provider in regard to treatment, issues of protocol involving medical history concerns and patient confidentiality, peer relationships, and personnel practices in regard to employee discrimination.

The first noticeable problem comes as a result of the poor communication that exists between Dr. Hastings and Mr. Cook. Both parties share

the negligence, as neither fulfills his responsibilities in the usual patient-doctor contractual relationship. Dr. Hastings needs to be more careful to go over treatment planning with his patient as well to document missed appointments and unpaid bills. If a patient has been delinquent in these areas, it is important that the office send this patient a letter of termination from the practice before he or she tries to schedule another appointment. Failure of the dentist to follow these rules could result in charges of abandonment.

RESPONSE TO CASE STUDY—cont'd

When it comes to protocol involving medical history issues, Ms. Gale, the hygienist, was prudent to call Mr. Cook's cardiologist for more information concerning his heart condition. The transgression resides in the fact that the patient was able to convince the educated professional that his health and well-being should be compromised for the sake of his personal convenience. This mistake becomes more significant when Mr. Cook moves on to Dr. Warner's office and thinks that he has nothing to lose by not informing Dr. Warner's office of his cardiac condition.

Once Mr. Cook got to Dr. Warner's office, the unethical behavior continued. Recognizing that a colleague's judgment was in question; Dr. Warner would want to send for Mr. Cook's records to determine what exactly had transpired in the previous office in regard to dental treatment and financial considerations. Without more information, speaking negatively about the actions of a colleague and advising a patient to go to the state board are not the correct course of action for Dr. Warner.

While not enough communication takes place in the instances mentioned above, far too much occurs between the dental staffs of the two offices. The legal and ethical imperative for confidentiality surrounding a patient's medical and financial records should be a well-known fact. Without proper justification, no personal information should ever be disclosed.

Finally, Dr. Hastings' practices concerning the hiring of new staff need to be examined. If we compare the resumes of the applicants for the job of dental assistant, it does not appear that the most qualified applicant was hired. Because some dental offices employ only a few people and are somewhat isolated, it would be relatively easy for these events to occur and to go unnoticed.

Quite candidly, most of the unfortunate events that take place in this case could happen in any dental practice. It is important that clear guidelines be established for all members of the dental team and that they be reviewed frequently.

CASE STUDY QUESTIONS

1. Does a contract exist between Mr. Cook and Dr. Hastings?
2. Did the "waiver" Mr. Cook signed have any force of law?
3. Did Mr. Cook have the right to refuse antibiotic therapy?
4. Did Dr. Hastings abandon Mr. Cook, or was he within his legal rights not to treat him?
5. Does Mr. Cook have a claim against Dr. Hastings?
6. Does Mr. Cook have a claim against Ms. Gale?
7. Does Mr. Cook have a claim against Dr. Warner?
8. Does Dr. Hastings have a claim against Dr. Warner?
9. Is Ms. Charles suggesting that Dr. Hastings' office policy is to refuse to treat patients with AIDS?
10. What would you say to Ms. Jenret if she asked your advice regarding her loss of employment?
11. Do any applicants for Dr. Hastings' dental assisting position have a claim against Dr. Hastings?

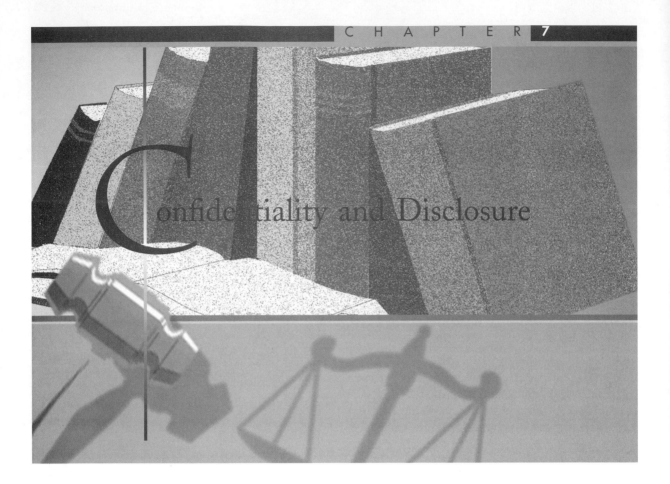

CHAPTER 7

Confidentiality and Disclosure

LEARNING OUTCOMES

After reading this chapter, you should be able to:

- Recognize when a breach of confidentiality may be a breach of ethics.
- Discuss what action a patient may take should information regarding his or her health be disclosed without his or her consent.
- Examine how "privilege" could determine whether information regarding an individual's health could be introduced as evidence in a court of law.
- Discuss several situations in which a health care professional must disclose information regarding a patient's health.

KEY WORDS

CONFIDENTIALITY
DISCLOSURE
HIPPOCRATIC OATH

PRIVILEGE
WAIVE

As stated in Chapter 3, there is a close relationship between ethical and legal responsibilities. Numerous occasions exist in which ethical practice and the legal "standard of care" are inseparable. A health care professional's duty to maintain confidentiality with regard to a patient's medical information or treatment is one of those occasions.

RIGHT TO PRIVACY

The concept of **confidentiality** is founded in an individual's right to privacy, which is recognized in various forms in all states. Laws enacted by state legislatures and Congress created the right to privacy. For example, the Federal Privacy Act of 1994 requires consent of the individual "to whom the record pertains," prior to **disclosure** of any information by federal agencies (including federal hospitals). The right to privacy is articulated in numerous state and federal judicial decisions, such as *Hammonds v. Aetna Casualty & Surety Co.*,[1] Hammonds sued Aetna Casualty for inducing a physician to disclose confidential medical information. The court stated that a legal and ethical duty required the physician to keep patient information confidential and that the physician had breached that duty. Generally, however, in regard to medical information, the courts agree that in certain situations an individual's right to protect confidential information is outweighed by society's right to know. For example, in the case of a person who is a public figure, such as the President of the United States, the public has a right to know of illnesses that could impede his or her ability to govern.

The patient's right to privacy is coupled with the health care provider's duty to keep medical information confidential. This duty originated with the physician's duty in the **Hippocratic Oath.** In 1983 the World Medical Association revised the Hippocratic Oath,[2] which had been in language not easily understood. It now reads in part: "I will respect the secrets which are confided in me, even after the patient has died." The American Medical Association's Principles of Medical Ethics state: "The physician should not reveal confidential communications or information without the express consent of the patient, unless required to do so by law." All other health professions followed with official codes of ethics, with each code representing a consensus of a profession's membership. Each health profession has addressed the issue of confidentiality, creating an ethical as well as a legal basis for protecting a patient's medical record.

An individual seeking medical or dental treatment places his or her person and reputation in the hands of a health care provider. A medical record is created each time a person visits a health care professional. Medical records often contain very private information, and their disclosure could prove devastating to an individual.[3] For instance, these records may contain information relating to a patient's treatment for drug abuse, AIDS, or psychotherapy. As a result of wrongful disclosure, an individual could be denied credit or insurance. Loss of employment or loss of

CONFIDENTIALITY

The principle that a health care professional must hold in strict confidence all information gained regarding a patient in the course of treatment.

DISCLOSURE

The act of revealing facts that had been unknown or not understood.

HIPPOCRATIC OATH

An oath specifying standards of conduct for physicians, written by the Greek physician Hippocrates in the fourth century B.C.

[1]243 F.Supp. 793 (1965).
[2]*The handbook of medical ethics*, London, 1984, British Medical Association, p 69.
[3]Institute of Medicine: *Health data in the information age: use, disclosure, and privacy*, Washington, DC, 1994.

ability to be self-employed would be as devastating to the patient as loss of licensure would be to the health professional responsible for the breach. Thus, not only is the issue of releasing data from a patient's medical or dental record of concern to the patient, but the issue of liability in releasing such data should be of great concern to the health care provider.

LIABILITY FOR BREACH

A health care professional cannot disclose information regarding a patient's medical or dental record without statutory authority. However, a patient may authorize disclosure of all or part of his or her medical or dental record. A patient's consent to release of information should be written, unambiguous, and an act of his or her own free will. If the patient is not informed of all the facts surrounding the disclosure, the consent cannot be unambiguous or of his or her own free will. For instance, in the first case study for Section II, Dr. Roberts took photographs of a patient's condition. Although he obtained permission to take such photographs, the patient had no knowledge that they would be shown at a state dental meeting or would be published in a textbook. His consent was not free, voluntary, or unambiguous, since he simply did not have all of the facts. No information was available as to whether the patient's consent was oral or in writing. Oral consent is as valid as written consent. However, if litigation is initiated, written consent is a better form of evidence in a court of law. Several areas of liability should be considered in regard to unauthorized disclosure.

Should a breach of confidentiality occur, a patient may pursue several options. A patient may sue under a theory of defamation, invasion of privacy (see Chapter 5), or breach of contract. The patient may also report the health care provider to the appropriate professional organization for censure or to a licensing board for revocation of the health care provider's license.

Invasion of Privacy

Medical or dental records should be factual data. Truth is the only defense against claims of defamation. An action for defamation based on the unauthorized release of medical or dental records is unlikely. A charge of defamation would be more applicable if information from the patient's medical history were distorted and repeated to a third party. Invasion-of-privacy actions can be based on release of truthful information. All of the four tort claims within invasion of privacy are clearly applicable to the medical or dental setting:
1. Appropriation of the plaintiff's name or likeness
2. Unreasonable and offensive intrusion upon the seclusion of another
3. Public disclosure of private facts
4. Publicity that places the plaintiff in a false light in the public eye

In *Berthiaume's Estate v. Pratt*,[4] the court held that the unauthorized use of a photograph of a dying patient for documentation in the medical record was an intrusion upon seclusion. A specific agreement for nondisclosure of confidential infor-

---

[4]365 A.2d 792 (Me. 1976).

mation is required for the application of breach of contract. Courts have upheld actions for breach of express oral contract by a physician to maintain the confidentiality of a patient's HIV-positive status.[5] Some courts have implied the existence of a contract in order to determine whether a breach of confidentiality has occurred.

PRIVILEGE

Privilege is a legal tool to prohibit discovery of medical information or court testimony relating to a patient's medical record. Privilege is a patient's right whereby a doctor is prohibited from divulging information that the patient had disclosed to him or her with an expectation of privacy. However, privilege applies only to confidential disclosures made to a physician during the course of treatment and may be **waived** by the patient. A physician may assert privilege on behalf of the patient for the protection of the patient and the physician. Privilege does not exist in all states and does not apply to federal court proceedings unless the basis of the federal jurisdiction is diversity of citizenship (plaintiff and defendant are residents of different states). Some state statutes apply only to physicians, and many states have privilege in regard to psychiatrists only. If privilege does exist, it extends to written communication as well as oral statements.

> **PRIVILEGE**
>
> An advantage conferred on a person. In law, a privileged communication (such as a doctor-patient communication) is made under circumstances whereby a person cannot be compelled to disclose it in court.

> **WAIVE**
>
> To forfeit a right voluntarily.

DUTY TO DISCLOSE

Situations exist in which there is a legal duty to disclose information relating to medical care. For example, public health authorities must be notified in cases involving gunshot wounds, communicable or venereal diseases, or suspected child or elder abuse. Certain government agencies have the right, and the duty, to collect information normally considered confidential (e.g., Internal Revenue Service, Environmental Protection Agency, Department of Labor, Equal Employment Opportunity Commission, and Centers for Disease Control).

A number of legitimate requests for medical records are made with regularity by third parties; health care providers continuing the care of patients who have already been treated by other providers, insurance companies providing payment for services, and attorneys seeking medical records to establish claims for their clients are a few examples. Disclosure of medical information should occur only with a formal request and should be provided only with a patient's written authorization. Patients may consent to the release of information in their medical records. In some cases patient consent is presumed—for instance, if a patient is transferred from one provider to another or for emergency treatment. From an ethical and legal standpoint, the disclosure of confidential medical information should be based only on patient authorization, judicial decision, or state or federal statutes.

SUGGESTED READINGS

Hall MA, Ellman IM: *Health care law and ethics*, St Paul, 1990, West Publishing Co., Chapter 9, Patient confidentiality and the AIDS epidemic, p 376.

Thompson IE: The nature of confidentiality, *Journal of Medical Ethics* 5: 57-64, 1979.

---

[5]*Doe v. Roe*, 400 N.Y.S.2d 668 (N.Y. Supp. 1977).

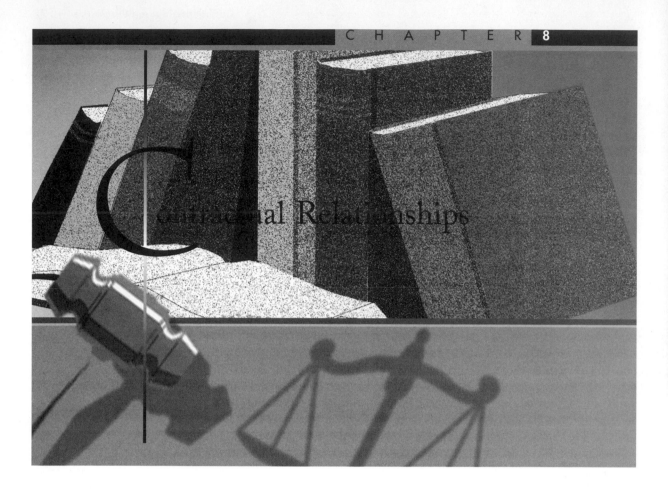

Contractual Relationships

After reading this chapter, you should be able to:
- Recognize the elements that legally define a contract.
- Differentiate express from implied contracts.
- Apply the concept of abandonment to contract law.
- Discuss which duties a patient is responsible for in a contractual relationship with a health care provider.
- Describe what circumstances must exist for a health care provider to dismiss a patient from his or her care.
- Differentiate "therapeutic assurances" from "express warranties" as they relate to dental health care services.

ABANDONMENT
CONSIDERATION
CONTRACT
DUTY
EXPRESS CONTRACT

IMPLIED CONTRACT
INCOMPETENT
MUTUAL ASSENT
OFFER AND ACCEPTANCE
PRUDENT

"A **contract** is a promise, or set of promises, for a breach of which the law gives a remedy, or the performance of which the law in some way recognizes as a duty."[1] When individuals make promises to one another and all of the elements of a contract are present, each party to the promise has a duty to the other. Should one party break the promise, a breach of the promise occurs. The party not in breach of the promise can have a court of law enforce the promise or provide a remedy by ordering money damages for the breach. The law of contracts determines what kinds of promises the courts will enforce.

ELEMENTS

The court will enforce an agreement made by a contract only if the following specific elements exist:

1. Mutual assent
2. Consideration
3. Two or more parties with legal capacity

Mutual assent occurs when the parties to a contract reach an agreement to which they "mutually assent." An **offer and acceptance** must transpire. The courts will not enforce mere mutual promises; the promises must represent a bargain between the parties. The offer is complete when one party proposes a bargain and the other party agrees to the proposed bargain. An agreement exists when one party accepts the offer of the other.

Consideration occurs when one party gives up something of value and the other party makes a promise, as part of the bargain, in exchange for that something of value. In a health care setting, a patient agrees to pay a fee for services that the health care professional promises to provide.

"Two or more parties with legal capacity" implies that at least two parties must be involved for the existence of mutual assent and consideration. All parties to a contract must have legal capacity in order for the contract to be legally enforceable. To have legal capacity, the parties must be at least the age of majority (18 or 21 years, depending on the jurisdiction in which the contract is made), and both parties must be mentally competent. In most states, an intoxicated person is considered **incompetent**. Both parties must understand the agreement and must have made the agreement voluntarily.

In general, if these three elements (mutual assent, consideration, and legal capacity) are present, a legally enforceable contract exists.

EXPRESS AND IMPLIED CONTRACTS

A contract may be either express or implied. **Express contracts** are stated orally or in writing. The patient may agree orally or sign a treatment plan in a health care setting. **Implied contracts** are agreed to by the actions of two or more people. In a health care setting, when a person seeks care for a particular health problem, he or she is offering to enter into a contract with the health care professional being consulted. When the health care professional examines the patient and proceeds

---

[1] *Restatement of the law of contracts*, St Paul, 1932, The American Law Institute.

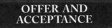

CONTRACT

"A contract is a promise, or set of promises, for a breach of which the law gives a remedy, or the performance of which the law in some way recognizes as a duty."

MUTUAL ASSENT

Agreement of the parties to the terms of a contract.

OFFER AND ACCEPTANCE

Requirements of a contract. Offer and acceptance are necessary in order for mutual assent to exist.

CONSIDERATION

A legal benefit received or a legal detriment suffered by one party to a contract, which represents the inducement to a contract.

INCOMPETENT

Lacking the capacity to discharge a legal duty.

EXPRESS CONTRACT

A contract that is either written or verbally agreed to by the parties.

IMPLIED CONTRACT

A contract assumed, under law, by the circumstances or facts of the situation.

with treatment, the offer is accepted and an implied contract exists. The health care professional is free to reject the offer and send the patient away, even under emergency conditions.[2] Implied contracts are valid under law, as long as they involve some consideration or compensation for services. Implied contracts are the usual basis of the relationship between a health care provider and a patient. The court may find an implied contract to exist in rather surprising circumstances. In *Weaver v. University of Michigan Board of Regents*,[3] a physician who spoke to a patient by phone was held to have an implied contractual obligation to the patient, since medical advice was given to the patient by the doctor.

DUTY

Under the law, a "no-duty" rule usually protects a private health care professional from liability for refusing to provide services for a member of the public, unless a duty exists. A **duty** exists when the professional begins treatment or a patient–health care professional relationship is established. Once a duty is recognized, the professional must act as a "reasonably **prudent** professional" and comply with the applicable standard of care in treating the patient. After the contractual relationship has been established between the patient and the health care professional, the health care professional has the duty to treat the patient and is not at liberty to terminate that relationship at will. The health care professional may not terminate the relationship or refuse to treat the patient without reasonable notice in advance; however, the patient may terminate the relationship at will. Notice of termination must give the patient adequate time to find the same services from another health care provider. Such notice should inform the patient of his or her medical or dental status and the need for future treatment. If no notice is given and any current treatment is completed, a health care provider owes a duty to the patient for emergency treatment. Failure to perform the duty, coupled with no reasonable notice, constitutes abandonment and breach of contract.

Abandonment

In *Longman v. Jasleh*,[4] an oral surgeon referring a patient to the family physician was held liable for not completing the patient's treatment. If a patient fails to pay or does not cooperate with treatment, abandonment on the part of the health care professional can still occur. The health care professional must complete all treatment started, even if the patient is not paying for services. If the patient suffers *any* injury as a proximate result of such wrongful abandonment, the health care professional is liable.[5] In *Lee v. The State Board of Dental Examiners*,[6] the court defined **abandonment** as "an unjustifiable renunciation by the dentist of his professional relationship with the patient and a repudiation of his responsibility for the patient's condition." In this case a dentist failed to diagnose a child's cavities and simply told

---

DUTY

An obligation, in law, that one owes to another person or a business.

PRUDENT

Sensible, careful.

ABANDONMENT

Once a health care professional establishes a relationship with a patient, services must continue to be provided for the patient, or a legal action of abandonment may be commenced against the health care provider. There are specific conditions under which the relationship may be terminated and no action may be taken.

---

[2]*Hiser v. Randolph*, 617 P.2d 774 (Ariz. App. 1980).
[3]506 N.W.2d 264 (Mich. App. 1993).
[4]414 N.E.2d 520 (1980).
[5]*Ascher v. Gutierrez*, 533 F.2d 1235 (1976).
[6]654 P.2d 839 (Colo. 1982).

the mother to bring the child back in six months for his regular examination. The court found the dentist guilty of negligent malpractice, but not abandonment.

For a court to find abandonment, the patient–health care professional relationship must be an ongoing, continuous, developing, and dependent one.[7] Treatment obligations cease if the health care professional can do nothing more for the patient.[8,9] However, if follow-up care is needed, a practitioner must continue to care for the patient until the threat of postoperative complications has passed.[10]

Use of "on-call" substitutes for professional services is not abandonment when such arrangements are commonly known or explained to patients in advance. Should a health care professional be unavailable for an extended period of time, arrangements should be made for patient care during the professional's absence, or a patient may charge abandonment. If the original practitioner arranges for another to "cover" his or her patients, with the patient's agreement, the original practitioner is not vicariously liable for any malpractice of the covering practitioner.[11]

Patient Duty

With respect to contractual obligations, patients have the duty to pay reasonable fees for services received. Patients also have the duty to comply with treatment recommendations—for example, keeping scheduled appointments, following instructions regarding medications, or informing the person providing treatment of accurate health status. Breach of these duties can be cause for terminating the relationship with the patient. As stated previously, no termination should take place prior to the completion of current treatment. The health care professional must have reasonable justification for termination and must provide the patient sufficient opportunity to secure an alternative source of care. Certain protocols must be met to ensure that the health professional is not charged with abandonment.

Terminating the Relationship With a Patient

The health professional should, if possible, verbally notify the patient of termination and then send written notification in the form of a letter sent by certified mail with return-receipt requested. Reasons for termination should be stated in the letter. A reasonable time period (30 to 60 days) should be available to the patient for emergency service and an opportunity to secure the services of another health professional. Patients should be told that copies of their records and radiographs will be sent to the new individual providing treatment. Because of the possibility that a legal record of the treatment may be necessary at a later date, originals should never be sent; original documents may be critical in a legal case. Although it is the patient's duty to pay fees and the professional can officially dismiss the patient for

---

[7]*Sander v. Gelb, Elston, Frost Professional Association,* 506 N.W.2d 107 (S.D. 1993).
[8]*Jewson v. Mayo Clinic,* 691 F.2d 405 (8th Cir. 1982).
[9]*Wells v. Billars,* 391 N.W.2d 668 (S.D. 1986).
[10]*Wells,* supra).
[11]*Shirk v. Kelsey,* 617 N.E.2d 152 (Ill. App. 1 Dist. 1993).

nonpayment of fees, the patient's records cannot be withheld for nonpayment. Once the letter is sent, the action should be noted in the patient's record and a copy of the letter should be placed in the patient's file.

There are circumstances under which a health care professional cannot terminate a patient. In addition to not being able to terminate a patient whose treatment has not yet been completed, the law prohibits a health care provider from refusing to treat or dismissing a patient solely on the basis of disability, race, color, creed, ethnicity, gender, or age. This does not mean that a health care provider cannot terminate patients who are members of minority groups; it does mean that a provider must treat members of these groups the same as all other patients. If patients who are members of these groups comply with office policies and treatment recommendations, they must be treated. If they do not comply, they can be dismissed in the same manner as other patients.

The health care professional is under no legal obligation to provide services for a new patient. However, the creation of a contract imposes a duty on the health care professional treating the patient to apply skills and abilities in a reasonable and prudent manner. Exercising reasonable care in performing health care services is a duty that the law recognizes and is not necessarily excused by a patient's signing of a waiver.

BREACH OF CONTRACT

Breach of contract is a material failure of performance of a duty arising under or imposed by an agreement or promise. Breach of contract not only includes a failure to perform on the part of the breaching party, but also may include the failure to perform at a proper time. A suit for contract damages is a demand that a sum of money be granted as compensation for injury caused by the breach of contract. Courts allow money damages as recovery for breach of contract if one party is found liable for the breach. Courts differ in measuring damages in cases in which liability is found. Remedies for breach of contract generally fall into three categories:

1. *Expectancy damages:* money awarded as compensation for injury caused by the breach
2. *Restitution damages:* the value in money of performance rendered by one party and received by another
3. *Reliance damages:* usually the value of the contract

Courts will find a breach of contract in medical or dental cases in which a patient shows that a health care professional affirmatively promised a particular result. In *Guilmet v. Campbell,*[12] a physician promised a patient with a bleeding ulcer that an operation would take care of all his troubles. The patient suffered serious after-effects, and the court found that the physician had breached his contract with the patient. In *Sullivan v. O'Conner,*[13] a plastic surgeon promised a specific result for

---

[12]188 N.W.2d 601 Mich. 1971).
[13]296 N.E.2d 183 (Mass. 1973).

nose surgery. After surgery the condition of the nose worsened, and the court awarded the patient:

1. The fee that had been paid
2. The difference between the value of the patient's nose before the operation and the value afterward
3. The value of pain and suffering and mental distress

Courts do distinguish "therapeutic assurances" from express warranties to effect a cure.[14] In *Ferlito v. Cecola*,[15] the court held that a dentist's statement that crown work would make a patient's teeth "pretty" did not constitute a guarantee or warranty. In some states the statute of frauds specifically requires agreements guaranteeing therapeutic results to be in writing and signed to be enforceable.[16]

SUGGESTED READINGS

Beatty v. Morgan, 317 S.E.2d 662 (Ga. App. 1984).
Lopez v. Southern Calif. Permanente Group, 171 Cal. Rptr. 527 (1981).
Perna v. Pirozzi, 457 A.2d 431 (N.J. 1983).
Powers v. Peoples Community Hosp. Auth., 455 N.W.2d 371 (Mich. App. 1990).
Restatement of the law of contracts, second, St Paul, 1981, The American Law Institute.

---

[14]*McKay v. Cole*, 625 So.2d 105 (Fla. App. 3 Dist. 1993).
[15]419 So.2d 102 (La. App. 1982).
[16]*Rogala v. Silva*, 305 N.E.2d 571 (Ill. App. 1973).

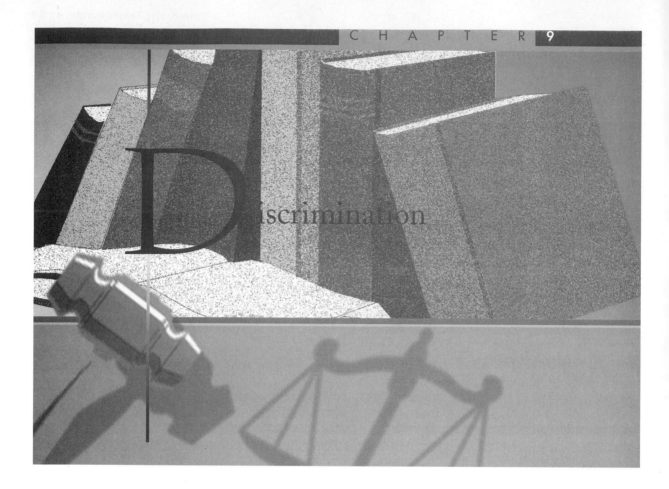

D iscrimination

LEARNING OUTCOMES

After reading this chapter, you should be able to:
- Discuss several means of discrimination that exist in American society.
- Identify which laws have been enacted to eliminate discrimination throughout the United States.
- Discuss how discrimination in regard to disability, race, age, sex, religious beliefs, or sexual preference can occur in the dental setting.

KEY WORDS

DISABILITY

DISCRIMINATION

HISTORICAL PERSPECTIVE

We tend to view discrimination as evil, an act of bigotry against a person because of his or her race, sex, religion, age, or nationality. Nevertheless, there is an up side to the word: it also refers to one who is fastidiously selective. In fact, the word has several meanings. For our purposes we shall limit discussion to the definition "to act on the basis of prejudice."[1] The word "prejudice" has several meanings. Health professionals and the majority of Americans are most affected by two of its meanings: "the irrational suspicion or hatred of a particular group" and "a detriment or injury caused to a person by the preconceived and unfavorable conviction of another or others."[2] The law tends to define **discrimination** as the unfair treatment of, or denial of normal privileges to, persons because of their race, sex, age, religion, or nationality; it is a failure to treat all persons equally when no reasonable distinction can be found between those favored and those not favored.[3] But what has this to do with me?" you ask. "I'm performing a health service for my patient," says the dentist. "I'm assisting him," says the assistant. "I'm performing an oral preventive service," says the dental hygienist.

This chapter will explore areas that will assist the health professional in avoiding acts of discrimination that discredit our professions. In the twentieth century we have learned to conquer space and walk on the moon. We have learned to control many diseases, as well as prevent many cases of premature death. However, we seem to dwell in the Ice Age with respect to our handling of human relationships. Every part of our world has its own special animosities. Jewish people reside in Israel surrounded by nations that harbor hostility toward them. Refugees wander in inhospitable countries. Many Irish Catholics and Protestants despise and kill each other in the name of religious dogma. Many people of color suffer indignities to justify behavior based on racist doctrines. The fabric of prejudice in the United States is the most intricate. Continuous antagonism is based on insecurity and unfounded, imaginary fears. Yet the philosophy of every religion emphasizes brotherhood among the peoples of the world. What is the secret of our irrational nature? It has been said that smashing an atom is easier than smashing prejudice. Discrimination remains with us. Why?

The simplicity of the concept of "race" gives us a quick and easy way to identify and designate the victims of our dislike. Added to this is the false concept of racial inferiority, which gives the racist a justification for prejudice. Such fiction spares us the pain of examining the complex economic, political, psychological, and cultural conditions that exist in group relations. Prejudice and discrimination gain power from many sources: economic exploitation, fear, social structure, aggression, and so on. The overall effect of prejudice is to place the object of prejudice at a disadvantage not merited by any misconduct on his or her part.

To distinguish attitude from behavior is useful. Designed to reduce or eliminate

> **DISCRIMINATION**
>
> Bias against a person or group on the basis of race, gender, religion, age, physical infirmity, or sexual preference.

---

[1]Black HC: *Black's law dictionary,* ed 5, St Paul, 1971, West Publishing Co.
[2]Morris W, ed: *American heritage dictionary,* New York, 1971, American Heritage Publishing Co and Houghton Mifflin Co.
[3]*Baker v. California Land Title Co.,* 349 F.Supp 235 (1972).

prejudice, laws and court decisions have succeeded in altering particular types of behavior but not in changing overall attitudes. For example, a dental health care provider may treat a minority patient out of fear of violating the law. But does this experience change the provider's overall attitude? This chapter is not designed to resolve these issues; it is designed to illustrate how laws were created to overcome discrimination. Everyone must fight and conquer his or her own prejudices, which often cause others to suffer needlessly.

DISABILITY DISCRIMINATION

Discrimination has existed in America since the earliest days, and we are just beginning to recognize its various forms and legally prohibit them. In this section, we will specifically examine discrimination against disabled persons in regard to employment and in other areas.

The Equal Employment Opportunity Act and the Americans with Disabilities Act

DISABILITY

A condition that incapacitates an individual in some manner; an impairment that renders a person unable to work for an extended period of time.

Approximately 45,000,000 Americans have some form of physical or mental **disability,** and the number is growing as Americans age. In the past, society tended to shun people with disabilities. Although some improvement has been made, disability discrimination continues to be a pervasive and serious problem. To remedy this situation, Congress passed the Americans with Disabilities Act (ADA) and the Equal Employment Opportunity Act (EEOA). The Equal Employment Opportunity Act prohibits discrimination in employment practices on the basis of race, color, religion, sex, national origin, or age. The Americans with Disabilities Act prohibits discrimination in employment, in public services, and in public accommodations and services operated by private entities, on the basis of a person's disability.

The ADA also prohibits programs that receive federal financial assistance from discriminating against qualified handicapped people. The Act also requires affirmative action on behalf of handicapped individuals. The EEOA prohibits programs that receive federal financial assistance from discriminating against program participants on the basis of race, color, or national origin.

A majority of states also have antidiscrimination statutes. In addition, some cities have ordinances that prohibit certain forms of discrimination.

The Rehabilitation Act of 1973 and the Americans with Disabilities Act

Section 504 of the Rehabilitation Act of 1973 and the Americans with Disabilities Act prohibit discrimination in employment on the basis of disability. Both Acts prohibit discrimination based solely on the disability of a qualified individual. The Equal Employment Opportunity Commission enforces the ADA in relation to employment discrimination.

In regard to employment of persons who have impairments or physical limitations other than infectious or communicable diseases, court decisions have brought about substantial litigation under the Rehabilitation Act.[4,5] In addition, many

---

[4]*Landefield v. Marion General Hospital*, 994 F.2d 1178 (1993).
[5]*Carter v. Casa Central*, 849 F.2d 1048 (1988).

HIV-positive and AIDS patients have tested the applicability of Section 504 of the Rehabilitation Act. An article by Lawrence O. Gostin, "The AIDS Litigation Project: A National Review of Court and Human Rights Commission Decisions" (part II, "Discrimination"),[6] provides a review of cases and settlements, under state and federal statutes.

In *School Board of Nassau County v. Arline*,[7] the United States Supreme Court considered the application of Section 504 to a teacher who had tuberculosis. The Court held that the plaintiff teacher was handicapped within the meaning of Section 504 because the medical condition "gave rise both to a physical impairment and to contagiousness." The Court's opinion established a basis for analyzing the application of Section 504 in the context of transmissible disease that has been adopted consistently in cases involving HIV. Since the Arline case, several cases have held that Section 504 prohibits discrimination against HIV-positive persons or persons who have AIDS.[8-10]

Disability Discrimination Case Example

One of the leading cases relating to disability discrimination is *Abbott v. Bragdon*.[11] Plaintiff Sidney Abbott, an individual with human immunodeficiency virus (HIV) infection, filed this action against defendant Randon Bragdon, a dentist with a practice in Bangor, Maine. The plaintiff's complaint alleged violations of Title III of the Americans with Disabilities Act and the Maine Human Rights Act (MHRA), based on the defendant's refusal to treat the plaintiff in the defendant's office. The defendant offered the plaintiff alternative treatment in a hospital setting. With respect to the ADA, the dispute involved two issues:

1. Whether the plaintiff's asymptomatic HIV constituted a disability under the statute
2. Whether treatment of the plaintiff in the defendant's office posed a direct threat to the health and safety of others such that the defendant could lawfully refuse such treatment

With respect to the MHRA, the parties disputed whether the defendant's office constituted a place of public accommodation. Under Title III a place of public accommodation may not discriminate against an individual on the basis of a disability in the full and equal enjoyment of services. However, places of public accommodation may deny full and equal enjoyment of services to an individual who poses a direct threat to the health or safety of others.

To have found a violation of Title III, the Court would have had to determine that:

1. The defendant's office constituted a place of public accommodation.
2. The plaintiff had a disability for purposes of the ADA.

[6]Gostin LO: The AIDS Litigation Project: a national review of court and Human Rights Commission decisions. II: Discrimination, *JAMA* 263:2086, April 18, 1990.
[7]480 U.S. 273 (1987).
[8]*Severino v. North Fort Myers Fire Control District*, 935 F.2d 1179 (1991).
[9]*Chalk v. United States District Court*, 840 F.2d 701 (1988).
[10]*Harris v. Thigpen*, 941 F.2d 1495 (1991).
[11]163 F.3d 87 (1998).

3. Treatment of the plaintiff in the defendant's office did not pose a direct threat to the health or safety of others.

The defendant did not dispute that his office constituted a place of public accommodation under the ADA.

Under the ADA, "disability" means that the following three conditions must exist:

1. A physical or mental impairment that substantially limits one or more of the major life activities
2. A record of such impairment
3. Being regarded as having such an impairment

The defendant contended that asymptomatic HIV did not constitute a disability and that the plaintiff had failed to offer evidence to show that her asymptomatic HIV substantially limited any major life activity. The Court, however, was persuaded that asymptomatic HIV did constitute a physical impairment for the purposes of the ADA. Also, the Court concluded that the plaintiff was disabled as a matter of law under the ADA.

The defendant asserted that performance in his office of invasive dental procedures, such as filling a cavity, for HIV patients posed a significant risk to the health and safety of others and that the risk could not be eliminated.

The plaintiff provided evidence, from the Centers for Disease Control (CDC), that the reasonable medical judgment of public health officials, based on current medical knowledge, was that treating HIV-positive patients, such as the plaintiff, in a dental office did not pose a direct threat to the health and safety of others.

The Court concluded that the risk of transmission from patient to dentist[12] did not rise to the level of a direct threat to the health or safety of others and that refusing to treat HIV-positive patients in the dental office therefore constituted unlawful discrimination under the ADA.

Like the ADA, the MHRA prohibits public accommodations from discriminating on the basis of disability. The MHRA defines a place of public accommodation as "any establishment that caters, offers its goods, facilities or services, or solicits or accepts patronage from the general public, including, but not limited to, clinics and hospitals."

This case was appealed to the U.S. Supreme Court, where the decision of the lower court was affirmed.[13]

Societal Progress

Not long ago, members of society who were afflicted with some form of disability were not able to join others in daily activities. Some were restricted to isolated groups or geographic areas for disabled people, such as tuberculosis sanitariums or leper colonies. However, as a consequence of education and the law, various infirmities and their causes began to be better understood. Gradually, society has ac-

---

[12]This particular case involved a dentist's refusal to treat an HIV-positive patient; however, the court's decision is applicable to all health care providers.
[13]*Abbott v. Bragdon*, 118 S.Ct. 2196 (1998).

cepted people with disabilities into the work place. Now the law requires barrier-free architecture for new construction and major remodeling of public places to enable persons with disabilities to participate fully in society.

SEX DISCRIMINATION
History
Before and during the early lives of our grandparents, women in America were generally relegated to childbearing and to duties in the home—cooking, mending, cleaning, washing, child raising, and so forth. After much prodding by women's rights groups, the American male gave women the right to vote in 1920. (Be assured, however, that the right to vote did not break or even dent the "good ole boy" network.) Employers gradually allowed more women into the work place, generally in front of the sewing machine (sweatshops) or the typewriter. Slowly, other areas of employment were opened to women, but a "ceiling" remained firmly in place, usually keeping women out of positions of authority and limiting them to certain kinds of work.

World War II forced women into positions that had been exclusively men's province. Slowly, the universities allowed women to pursue professions. Even more slowly, the professionals allowed qualified women to join their ranks.

Vestiges of that bygone era remain. Note the small numbers of men, compared to women, in nursing, dental assisting, and dental hygiene. Place those statistics next to the small numbers of women doctors, dentists, lawyers, and engineers. Ask yourself, "When was the last time, if ever, I saw a male receptionist or secretary?" Admittedly, the wide discrepancies are narrowing. Again, education, societal changes, and the law have brought about changes and improvements for women in the work place.

Sex Discrimination Case Example
Consider the case of *Kolstad v. American Dental Association*.[14] In September 1992, Jack O'Donnell announced his retirement as a director in the Washington offices of the American Dental Association (ADA). Two attorneys, Carole Kolstad, ADA Director of Federal Agency Regulations, and Tom Spangler, the ADA's legislative counsel, expressed interest in the position. Both received "distinguished" performance evaluations from the ADA's Washington offices director, Leonard Wheat. However, Wheat deferred the naming of O'Donnell's replacement to Dr. William Allen, the ADA's Executive Director. Allen drafted a revised position description questionnaire (PDQ) for O'Donnell's job, which followed verbatim many of the responsibilities for legislative counsel (Spangler's current position). Spangler and Kolstad both formally applied when the job was posted. Kolstad claimed that Wheat refused to meet with her during this time. After interviewing both candidates for the position, Wheat recommended Spangler. Allen offered the position to Spangler, and he accepted. Kolstad was informed that she did not receive the position because she was too valuable to the ADA where she was.

---

[14]108 F.3d 1431 (1997).

Kolstad exhausted her administrative remedies with the Equal Employment Opportunity Commission before filing suit for unlawful employment discrimination. The plaintiff demanded a jury trial. The ADA moved for summary judgment. The district court denied the ADA's motion and also dismissed Kolstad's compensatory and punitive damages claims because of insufficient evidence. The jury found that the ADA had discriminated against Kolstad on the basis of gender and awarded her $52,718 in back pay. Kolstad moved for instatement into Spangler's present position and for attorneys' fees. The ADA again moved for summary judgment. The trial court ruled that there was sufficient evidence for finding unlawful discrimination, held that the jury's finding regarding back pay was binding, and decided that the plaintiff was not entitled to further equitable relief or attorneys' fees. Kolstad appealed and the ADA cross-appealed.

The remaining issue was whether the plaintiff was entitled to punitive damages. The U.S. Supreme Court held that she was so entitled. The Court further held that punitive damages were available in claims under the terms of the Civil Rights Act of 1999 and under the Americans with Disabilities Act of 1990. Punitive damages are limited, however, to cases in which the employer has engaged in intentional discrimination and has done so "with malice or reckless indifference to the federally protected rights of an aggrieved individual."[15]

RACE DISCRIMINATION

Race discrimination is perpetuated through myth and ignorance. Unfortunately, many Americans continue to teach it to their children, often in indirect ways. Although free "men of color" were in America with French fur traders and the Conquistadors, blacks generally were brought to America to serve as slaves. As a result, they were considered property, even after our Declaration of Independence stated, "All men are created equal." The feeling that African Americans were inferior did not end with the Civil War but continued unabated in every field, particularly employment. In the 1960s the civil rights movement produced major federal legislation aimed at racial discrimination in employment practices. A great change came with the enactment of Title VII of the 1964 Civil Rights Act, which prohibited discrimination based on race, color, sex, religion, or national origin by both employers and labor unions.

Challenges to the Civil Rights Act

The Civil Rights Act withstood its first major challenge in *Griggs v. Duke Power Co.*[16] Unanimously, the Supreme Court held that the Act bars the use of employment practices that exclude African Americans if the practices are unrelated to job performance. African American employees of the Duke Power Company contested a system that "conditioned" employment: completion of high school or passing a

---

[15]*Carole Kolstad, Petitioner, v. American Dental Association,* Supreme Court of the United States, 1999, U.S. Lexis 4372, decided June 22, 1999. As of this writing, this recently decided case has not yet been published; the full case is available through Lexis-Nexis, a legal research computer service.
[16]401 U.S. 424 (1971).

standardized intelligence test was required for employment or for transfers to other jobs within the company. The practical effect of this requirement was to preclude African Americans from employment in or promotion to jobs in the highest paying departments of the company.

Later, in *McDonnell Douglas Corp. v. Green*,[17] the Court established some of the factors that a complainant could use in establishing a prima facie case of racial discrimination. These factors include:

1. The complainant belongs to a racial minority.
2. The complainant applied and was qualified for a job for which the employer was seeking applicants.
3. The complainant was rejected despite his or her qualifications.
4. The employer continued to accept applications for the position from persons with similar qualifications.

An African American, employed by the defendant as a mechanic, was laid off in the course of a general reduction in the defendant's work force. Later he participated in a protest against alleged racial discrimination in the defendant's employment practices. The protest included a "stall-in." The plaintiff and others stopped their cars along roads leading to the defendant's plant to block access to the plant during the morning rush hour. When the defendant advertised for replacement mechanics, the defendant rejected the plaintiff on the asserted ground of his participation in the "stall-in." The plaintiff filed a complaint with the Equal Employment Opportunity Commission, claiming that the defendant had violated § 703(a)(1) of the Civil Rights Act of 1964 by refusing to rehire him because of his race, and also that the defendant had violated § 704(a) of the Act by refusing to hire him because of his activities in the racial discrimination protest.

The Court concluded that the plaintiff, a long-time activist in the civil rights movement, had proved a prima facie case:

1. The evidence showed that the defendant sought to employ mechanics and continued to do so after rejecting the plaintiff's application for reemployment.
2. The defendant did not dispute the plaintiff's qualifications and acknowledged that the plaintiff's past work performance as a mechanic in the defendant's employ was satisfactory.

Note: The case started as *Green v. McDonnell Douglas Corp.* However, when a case is appealed and winds up in the Supreme Court, it is not unusual that the name of the case comes out in reverse order. The plaintiff was Mr. Green.

Race Discrimination Case Example

The subject of racial discrimination would not be complete without reference to a well-known case, not directly related to employment or health care, that set the standard for civil rights, *Plessy v. Ferguson*.[18] In 1896 the general assembly of the

---

[17]411 U.S. 792 (1973).
[18]163 U.S. 537 (1896).

state of Louisiana enacted legislation to provide for separate railway carriages for "whites and coloreds." The first section of the statute specified "that all railway companies, carrying passengers in their coaches in this state, shall provide equal but separate accommodations for the white and colored races. Two or more passenger coaches must be provided for each passenger train. The passenger coaches could be divided by a partition to secure separate accommodations." The state claimed that such legislation was authorized in the exercise of its police power, to protect the public good, and mandated that any passenger violating this law would be subject to a fine of twenty-five dollars or twenty days of imprisonment. Plessy, who was reportedly one-eighth African American, a passenger on a train in the state of Louisiana, was assigned by officers of the company to the black section but insisted on riding in the coach designated for white passengers. In affirming the doctrine of "separate but equal," the U.S. Supreme Court referred to judicial decisions that forbade intermarriage of the two races and decisions that established separate schools for black and white children. The Court pronounced that "legislation is powerless to eradicate racial instincts or to abolish distinctions based upon physical differences . . . . If the civil and political rights of both races be equal, one cannot be inferior to the other civilly or politically." History demonstrated how misguided Justice Brown's opinion turned out to be in this case.

The *Plessy* decision remained the law of the land until the Supreme Court proclaimed, in *Brown v. Board of Educaion*,[19] that in the field of public education, the doctrine of "separate but equal" had no place. Separate educational facilities were found by the Court to be inherently unequal. Over the years, several additional cases, based on *Brown*, were brought to the Court. This kept the issue before the public.

Legislation in Other Areas of Race Discrimination

Society gradually examined other facets of our culture in which segregation and discrimination regularly occurred. In real estate, the practices of "redlining," "blockbusting," and "steering" were outlawed. Redlining is the practice of refusing to make mortgage loans or issue insurance policies to specific individuals or in specific areas, without regard to qualifications of the applicant. Blockbusting is inducing homeowners to sell by making representations that minority persons are entering the neighborhood to live. Steering is directing home seekers to particular areas, either to maintain homogeneity of an area or to change the area and to create a situation in which homeowners would sell their property at a price well below its market value. All three practices were common until the Federal Fair Housing Act of 1968 and the Home Mortgage Disclosure Act of 1975 were passed by Congress.

Health care was not always available to members of minority groups in the United States. Health care providers and hospitals often refused to provide services for members of the black race. Passed in 1945, the Hill-Burton Act provided federal financing for construction and expansion of health care facilities. The statute requires that the states provide hospitals for all persons within their borders, regardless of ability to pay. Some states have since insisted that hospitals provide

---

[19]347 U.S. 483 (1954).

emergency care on a nondiscriminatory basis or be faced with loss of licensure. Judicial decisions and other statutes have also addressed medical care doe all Americans. Today, however, economic barriers to health care services remain.

As noted previously, discrimination takes many forms and invades every facet of American society. Accordingly, most members of society feel that law must intercede to bring about justice.

AGE DISCRIMINATION

The Age Discrimination in Employment Act (ADEA) of 1967 is the most significant federal statute outlawing age discrimination in employment. The ADEA covers employers, including the federal government, as well as the states, their political subdivisions, and any interstate agencies, employment agencies, and labor unions.

Before the passage of this law, an employee who reached age 65 could be given a gold watch and a five-minute farewell party by his or her employer and escorted off the employer's property. People who, because of their age, were no longer employed were sometimes shunned or placed in "old folks" homes unnecessarily. But Americans were now living longer. Forcing someone to retire at age 65, based on that fact alone, came to be seen as an act of discrimination. That person was being placed at a disadvantage economically. Because people were living longer, the need for greater legal protection from age discrimination became evident, and thus the ADEA was born.

The ADEA makes it unlawful for employers "to fail or refuse to hire or to discharge any individual or otherwise discriminate against any individual with respect to his compensation, terms, conditions or privileges of employment, because of such individual's age." Any person who is at least 40 years of age and is discriminated against on the basis of age may commence a civil action for legal relief.

Despite this law, older people's participation in the work force is declining. Unless strategies are developed to keep older people in the work force, economic issues (as well as other issues) will force a "second look" regarding our practice of forcing older individuals out of the work place. One example is the viability of our social security system. As a greater proportion of Americans retire, there will be fewer members of the work force to keep the system solvent.

Age Discrimination Case Example

Frank Spulak sued K-Mart Corporation, alleging that he had been constructively discharged from his employment with K-Mart as a result of illegal age discrimination. A constructive discharge occurs when an employer, by its illegal discriminatory acts, makes working conditions so difficult that a reasonable person in the employee's position would feel compelled to resign. In constructive discharge cases an employee resigns rather than waiting to be fired, because of unreasonably harsh conditions that have been applied to him or her in a discriminatory fashion.

In an age discrimination case a plaintiff/employee must establish a prima facie case by showing the following:

1. He or she is within the protected age group.
2. He or she is doing satisfactory work.

3. He or she was discharged despite the adequacy of his or her work.
4. The position was filled with someone younger than him or her.

Should the plaintiff/employee show that the above elements have been met, the burden of showing a legitimate, nondiscriminatory reason for the challenged action shifts to the defendant/employer.

Spulak presented evidence that he was 58 years of age at the time he left K-Mart and that he was replaced by a man in his late twenties or early thirties. The record showed that Spulak rated average or above in the two previous yearly performance reviews and had received average or above average annual merit raises. K-Mart contended that the evidence was insufficient to establish that age was a determining factor in the actions it took and that there were legitimate nondiscriminatory reasons for its action. Price, the district manager, had informed Spulak that he was going to fire him for violating company policy by using the store's back door, failing to sign in and out properly, using improper invoice procedures, and so forth. Spulak showed that the rules were not uniformly enforced, that the employer had selectively enforced its rules against Spulak, and that the rules were a pretext for age discrimination. Another employee testified that Price had stated to him, "These old fogies are either going to have to comply or get out." Other former K-Mart employees testified to substantially similar treatment by K-Mart, and to having been replaced with younger people.

The jury returned a verdict in favor of Spulak, and K-Mart appealed. The appeals court affirmed the judgment of the district court.[20]

OTHER ANTIDISCRIMINATION LAWS

Prior to 1964, there were some court decisions based upon specific instances of discrimination. Federal legislation dealing with many aspects of discrimination was not enacted until 1964.

Today's antidiscrimination laws are based on three major pieces of federal legislation:
1. Title VII of the Civil Rights Act of 1964
2. The Equal Pay Act of 1963
3. The Age Discrimination in Employment Act of 1967 (Please see further discussion in Chapter 16, p. 205.)

Society has recognized that although discrimination may appear to be a fairly straightforward concept, it can and does manifest itself in subtle, inconspicuous ways. The following is an overview of the antidiscrimination laws, all enforced by the Equal Employment Opportunity Commission (EEOC):
1. The Pregnancy Discrimination Act of 1968. "An employer cannot refuse to hire, promote, fire or force a leave at an arbitrary time because of pregnancy."
2. Sexual harassment is deemed a form of discrimination and is prohibited under Title VII.
3. Religious discrimination. When an employee's religion or religious beliefs are

---

[20]*Spulak v. K-Mart Corp.*, 894 F.2d 1150 (1990).

an issue, the employer may not discriminate and must reasonably accommodate expression of those beliefs.

4. The Equal Pay Act of 1963 forbids local, state, and federal governments and almost all private employers from paying different wages for equal jobs because of the sex of the employee.

5. Executive Order 11141 prohibits age discrimination by federal contractors.

6. The Civil Rights Act of 1991 expands the rights and remedies that are available under the federal antidiscrimination laws. It establishes the right to a jury trial under Title VII, and it allows for recovery of compensatory and punitive damages for intentional discrimination and eases the burden of proof for plaintiffs in such cases.

7. The Fair Labor Standards Act sets the national minimum wage, determines overtime pay standards, and regulates the employment of minors. Many other federal and state laws provide employees with certain protections and/or benefits.

SUGGESTED READINGS

Employee Rights Handbook for Dental Hygienists, Chicago, 1993, American Dental Hygienists' Association.

Parmet W: Discrimination and disability: the challenge of the ADA, *Law, Medicine & Health Care* 18:331, 1990.

AUTHOR'S CASE STUDY COMMENTS

Reread Case Study 2 and the Accompanying Study Questions
Questions 1 through 11 are examined in the following analysis:

1. Does a contract exist between Mr. Cook and Dr. Hastings?

The stated elements of a contract are mutual assent, consideration, and the presence of two competent parties. Mr. Cook was injured. He requested treatment from Dr. Hastings. Dr. Hastings accepted Mr. Cook's request and treated his tooth for a $1,000 fee. Mr. Cook proceeded with treatment, agreeing to pay the $1,000 fee. Mutual assent (the offer by Mr. Cook and the acceptance by Dr. Hastings) and the consideration (a $1,000 fee for treatment) were present. Mr. Cook and Dr. Hastings had legal capacity. No information that either one was a minor, mentally incapacitated, or intoxicated was available. Therefore, an express legal contract exists.

2. Did the "waiver" Mr. Cook signed have any force of law?
3. Did Mr. Cook have the right to refuse antibiotic therapy?

Although Mr. Cook had the right to refuse antibiotic therapy, he could not legally authorize Dr. Hastings or Ms. Gale to breach their duty to provide reasonable and prudent care. A waiver, signed by a patient, requesting or permitting either a doctor or a hygienist to commit malpractice is invalid. If antibiotic therapy is necessary for safe treatment of a patient, and the patient refuses the antibiotic, the patient should be dismissed by the health care professional to avoid any risk of liability. If treatment proceeds and the patient is injured, the health care professional could be held liable for such injuries. In this particular case we know that Mr. Cook was in the hospital following his initial treatment at Dr. Hastings' office. We do not know if the reason for his hospitalization was related to his dental treatment. If it could be proven that the hospitalization was a result of dental treatment, Dr. Hastings, Ms. Gale, or both could be held liable.

4. Did Dr. Hastings abandon Mr. Cook, or was he within his legal rights not to treat him?
5. Does Mr. Cook have a claim against Dr. Hastings?
6. Does Mr. Cook have a claim against Ms. Gale?

Dr. Hastings did not complete Mr. Cook's treatment. Mr. Cook did not return to the office. Dr. Hastings had not previously treated tooth #18. Mr. Cook had not paid Dr. Hastings for services rendered to him nine months prior to his second emergency visit. It appears as though Mr. Cook should have no claim for abandonment. However, Mr. Cook was still a patient of record of Dr. Hastings: Dr. Hastings never notified Mr. Cook that he was terminating him as a patient. Treating an abscess is considered an emergency situation; so Mr. Cook has a claim of abandonment against Dr. Hastings. Should Mr. Cook discover that the condition that required his hospitalization was causally connected to his dental treatment, he may have a claim of malpractice against both Dr. Hastings and Ms. Gale.

AUTHOR'S CASE STUDY COMMENTS—cont'd

The public conversation between Ms. Charles and Ms. Lane also could be the basis for legal action by Mr. Cook against Ms. Charles and Dr. Hastings. To keep patient information confidential is a legal and ethical duty. Such information may not be disclosed without legal authority or patient consent. Mr. Cook would have an action for defamation, based on Ms. Charles' allegations that he was a deadbeat and had a bad temper. No information is provided that Mr. Cook has AIDS or is HIV positive. Assume that he has AIDS. Since truth is a defense to an allegation of defamation, Mr. Cook would have another alternative—a lawsuit based upon invasion of privacy (public disclosure of private facts). Alternatively, if Mr. Cook does not have AIDS, he has a reasonable basis for a defamation suit.

7. Does Mr. Cook have a claim against Dr. Warner?

If Mr. Cook was hospitalized with bacterial endocarditis after his treatment with Dr. Warner and it was determined that his dental treatment with Dr. Warner was the cause of his illness, would he have a claim against Dr. Warner? When Mr. Cook presented himself to Dr. Warner's office, he was asked to provide information regarding his medical history. At this point Mr. Cook chose not to include any information regarding his heart condition. It was his duty to provide Dr. Warner with accurate information regarding his health status. Dr. Warner was not informed that Mr. Cook had a condition that required premedication with an antibiotic. Dr. Warner did not breach his duty to his patient.

8. Does Dr. Hastings have a legal claim against Dr. Warner?

From the facts presented, Dr. Warner suggested to Mr. Cook that he report Dr. Hastings to the state board of dental examiners. If he made this suggestion in good faith, as he believed Dr. Hastings had committed a wrong against Mr. Cook, Dr. Hastings has no claim against Dr. Warner. Defamatory words used against Dr. Hastings were not indicated.

9. Is Ms. Charles suggesting that Dr. Hastings' office policy is to refuse to treat patients with AIDS?

If this is the case, Dr. Hastings could be in line for a lawsuit based on discrimination. If we find that Ms. Charles' comments are exclusively defamatory, Dr. Hastings could also be held liable as her employer, on the basis of vicarious liability. Vicarious liability, or respondeat superior, is discussed in Chapter 4.

10. What would you say to Ms. Jenret if she asked your advice regarding her loss of employment?

Ms. Jenret should go to her state department of labor or the office of the state attorney general to find out what statutes regarding age discrimination exist in her state. The Equal Employment Opportunity Commission investigates complaints to permit an individual to bring a lawsuit under federal law. Dr. Hastings informed her that he was eliminating her position and then filled that position one month later with a much younger woman who had no dental office experience or dental assisting education. No evidence of poor job performance was found. Ms. Jenret may have a claim of age discrimination.

11. Do any applicants for Dr. Hastings' dental assisting position have a claim against Dr. Hastings?

Since Dr. Hastings passed over several qualified applicants in order to hire someone with no qualifications, each should be able to claim discrimination. However, these cases are difficult to prove, which is why discrimination continues in many facets of our lives—no real proof. We need laws to protect individuals from such senseless treatment. Remember, though, that the only person who knows the qualifications and characteristics of the individuals who applied for this position is Dr. Hastings, who may legally hire whomever he wishes.

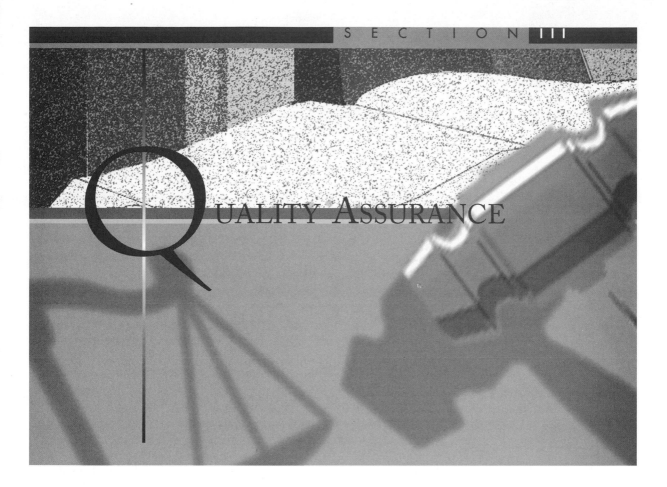

QUALITY ASSURANCE

CASE STUDY

As discussed in the Case Study for Section I, Ms. Jean Casey, R.D.H., and Ms. Sara Smythe are employed by Dr. James Albright, whose office is in Brown, Indiana. Both enjoy their employment with Dr. Albright, primarily because of the variety of duties they perform on a daily basis. Both women are competent in condensing, carving, and finishing amalgam restorations. Each spends a portion of each day performing this duty, as well as more traditional dental assisting and dental hygiene functions.

Ms. Casey's patients were all completed early one day, and she took a seat in the front office to review the records for the next day's patients. Next to her was a stack of insurance forms that represented the billing for the day's services. Remembering that she may have neglected to include the radiographs taken for her last patient of the morning, she reached to find the billing and check to see if it was completed correctly. Ms. Casey noticed several insurance bills for prophylaxis for patients she had not seen that day. Upon asking the receptionist about the bills, she was told not to worry about it; these were just patients who were recipients of the Medicaid program. The receptionist further explained that they never keep their appointments anyway, so no one will know the difference.

Ms. Smythe and Ms. Casey are roommates, and both love to travel. One evening as they were planning their trip to the East Coast, Ms. Smythe suggested that during their travels they search for possible opportunities for employment. Neither had

lived outside of the state of Indiana, and the prospect of exploring new territory was an exciting thought to both women.

While visiting Ms. Casey's Aunt Gloria in Portland, Maine, they told her of their desire to find new positions. Aunt Gloria told them of a friend of hers who practiced dentistry in a nearby town, and she called the friend as a favor to her niece. The next day Ms. Casey and Ms. Smythe found themselves in the office of Dr. Robert Kemper in Falmouth, Maine. They explained their goals, talked about the expanded functions each could perform competently, and discussed how they could increase the productivity of Dr. Kemper's dental office. Dr. Kemper had a very busy practice, and he was very impressed with both Ms. Casey and Ms. Smythe. He told them that he would consider hiring them and that he would contact them by the end of the week, when they were going to leave to return home. The next day Dr. Kemper telephoned them and offered them both positions, a more than adequate salary, and the stipulation that they must begin their employment with him in one month. They both accepted the positions immediately.

Ms. Smythe and Ms. Casey returned home the next day and notified Dr. Albright that their employment with him would terminate in two weeks because of a new opportunity for both of them. The move was uneventful, and Aunt Gloria offered her home to them for a few weeks until they located suitable living quarters. The third day in Portland, Ms. Casey found a beautiful home near Dr.

100

Kemper's office and signed a lease for one year. The next week was spent settling in to their new home; they were now ready for a new work setting.

Ms. Casey and Ms. Smythe arrived at the office at 7:45 A.M. Ms. Casey was handed a schedule that indicated that her first patient was at 8:00 A.M. Ms. Casey explained that she had been able to apply for a dental hygiene license but had not yet completed the process. She assumed that she was to perform other duties in the interim.

Dr. Kemper stated that he would assume responsibility, and that it was perfectly fine for her to practice dental hygiene; after all, she had practiced for many years and was a graduate of an accredited dental hygiene program. Ms. Casey provided dental hygiene services for her patients. Ms. Smythe spent her first day placing amalgam restorations after Dr. Kemper completed the cavity preparations. Several weeks passed. Ms. Smythe, Ms. Casey, and Dr.

Kemper were all quite happy with the employment arrangements.

Ms. Casey was then notified that she must appear before the Maine Board of Dental Examiners and complete an examination on the dental laws in order to obtain her license. As she read the rules and regulations in preparation for the examination, she discovered that both she and Ms. Smythe were violating the law. The next day she explained to Dr. Kemper that she could not continue to treat patients until she received her license. Furthermore, neither she nor Ms. Smythe could continue completing amalgam restorations, as that too was in violation of the law. Dr. Kemper again stated that he would take full responsibility. He explained that the only reason they had been hired was their competence in expanded dental functions. If they could not perform these tasks as he requested, they would need to find employment elsewhere.

RESPONSE TO CASE STUDY — Morris L. Robbins, D.D.S.

The omnipresent issue in health care is "doing the right thing." The decisions you must face to do the right thing are based upon two important issues. One is the state laws that govern the healing arts profession in which you are allowed to practice. This allowance to practice is governed by the law of the state you practice in and is managed by the respective board of health arts that relates to your profession. The second issue is the more subjective professional code of conduct or ethics of the profession. When a dentist or dental hygienist enters the practicing profession by passing the proper credentialing examination and understands the ethical purpose of his or her profession, the burden of doing the right thing shifts directly to that person. A responsible dentist-employer must also ensure that dental assistants meet the criteria of the state to provide care. Finally, in addition to being cogni-

zant of the federal, state, and local laws that control the practice, the dentist must instill in all the staff the desire and will to do the right thing.

In this case study, Ms. Casey found that Dr. Albright appeared to be billing Medicaid for prophylaxis care not rendered by her and that the patients had not been seen in the office. The duty of trust and ethical behavior had been breached by at least the receptionist. It is implied, although not clearly stated, that Dr. Albright had approved this billing; possibly, only the receptionist had been billing for these services, and she had not informed Dr. Albright that she was doing so. Nonetheless, a suspicion was raised in the mind of Ms. Casey.

Upon the trip to the East Coast, Ms. Casey and Ms. Smythe decided to move and take another position. Some of this move could have been predicated on the fact that Dr. Albright's

RESPONSE TO CASE STUDY—cont'd

office was illegally billing Medicaid and that they did not want any further association with this practice—an example of not doing the right thing.

With the move to Maine, disaster occurs because neither Ms. Casey, Ms. Smythe, nor Dr. Kemper does the right thing. No matter the circumstance, all health professionals are charged with knowing and practicing within the laws of the state. In addition, breach of public trust is a major example of not following the law of the state.

Each individual will now have to answer directly to the state board and defend his or her practices. Imagine, for a moment, that you were each of these people: a dentist who knowingly hired a dental hygienist and a dental assistant who were not yet properly licensed and put them

to work in his practice treating patients in violation of the law; a dental hygienist who practiced her profession prior to being licensed in the state; and a dental assistant who performed duties that may have been in the realm of expanded duties for dental assistants and was not certified by the board for those duties.

Here are three individuals who have made independent decisions to provide health care without the sanction of the state, to compromise their ethical behavior, and to risk monetary fines and the possibility of actions against their abilities to practice in the state.

It is evident that each person in this scenario did not do the right thing. Obeying the law and practicing ethically are critical to the health professions and are clearly individual responsibilities.

RESPONSE TO CASE STUDY   Jonathan Shapiro, Esq.

As an attorney who regularly counsels medical and dental providers and practice groups regarding the recruiting and hiring of employees, I would counsel all dental hygienists to take very seriously state licensing and practice requirements. For example, dental hygienists must educate themselves about state licensing and regulatory requirements (i.e., contact the state board of dental examiners and become familiar with the state rules for practicing "dentistry") *before* considering to move to another state—and certainly before accepting a position in another state. Despite representations to the contrary, *no* employer or prospective employer can exempt a dental hygienist or a dental assistant (or any other professional) from the licensing and prac-

tice requirements of the state in which he or she works. Similarly, *no* employer or prospective employer can protect or insulate a dental hygienist from the hygienist's own violations of state licensing and practice requirements. I also would counsel dental hygienists or dental assistants to seek legal counsel regarding their own exposure to liability if they find themselves working for a dentist who is engaging in unlawful or potentially unlawful conduct (e.g., submitting fraudulent insurance or Medicaid bills). Depending upon the circumstances of a situation, a dental hygienist, dental assistant, or other professional could have exposure to liability for knowingly participating in or assisting the employer's unlawful acts.

CASE STUDY QUESTIONS

1. Are both Ms. Casey and Ms. Smythe in violation of the Maine Dental Practice Act? If so, explain.
2. Should a violation be found, will their punishment be the same?
3. Is Dr. Kemper in violation of the Maine Dental Practice Act?
4. What are the possible consequences if one is in violation of the dental practice act?
5. What rights do Ms. Smythe, Ms. Casey, and Dr. Kemper have regarding any action against them by the Maine Board of Dental Examiners?
6. What if Dr. Kemper's office was located in Casper, Wyoming, rather than Maine; would there be any different outcome?
7. What would the outcome be if Dr. Kemper's office was located in your state?
8. Has Dr. Albright committed any violations?

There are additional ethical considerations that have no black and white answers. Each of us needs to arrive at his or her own determination. There are often legal ramifications connected to personal decisions. To examine just a few presented with this case:

1. Do you believe that Dr. Kemper should be reported to the board of dental examiners? If so, whose duty is it to report him?
2. What about Dr. Albright? Whose responsibility is it to monitor his behavior? What, if anything, would you do?
3. What should Ms. Casey and Ms. Smythe do? Should they sacrifice their employment for their principles?
4. Is it justified to ignore the dental practice acts when, as a professional, you believe that the rules and regulations are not necessarily protecting the public's health?
5. Do you believe that the dental practice acts truly protect the quality of dental health care, or do they protect the income of dentists?

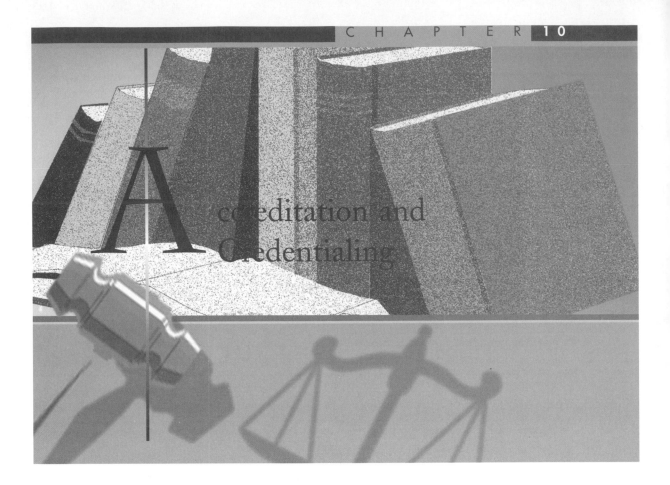

C H A P T E R 10

Accreditation and Credentialing

LEARNING OUTCOMES

After reading this chapter, you should be able to:

- Explain how accreditation relates to dental, dental assisting, dental hygiene, and dental laboratory technology education.
- Discuss licensure and explain its purpose.
- Discuss certification, explaining how it is utilized in the dental professions.
- Explain the purpose of a dental practice act.

KEY WORDS

ACCREDITATION
CERTIFICATION
CREDENTIALING

LICENSURE
OPEN DENTAL PRACTICE ACT
REGISTRATION

Education and credentialing are the primary means utilized to maintain quality assurance for dental health care providers. Appendixes H and I include the dental practice acts and the rules and regulations for the states of Maine (Revised Statutes, Title 32, Chapter 16 of Maine Statutes) and Wyoming (Title 33, Chapter 15, Sections 33-15-101 through 33-15-130 of Wyoming Statutes). The similarities and differences between the two are typical of all fifty states. However, the larger and more populated states tend to have more rules and regulations regarding the dental professions. The discussion in this chapter will frequently refer to the Maine and Wyoming documents for further clarification of the statutes, rules, and regulations that affect the professional lives of dental health care providers. It should be mentioned that a few states have an "open provision" approach to their dental laws. Under this situation a dentist may delegate any duty that a dental auxilliary is competent to perform. The only limitation is a list of duties that require the knowledge and skill of the dentist. Usually, there can be no delegation of diagnosis and treatment planning, writing authorizations for restorative, prosthetic, or orthodontic appliances, writing prescriptions for drugs, or cutting hard or soft tissue (Figure 10-1). Dental practice acts are opened for periodic review. The number of years between each review is set by each state. The many new provisions in dental practice acts, the fact that legal duties of dental personnel vary from state to state, and the ambiguity of terminology all produce a great deal of confusion regarding provisions in state dental practice acts.

ACCREDITATION

Legislative bodies have the responsibility of protecting the public welfare. This includes maintaining quality assurance in our health care system. As a society we utilize several means to protect the public from poor-quality health care. **Accreditation** is one of these means. Private agencies accredit educational institutions and

OPEN DENTAL PRACTICE ACT

A state dental practice act that permits a supervising dentist to delegate tasks to other dental personnel on the basis of his or her judgment.

ACCREDITATION

The processes of approving, certifying, or endorsing. For example, a dental education program can be accredited by the American Dental Association.

SECTION 51. DENTAL HYGIENISTS, PARAGRAPH 3

A dental hygienist may perform all acts which may be performed by a dental assistant and may under the appropriate supervision of a dentist perform acts or services on teeth and related structures that are educational, therapeutic, prophylactic and preventive in nature but may not perform acts or services which require the knowledge and skill of a dentist such as diagnosis, treatment planning, surgical or cutting procedure on hard or soft tissue, and the prescription of medications; provided, however, that the term "therapeutic," as used in this section, shall include gingival curettage and root planing in accordance with rules and regulations adopted by the board.

FIGURE 10-1
The Commonwealth of Massachusetts Dental Laws. Chapter 112, General Laws. Section 51, paragraph 3.

specific programs within most institutions. Regional accrediting agencies accredit an institution as a whole.

The Commission on Accreditation of Dental and Dental Auxiliary Educational Programs is the agency recognized by the Council on Post-secondary Accreditation and the United States Office of Education as having the authority for accreditation of dental, dental hygiene, dental assisting, and dental laboratory technology programs.

The Commission publishes standards for evaluation of new and existing programs. All programs must meet these standards to be accredited by the Commission. This accrediting body has almost total control over defining each profession in terms of what skills are taught and what body of knowledge is contained within the curriculum. Periodic visits by accrediting teams are utilized to ensure that each program remains in compliance with the standards set by the Commission. A different model is utilized in medicine, as the American Medical Association controls accreditation for medical educational programs, and the state boards of nursing, established within each state, accredit educational programs for nurses.

LICENSURE

Generally, licensed professionals such as dentists, dental hygienists, physicians, and nurses must graduate from an accredited program in order to obtain **licensure.** See sections 33-15-108 and 33-15-120 of The Dental Practice Act of Wyoming and Sections 1082 and 1096 of the Maine Dental Practice Act.

State law governs the requirements for licensure of health care professionals. The state's authority to control the practice of health care professionals resides in its police power—that is, the power to protect the health, safety, and welfare of the community. Laws are enacted to control the practice of various professional groups. Such laws are meant to prevent incompetent individuals from practicing in health care professions. They do so by establishing minimum qualifications for entry, the scope of practice, and disciplinary actions for each profession. An example of such a law enacted by a state legislature is a state dental practice act. This body of law empowers the state board of dental examiners to regulate the dental professions. The state board creates rules and regulations for the practice of the dental professions. For example, in the Maine Dental Practice Act, Section 1073 gives the board the power to adopt rules necessary to implement the law, and Sections 1084 and 1098-B stipulate that dentists and dental hygienists must have 40 and 20 hours of continuing education, respectively, for biennial license renewal. Now examine Chapter 12 of the rules and regulations adopted by the board. Chapter 12 stipulates requirements, definitions and categories, evidence of completion, monitoring procedure, and exceptions or waivers to the requirements.

We **credential** health professionals by certification or licensure. Licensure is a process by which an agency of the state government grants permission to an individual to engage in a certain profession and/or use a specific title. Therefore, minimum standards are set for licensure or certification, and the agency certifies that those licensed or certified have attained the minimum degree of competence required. As mentioned earlier, it is the state board of dental examiners that regulates the practice of dentistry, dental hygiene, dental assisting, and dental laboratory technology. In general, the board stipulates the qualifications for licensure and mandates what procedures each dental professional may legally perform. In many states, tasks that are identified as being legal for a specific provider are further categorized according to the conditions under which each task may be legally performed (i.e., under the general, direct, or indirect supervision of a dentist). In 1986, the Colorado state legislature revised the state's dental practice law. The new law permitted dental hygienists to choose to practice in an unsupervised setting and to be the "proprietor of a place where supervised or unsupervised dental hygiene is performed and may purchase, own, or lease equipment necessary to perform supervised or unsupervised dental hygiene."[1] The law does not permit dental hygienists to take radiographs, remove live tissue, perform root planing, or administer local anesthesia, all of which require a dentist's supervision.

This law requires that a hygienist recommend to patients that they see a dentist for an examination. The law further states, "Failure of a dental hygienist to refer a patient to a dentist when the dental hygienist detects a condition that requires care beyond the scope of practicing supervised or unsupervised dental hygiene" would be cause for disciplinary action. The state boards determine criteria for disciplinary action, including suspension or revocation of licensure.

State laws, rules, and regulations vary from state to state. For instance, it may be legal in one state for a dental assistant to take impressions and not in another. Administering local anesthesia is a legal procedure for dental hygienists to perform in many states, but not all. The rules and regulations of both Maine's and Wyoming's boards of examiners lists duties that may be performed by each profession. (See Appendixes H and I.)

The model used in medicine (physicians and nurses) differs from that used in dentistry. The state board of nurse examiners is the administrative agency in each state that has been given the power to make regulations related to the practice of nursing. For physicians the state board of medical examiners performs this function. An exception to the model used in dentistry is the New Mexico Dental Practice Act. In 1994 New Mexico became the first state to establish self-regulation for dental hygienists. The law established a committee, within the New Mexico Board of Dental Healthcare, that is composed of five dental hygienists, one dentist, and one public member. This dental hygiene committee has the power to promulgate rules and formulate regulations related to dental hygiene practice (Figure 10-2).

An examination of when these health professions founded their professional associations reveals that the American Dental Hygienists' Association is the youngest of the four. The American Dental Hygienists' Association was established in 1923, the American Dental Association in 1854, the American Nurses' Association in 1896, and the American Medical Association in 1847.[2]

Organizations and their relationships to each other will change with time as the

---

[1]Colorado Revised Statutes, Dental Practice Law, Title 12-35-100, 1986.
[2]Woodall LR: *Legal, ethical, and management aspects of the dental care system,* St Louis, 1987, Mosby.

SECTION 61-5A-9. COMMITTEE CREATED.

A. There is created the seven-member "New Mexico dental hygienist committee." The committee shall consist of five dental hygienists, one dentist and one public member. The dental hygienists must be actively practicing and have been licensed practitioners and residents of New Mexico for a period of five years preceding the date of their appointment. The dentist and public member shall be members of the board and shall be elected annually to sit on the committee by those members sitting on the board.

B. The governor may appoint the dental hygienists from a list of names submitted by the New Mexico dental hygienists' association. There may be one member from each district. The list submitted shall consist, whenever possible, of names of dental hygienists in the district being considered but may also include names of dental hygienists at-large. No more than two dental hygienists shall serve from the same district at one time. All members shall serve until their successors have been appointed. No member shall be employed by or receive remuneration from a dental or dental hygiene educational institution.

C. Appointments shall be for terms of five years. Appointments shall be made so that the term of one dental hygienist expires on July 1 of each year.

D. Any committee member failing to attend three committee or board meetings, either regular or special, during the committee member's term shall automatically be removed as a member of the committee unless excused from attendance by the committee for good cause shown. Members of the committee not sitting on the board shall not be required to attend board disciplinary hearings.

E. No committee member shall serve more than two full terms.

F. In the event of any vacancy, the secretary of the committee shall immediately notify the governor, the committee and board members and the New Mexico dental hygienists' association of the reason for its occurrence and action taken by the committee so as to expedite appointments of a new committee member.

G. The committee shall meet quarterly every year. The committee may also hold special meetings and emergency meetings in accordance with the rules and regulations, upon written notification to all members of the committee and the board.

H. Members of the committee shall be reimbursed as provided in the Per Diem and Mileage Act and shall receive no other compensation, perquisite or allowance.

FIGURE 10-2
New Mexico Statutes. Chapter 61, Professional and Occupational Licenses, Part I. Section 61-5A-9.

I. A simple majority of the committee members currently serving shall constitute a quorum, provided at least one of that quorum is not a hygienist member.

J. The committee shall elect officers annually as deemed necessary to administer its duties and as provided in rules and regulations. Section 61-5A-10. Powers and Duties of the Board and Committee.

In addition to any other authority provided by law, the board or the committee shall have the power to:

A. Enforce and administer the provisions of the Dental Health Care Act (61-5A-1 to 61-5A-29 NMSA 1978).

B. Adopt, publish and file and revise, in accordance with the Uniform Licensing Act and the State Rules Act, all rules and regulations as may be necessary to:
    1. Regulate the examination and licensure of dentists and through the committee, regulate the examination and licensure of dental hygienists.
    2. Provide for the examination and certification of dental assistants by the board.
    3. Provide for the regulations of dental technicians by the board.
    4. Regulate the practice of dentistry, dental assisting and through the committee, regulate the practice of dental hygiene.

C. Adopt and use a seal.

D. Administer oaths to all applicants, witnesses and others appearing before the board or the committee, as appropriate.

E. Keep an accurate record of all meetings, receipts and disbursements.

F. Grant, deny, review, suspend and revoke licenses and certificates to practice dentistry, dental assisting and through the committee, dental hygiene and censure, reprimand, fine and place on probation and stipulation dentists, dental assistants and through the committee, dental hygienists, in accordance with the Uniform Licensing Act (61-1-1 to 61-1-31 NMSA 1978) for any cause stated in the Dental Health Care Act.

G. Maintain records in which the name, address and license number of all licensees shall be recorded, together with a record of all license renewals, suspensions, revocations, probations, stipulations, censures, reprimands and fines.

H. Hire staff and administrators as necessary to carry out the provisions of the Dental Health Care Act.

I. Establish ad hoc committees whose members shall be appointed by the chairman with the advice and consent of the board or committee, as it deems necessary for carrying on its business.

FIGURE 10-2, cont'd
For legend see opposite page.

Continued

J. Have the authority to pay per diem and mileage to individuals who are appointed by the board or the committee to serve on ad hoc committees.

K. Have the authority to hire or contract with investigators to investigate possible violations of the Dental Health Care Act.

L. Have the authority to hire an attorney to give advice and counsel in regard to any matter connected with the duties of the board and the committee, to represent the board or the committee in any legal proceedings and to aid in the enforcement of the laws in relation to the Dental Health Care Act and to fix the compensation to be paid to such attorney; provided, however, such attorney shall be compensated from the funds of the board.

M. Have the authority to issue investigative subpoenas prior to the issuance of a notice of contemplated action for the purpose of investigating complaints against dentists, dental assistants and, through the committee, dental hygienists licensed under the Dental Health Care Act.

N. Establish continuing education or continued competency requirements for dentists, certified dental assistants in expanded functions, dental technicians and, through the committee, dental hygienists.

Section 61-5A-11. Ratification of Committee Recommendations

A. The board shall ratify the recommendations of the committee unless the board makes a specific finding that a recommendation is:
   1. Beyond the jurisdiction of the committee.
   2. An undue financial impact upon the board.
   3. Not supported by the record.

B. The board shall provide the necessary expenditures incurred by the committee and the board in implementing and executing the ratified recommendations.

FIGURE 10-2, cont'd
For legend see p. 108.

numbers of members of each profession grow or decline. Each group's experience with the health care system as a whole will also bring about change. Our health care system often seems to be at odds with those who are seeking answers to problems of cost containment and quality assurance. New technology has forced us to examine not only the traditional modes of treatment, but the ethical and philosophical aspects of treatment as well.

Professional groups often view practice acts as solutions to their perceived problems. Those who are involved in public policy issues relating to amendments to our state statutes must distinguish between practice act amendments that promote economic self-interest and impede the availability of affordable care and those that further high-quality care and the availability of services. Future changes in the delivery of dental health care are inevitable.

CERTIFICATION

Licensure is granted by state authority; however, **certification** is the process by which a nongovernmental agency grants recognition to individuals who meet certain requirements. The Dental Assistants' National Board certifies dental assistants after graduation from an accredited dental assisting program. However, dental assistants may learn their profession through either on-the-job-training or professional educational programs. Dental assistants with only work experience and no formal education may challenge the national certification examination. Some states recognize more than one category of dental assistants. Expanded functions such as orthodontics and radiology are typical types of certifications that a dental assistant might hold. Laboratory technicians may also be certified. For certification they must pass an examination administered by the National Board for Certification.

CERTIFICATION

The formal documentation of recognition. For instance, a certification of proficiency in a specific skill.

REGISTRATION

Registration is separate from credentialing. Registration indicates that one's name is included on an official list of persons with specific credentials. A governmental or nongovernmental agency can hold this list. Registration may refer to both licensure and certification. Boards of licensure and certification are both often referred to as boards of registration or "registries." Also, "license" and "certificate of registration" are sometimes used interchangeably.

REGISTRATION

The process of entering or recording in some official register, record, or list.

CONTINUING EDUCATION

Many state boards of dentistry, through their rules and regulations, have adopted mandatory continuing education for dental professionals. This is an attempt to ensure the quality of dental care by requiring those who are licensed to continue their education in order to maintain their licenses and to continue to practice as dental health care providers. Maine law mandates continuing education for license renewal. The Wyoming Practice Act states that the board may require continuing education for relicensure.

MAINE AND WYOMING LAWS, RULES, AND REGULATIONS

The practice acts of both Maine (Section 1071) and Wyoming (Section 33-15-101) begin by defining the membership of the board of dental examiners. Both address disciplinary action. Wyoming Rules and Regulations contain a code of ethics for dentists and dental auxiliaries (Chapters 5 and 6, respectively). Maine has no code of ethics but discusses confidentiality and privilege (Section 1092-A). Maine's board has authority to license denturists (Section 1100-D) and dental radiographers (Section 1100-1). Wyoming's board issues a radiographic use permit (Section 33-15-129). There are numerous similarities and differences; however, the essential point of this discussion on dental laws is that each dental professional must become familiar with the laws, rules, and regulations of the jurisdiction in which he or she practices. Each professional is to abide by these mandates or participate in the process of changing them. Until changes occur, a professional must observe the laws of the state in which he or she practices.

SUGGESTED READINGS

American Dental Hygienists' Association: Colorado dental hygienists win precedent setting legal battle, *Access* 2:10, September 1988.

Astroth D, Cross-Poline G: Pilot Study of six Colorado dental hygiene independent practices, *Journal of Dental Hygiene* 72(1):13-22, 1998.

Colorado Revised Statutes, Dental Practice Law, Title 12-35-100, 1986.

Leland H: Quacks, lemons, and licensing: a theory of minimum quality standards, *Journal of Political Economy* 87(6):1328, 1979.

To keep informed on the latest changes and proposed changes in all state dental laws relating to the practice of dental hygiene, review STATELINE, a section appearing in *Access*, a monthly publication of the American Dental Hygienists' Association.

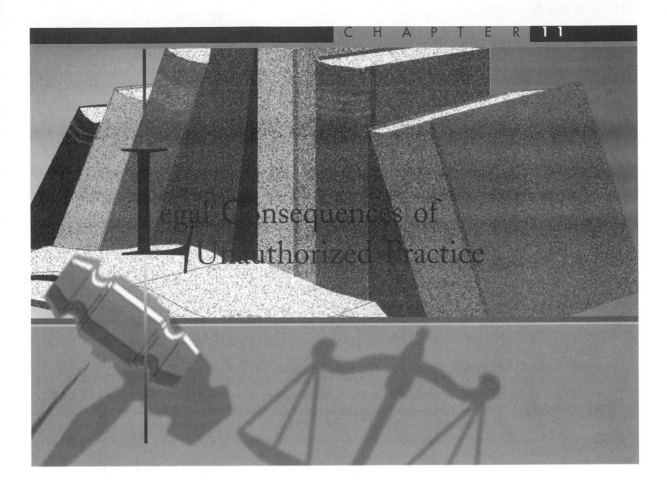

Legal Consequences of Unauthorized Practice

LEARNING OUTCOMES

After reading this chapter, you should be able to:
- Discuss the possible consequences of violating a medical or dental state practice act.
- Describe the National Practitioners Data Bank, explaining why it was created.
- Discuss general grounds for discipline in various state dental practice acts.
- Discusss, in general, the variations in the legal duties of dental hygienists and dental assistants from state to state.

KEY WORDS

DELEGATION
DOCTRINE OF VICARIOUS
   LIABILITY
DISCIPLINARY ACTIONS
FELONY

GROUNDS FOR DISCIPLINE
JUDICIAL REVIEW
MISDEMEANOR
PUNITIVE

UNAUTHORIZED PRACTICE

Unauthorized practice includes the practice of medicine or dentistry by unlicensed individuals or by licensed health care providers who are practicing outside the scope of their licenses. Disciplinary, civil, or criminal action may be taken against a physician or a dentist for aiding the unauthorized practice of medicine or dentistry. Statutes prohibiting the unauthorized practice of medicine or dentistry generally have a "holding out" requirement within the statute. In other words, one must have held oneself out as any of the following:

1. Offering services permitted only by a licensed professional
2. Having a professional license and failing to actually have one
3. Using a licensed title one does not possess

See Section 33-15-114 of the Wyoming Dental Practice Act and Section 1081 of the Maine Dental Practice Act. (See Appendixes H and I.)

Some states will not prosecute individuals who provide unauthorized services unless they receive a fee for such services. However, the Maine Dental Practice Act clearly states, "A person is considered to be practicing dentistry when that person performs, or attempts or professes to perform, a dental operation or oral surgery or dental service of any kind, gratuitously or for a salary, fee, money or other remuneration paid. . . ." The identical wording is in the Wyoming Dental Practice Act.

ARE DOCTORS SELF-MADE MEN?

Prosecution for unlicensed practice does not necessarily proceed as we anticipate. Robert C. Derbyshire, M.D., tells stories of make-believe doctors in a book entitled *The Health Robbers*. One of his tales is of Freddie Brant, alias Reid L. Brown, M.D.:

Freddie Brant was born in Louisiana in 1926 and was forty-three years old at the time of my tale. Reared in poverty, he quit school after the fifth grade. After four years in the army during World War II he found that jobs were scarce for a man with only a fifth-grade education, so he joined the paratroops. In 1949, along with a fellow paratrooper, Brant was sentenced to seven years in the penitentiary for bank robbery. He began his "medical education" working in the prison hospital. After he was released, Brant continued his education by working for four years as a laboratory and x-ray technician for Dr. Reid L. Brown of Chattanooga, Tennessee. There he picked up not only more medical lore but also the diplomas of his employer.

Brant was now ready to begin the practice of medicine. Assuming the identity of Dr. Reid L. Brown, he moved to Texas where he obtained a license by endorsement and served for three years on the staff of the state hospital at Terrell. He then resigned and took his wife on a vacation trip. Stopping for a Coca-Cola in the small village of Groveton, Texas, Brant treated the injured leg of a child. He found that Groveton had been without a doctor and its people were clamoring for medical care. "Dr. Brown" soon became established as the town physician and as a community leader.

Freddie Brant, alias Reid L. Brown, M.D., might still be carrying on his thriving practice in Groveton, Texas, had he not run afoul of a computer. By coincidence he ordered drugs from the same pharmaceutical firm in Louisiana that was used by the real Dr. Reid Brown. The computer gagged when it discovered orders on the same day from physicians with identical names in Groveton and Chattanooga. Following an investigation, Freddie Brant was charged with forgery and with false testimony that he was a doctor.

The exposure of Freddie Brant caused great consternation in Groveton, but its citizens still rallied around their "doctor." Many were the testimonials to his skills. According to one news report, the list of patients included some of Groveton's leading citizens as well as farmers, loggers, and welfare patients. The druggist said that many cases of hardship were caused by Freddie's arrest. A particularly glowing testimonial came from a farmer who said: 'My wife has been sick for fourteen years, we've been to doctors in Lufkin, Crockett, and Trinity, and he did more good than any of 'em. She was all drawed up, bent over, you ought to have seen her. He's brought her up and now she's milking cows and everything.'

The citizens of Groveton remained loyal to Brant, and a grand jury refused to indict him. Authorities then brought him to trial in another county for perjury, but the case ended with a hung jury with eight members voting for acquittal.[1]

Groveton's citizen's had no way of knowing how to identify those who engage in unprofessional behavior or how to restrict the ability of incompetent physicians to move from state to state to avoid discovery of their previous incompetent acts. Since stories similar to Freddie Brant's do occur throughout the United States, the National Practitioners Data Bank was designed to eliminate such situations.

NATIONAL PRACTITIONERS DATA BANK

The United States Department of Health and Human Services opened the National Practitioners Data Bank in September 1990. The United States Congress established the Data Bank through the Health Care Quality Improvement Act of 1986. The Data Bank was established primarily to improve communication regarding licensure, qualifications, staff privileges, and disciplinary actions. Clearly, communication needed to be improved to protect the public's health. By facilitating the identification and disciplining of those engaging in unprofessional behavior, the Data Bank has restricted the ability of incompetent physicians, dentists, and other health care practitioners to move from state to state without discovery of their previous damaging or incompetent behavior.

At present, licensing boards are required to report license revocations, suspensions, censure, reprimands, probation, or surrender. Unless fines occur with licensure action, reporting of them is not required. Some state boards are redesigning penalties to avoid reporting these incidents. Licensed individuals are not required to report incidents to the Data Bank. However, licensed individuals may request their own records and may dispute any report against them. Medical and dental societies must report to the Data Bank any actions taken against members, and they may request information from the Data Bank for a peer review process to further high-quality care. At least every two years, hospitals are required to review their medical staff members against information in the Data Bank. State licensing boards have access to the Data Bank, but are not required to make inquiry prior to issuing a license. A plaintiff's attorneys who are filing a medical malpractice action

---

[1]Barrett S, Jarvis W, eds: *The health robbers: a close look at quackery in America*, Amherst, NY, 1993, Prometheus Books.

or claim in a state or federal court against a hospital may access the Data Bank. Although researchers may access the Data Bank, professional liability insurers may not.

In summary, except for licensed individuals requesting their own reports, only state licensing boards, researchers, health care entities, such as hospitals or HMOs, professional societies, and attorneys have access to information in the Data Bank. The public has no access. Members of the public cannot review the credentials of their current physicians or dentists. Access has been debated since the Data Bank was created.

VARIATIONS IN STATE LAWS

The functions that dental assistants are permitted to perform are regulated by each state's dental practice act. Yet dental assistants are not licensed or certified by the board of dental examiners, which creates the rules and regulations relating to the practice of dental assisting. An exception may be a certification for a specific function. The states of Arkansas, California, Minnesota, Michigan, and New Jersey require dental assistants who perform expanded functions to register, and they use the title Registered Dental Assistant.

DELEGATION

The giving of authority to act for another. For example, a duty can be delegated.

These states require testing, a clinical component, and continuing education. As with dental hygienists, functions **delegated** to dental assistants vary considerably from state to state. For instance, Kentucky permits a trained dental assistant (dental therapist) to place and condense amalgam restorations. New Hampshire permits a "qualified" dental assistant to place pit and fissure sealants and to perform various orthodontic duties, but not to place or condense amalgam restorations. (See Maine and Wyoming dental laws, Appendixes H and I, for examples of listings of dental assistants' legally performed duties.)

Unlike the situation in regard to the profession of dental hygiene, most states do not mandate formal education or credentialing for dental assistants. As of this writing, the only state that does not require a dental hygienist to have graduated from an accredited dental hygiene program in order to be licensed is Alabama. Education for dental assistants is required only for a permit or certification to allow the dental assistant to perform a specific function, such as exposing radiographs.

It is likely that a dental assistant will not understand what tasks may be legally performed in each state unless he or she has a formal education. There are approximately 260 dental assisting education programs accredited by the American Dental Association throughout the United States. Educational programs for dental assistants are found in community colleges and technical schools and are accredited by the American Dental Association's Commission on Accreditation. Yet most dental assistants are office trained. An office-trained dental assistant may not be aware of the state dental practice act or the state board of dental examiners. Even if he or she is aware, the lack of standardization from state to state regarding the legality of delegating specific functions to a dental assistant is enough to confuse almost anyone.

The American Dental Assisting Association provides information regarding various state laws and what functions can and cannot be performed in each state.

In all likelihood, if a dental assistant did not graduate from a formal education program, he or she is not a member of the American Dental Assisting Association.

The **doctrine of vicarious liability** may protect the dental assistant who is unwittingly violating the law. However, he or she is exposed to liability daily, and that liability increases when the tasks being performed are illegal delegations of a duty by the dentist.

VIOLATIONS OF THE PRACTICE ACTS

In most practice acts, the practice of medicine and dentistry is defined as "diagnosis, treatment, and prescribing medications," and such a definition operates to prohibit most unauthorized activities. The practice acts require individuals who violate provisions prohibiting the unauthorized practice of dentistry or medicine to be charged with a **misdemeanor** or a **felony.** A licensed health care provider who aids and abets an unlicensed individual to practice a licensed profession is subject to disciplinary action such as revocation of his or her license.

This is precisely what happened to a dentist from Sparta, Wisconsin. The doctor claimed that he tried every avenue to replace the dental hygienist who had left his practice. When his efforts were to no avail, he instructed his dental assistant to perform prophylaxis and place sealants. When the Wisconsin Board of Dental Examiners was alerted to these practices, it disciplined him for illegal delegation of duties under the Wisconsin State Practice Act and fined him $500 plus $150 in court fees. His dental license was suspended for seven days. However, if a serious injury or death is a result of illegal treatment, criminal charges may be brought.

As stated earlier, a licensed health care provider may be prosecuted for the unauthorized practice of medicine or dentistry. In response, a licensed professional may claim that the specific activity in question was within the scope of his or her license. Usually, boards governing the licensed health care professional will enforce such statutory provisions and discipline that individual if the activity is deemed not to be within the scope of his or her license.

Violation Case Examples

Giroux v. Board of Dental Examiners,[2] *State Department of Health v. Hinze,*[3] *State ex rel Medical Licensing Board v. Stetina,*[4] *Foster v. Georgia Board of Chiropractic Examiners,*[5] *State v. Hoffman,*[6] and *Graham v. State*[7] are cases that provide examples of violations of various states' practice acts.

In *Giroux,* Giroux had not graduated from a dental school as he claimed in his application for licensure. He practiced seven years prior to the board's revoking his license.

> **DOCTRINE OF VICARIOUS LIABILITY**
> The principle that legal liability can be acquired through another. Vicarious liability most often exists when employers are found liable for acts of their employees. See respondeat superior, Chapter 4.
>
> **MISDEMEANOR**
> A crime punishable by less than a year in prison; an offense committed in violation of a law that is less than a felony.
>
> **FELONY**
> Any offense punishable by death or by imprisonment for at least one year.

[2]76 N.E.2d 758 (Mass. 1948).
[3]441 N.W.2d 593 (Neb. 1989).
[4]477 N.E.2d 322 (Ind. App. 1985).
[5]359 S.E.2d 877 (Ga. 1987).
[6]733 P.2d 502 (Utah 1987).
[7]480 N.E.2d 981 (Ind. App. 1985).

In *State Department of Health v. Hinze*, Hinze, who had a doctorate in pharmacology, established a medical clinic and held himself out as a physician. Since he had no medical license, the court issued an injunction, closing the clinic until the matter could be litigated. Hinze then presented a public seminar on naturopathic remedies. During the seminar, a business associate sold various tonics and herbs after Hinze diagnosed each participant and recommended the remedy for his or her particular malady. The court then ordered Hinze not to practice medicine without a license, brought criminal contempt charges against him, fined him, and incarcerated him for 60 days.

In *State ex rel Medical Licensing Board v. Stetina*, Stetina was found to have held herself out as a medical professional. She performed a medical diagnosis through an iridology chart developed by a chiropractor from Los Angeles. This is a chart that purports to diagnose physical ailments through the eyes. Stetina's suggested treatment for this particular patient was colonic irrigation, which she performed in her home. The court issued a temporary restraining order until litigation was commenced. (The term *ex rel* means that legal proceedings were initiated by a state's attorney general on behalf of a state agency.)

In *Foster v. Georgia Board of Chiropractic Examiners*, Foster was sanctioned by the Board of Chiropractic Examiners for exceeding the statutorily authorized scope of his license to practice as a chiropractor. He was recommending vitamins and food supplements to correct physical ills. Foster appealed to a court of law. The court upheld the board's decision.

In *State v. Hoffman*, Hoffman asserted an interesting defense. He contended that he could not be prosecuted, as the state did not obtain permission of the physicians licensing board. State statutes do not bestow upon boards prosecutorial power over criminal conduct of an unlicensed person. Therefore, prosecution of an unlicensed individual requires no permission of a licensing board. Hoffman received a criminal conviction for selling "celestial water" and "special pillows" to cure stomach pain.

In *Graham v. State*, a physician discovered a lump on a patient's breast. Not wishing to have a mastectomy, the patient sought the services of Harry and Ellen Graham. The Grahams were devout Seventh Day Adventists and treated the patient with herbs and natural remedies. Some days they performed up to eleven colonic irrigations, utilizing coffee, carrot juice, aloe vera, caster oil, and pure water. Ellen Graham was a licensed registered nurse. When the patient worsened, Ellen took her to a doctor, who prescribed Laetrile. Then, in addition to her regular treatment, the Grahams also injected the patient with Laetrile daily. After the patient became extremely weak, her husband was able to get her to the hospital. At this point the patient was too weak for chemotherapy and the breast cancer had metastasized to the lungs. The patient died of respiratory failure.

The Grahams were charged with and convicted of involuntary manslaughter, reckless homicide, and unlawful practice of medicine. One of Ellen Graham's defenses was that she was practicing as a nurse. The court found that her actions were outside the scope of her license to practice nursing. The Grahams were both sentenced to six years in prison and fined $5,000.

DISCIPLINARY ACTIONS

All licensed health care providers are subject to **disciplinary actions,** but only by the boards that issued their licenses. Like findings in criminal cases, disciplinary actions do not compensate an injured party. Disciplinary actions are **punitive,** with the ultimate goal being to rehabilitate a health care provider or to remove an incompetent one from practice. There is no need for an injury to be alleged.[8] In *Kim v. Sobol*,[9] a patient was improperly touched during a medical examination, but did not claim injury as a result. The board suspended Sobol's license to practice medicine for a year. A court affirmed the board's decision.

DISCIPLINARY ACTIONS

Actions that regulate or punish, such as suspension of one's license to engage in a particular profession.

PUNITIVE

Involving punishment by legal authority.

PROCEDURAL REQUIREMENTS

Specific procedural requirements must be followed by a licensing board when dispensing disciplinary actions. These procedures are found in the enabling statutes, such as the dental practice act for dentistry. See Wyoming Dental Practice Act, Section 33-15-126, and Maine Dental Practice Act, Section 1077. A board's failure to comply with specific procedures can result in a court's reversing a board's decision.

A professional license is considered a "property right." The United States Constitution guarantees individuals some form of due process prior to the deprivation or loss of a property right. This is procedural due process, which requires:

1. Adequate notice of the charges
2. A right to discovery. The board must disclose all information that substantiates the charges.
3. A right to a hearing prior to any final action, unless action involves immediate suspension for patient safety

JUDICIAL REVIEW

After the board has completed disciplinary action, the licensee may seek **judicial review.** The court reviews the decision by examining the evidence on the record. The court does not try the case. Courts generally uphold boards' decisions, but do reject them on occasion. Courts may also review the penalties set by the board in view of the record. The penalty must be consistent with the authority granted to the board by statute. For instance, Section 33-15-124 of the Wyoming Dental Practice Act clearly states, "Any person who practices dentistry without being properly qualified and licensed, or who violates any provision of this act is subject to a fine, not to exceed one thousand dollars, or imprisonment of not more than two years." Therefore, under Wyoming law, one could not be fined $5,000 for a single violation of the Dental Practice Act.

JUDICIAL REVIEW

A court's review of a finding of an administrative body such as a state board of dental examiners.

GROUNDS FOR DISCIPLINE

All states list various **grounds for discipline,** which vary from state to state. For example, the New York statute provides for disciplinary action against any licensed

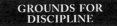

GROUNDS FOR DISCIPLINE

The basis or the real reason for punishment.

---

[8]*Colorado v. Hoffner*, 832 P.2d 1062 (Colo. App. 1992).
[9]580 N.Y.S.2d 581.

professional for refusing to provide professional services to a person because of that person's race, creed, color, or national origin. The most common grounds for discipline are as follows:

1. Gross negligence
2. Incompetence
3. Aiding and abetting the unlicensed practice of the profession
4. Conviction of a felony
5. Unlawful sale of drugs
6. Impairment due to drugs or alcohol
7. Unprofessional conduct
8. Immoral activities
9. Sexual activity with a patient

A single act, such as sexual misconduct, can subject one to disciplinary action by a licensing board, a legal claim of malpractice, criminal prosecution, or censure by or loss of membership in a professional association.

SUGGESTED READINGS

Eisenberg DM et al: Unconventional medicine in the United States, *New England Journal of Medicine* 328:246, 1993.

The National Practitioners Data Bank Guidebook Supplement, Washington, DC, United States Department of Health and Human Services, August 1992.

Furrow BR, Greaney TL, Johnson SH, Jost TS, Schwartz RL: *Health law*, St Paul, 1995, West Publishing Co.

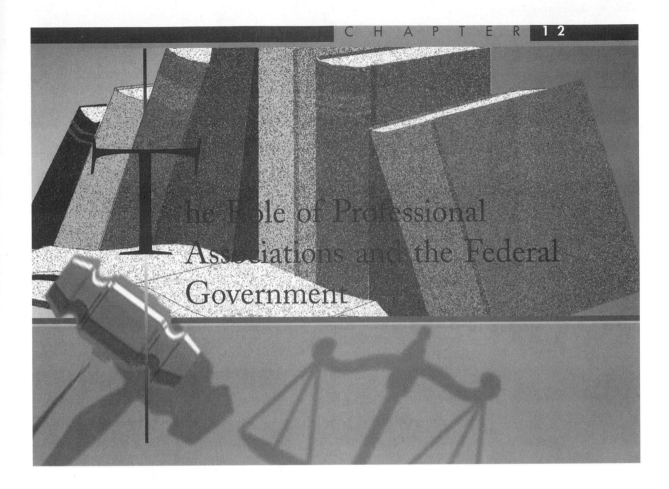

C H A P T E R **12**

The Role of Professional
Associations and the Federal
Government

LEARNING OUTCOMES

After reading this chapter, you should be able to:
- Discuss how professional associations affect health care delivery in the United States.
- List and define the purposes for the federal agencies involved in the delivery of health care.
- Explain the benefits and the abuses of the Medicare and Medicaid Programs.
- Describe how the False Claims Act is being utilized in health care today.

KEY WORDS

ALLEGATION
INDICTMENT
LITIGATE
MEDICAID

MEDICARE
PRECEDENT
REGULATORY POWER

PROFESSIONAL ORGANIZATIONS

One of the best discussions regarding professional organizations is found in *Community Health Today*, by Stephen E. Gray: It reads as follows:

There was once a guild of cobblers, which was very difficult to join and very costly once you did join. The apprenticeship time for nailing soles, gluing heels, cutting leather eyelets, and waxing laces was ten years. In fact, the apprenticeship could run much longer if the prospective cobbler didn't have a sharp eye, a skilled hand and a willing and energetic attitude. And the apprenticeship was just one step in being admitted to the guild. Several examinations had to be passed. The examination standards were quite high, so many candidates didn't pass. The public had to be protected, the cobblers argued. After all, you couldn't let just anyone make shoes. Man's health was involved. Walking was his main means of transportation, and his feet were intrinsically involved in his employment. There was plowing, there was mail delivery, there was housecleaning.

The king agreed with the guild. It really was performing a public service. And since cobblers were experts in shoemaking they should establish standards for the art, and only guild members should practice it. Most people in the kingdom went barefoot. but those who wore shoes wore the finest in the world. Then along came a machine, which made footwear for a quarter of the price that cobblers could. The guild, in panic, screamed that this was nonprofessional. The citizens' feet would never be able to tolerate such crude workmanship, and individual enterprise was what had built their kingdom into the thriving land that it was. The machine would destroy hard-won prosperity, and the entire country would become lazy and immoral, as well as poor. The cobblers had work slowdowns, went on strike, even tried to destroy the shoemaking machines. But the industrial revolution had come. Soon all in the kingdom wore shoes, even the lowliest of peasants. Cobblers, once upper-class entrepreneurs, were reduced to mere workers in shoe factories. Many looked on the change as progress. The cobblers, of course, didn't.

Some regard professional health organizations as holdovers from the old guilds. The doctor treats, or operates, on an independent basis, and is responsible only to other doctors. And the nature of his work resists most forms of organization and control. Any attempt at control, he claims, is a stride toward socialized medicine. The doctors' guild, say the critics, is the American Medical Association. It exercises total control over the type of training and apprenticeship needed to join this organization, how many can join, and the code of conduct that the members must adhere to. Isn't this total control of supply in a field that has an unlimited demand? Isn't this "monopoly" masquerading as "professionalism?" Similar criticisms are leveled at the American Nurses' Association, the American Dental Association, the American Dietetic Association, the American Pharmaceutical Association, the National Association of Sanitarians, and hundreds of others.

Others say this is nonsense. We have to have quality health care in this country. Americans demand it, Congress demands it, and common sense demands it. And health care isn't some kind of assembly-line effort. Organization charts, PERT diagrams, and time and motion studies are great for making automobiles and television sets. But health delivery is more of an art and science than a business. And individuals, not corporations, are artists and scientists. The only way you're going to assure quality in the health field is to assure that quality people practice the skills involved. Despite statistics that say Americans are sickly and death prone, despite critics who claim you can't afford to be sick in the United States, despite minority and consumer groups who claim that health is still more of a privilege than it is a right, Americans can get good health care—some of the finest in the world. The key reason is the high standards established by professional health organizations. You can't compare neurosurgery, radiology, and pathology to making shoes. It's ridiculous to imply that the guild that represented cobblers has, had, or ever will have a similarity to the American Medical Association, the American Dental Association, the American Nurses' Association, and others.

Are there answers to these arguments? No. That is, there aren't finite answers. Professional organizations, without a doubt, establish, maintain, and improve the quality of health care in this country. But even their strongest backers quietly admit that the organizations are primarily interested in improving the incomes of their members or assuring that nothing interferes with the fine incomes they already have. This makes them unresponsive to social reform, social need, and organizational and governmental control. To some extent they impede the progress of health care; to some extent they aid it. Like yesterday's cobblers, these organizations try to destroy the machine that keeps people from going barefoot. This can be both good and bad.[1]

Professional Associations and Health Care Delivery

Our health care system is often criticized as a system of professional self-regulation that is not responsive to the medical or dental needs of society. Professional associations dominate most aspects of health care delivery. First, they mandate uniformity in professional education by exercising authority over accreditation of professional education. They establish the levels of education required, and accreditation teams from professional associations evaluate educational programs. They examine each program in terms of: admissions policies, content of curriculum, facilities (clinical, classroom, laboratory, library, and so forth), qualifications of faculty, faculty-student ratios, evaluation criteria utilized, and financial support for each program, to name a few.

Second, professional associations control the selection of the people who serve on state boards of medicine, dentistry, nursing, and so forth. The selection process for board membership demonstrates this control. The professional organizations usually submit slates of several candidates to the entity (such as the governor of the state) making final appointments to the boards. The final appointments are made from these lists of names submitted. The state boards write rules and regulations pertaining to licensure. Boards establish rules designating which health care providers can perform specific procedures (see Maine and Wyoming rules and regulations, Appendixes H and I, for lists of duties for both dental hygienists and dental assistants), and the circumstances under which various procedures can be performed (e.g., direct supervision versus general supervision).

Third, members of the profession have power over the examinations that must be passed in order to become licensed to practice. For instance, in dentistry the Joint Commission on National Dental Examinations is composed of 15 members:

- Three appointed by the American Dental Association
- Three appointed by the American Association of Dental Schools
- Six appointed by the American Association of Dental Examiners
- One appointed by the American Dental Hygiene Association
- One appointed by the American Student Dental Association
- One public member

---

[1]Gray SE: *Community health today*, New York, 1978, Macmillan Publishing Co, Inc, pp 48-50.

The Commission is located at the American Dental Association headquarters in Chicago. This body sets policy relating to both dental and dental hygiene boards, reviews appeals for candidates who have problems with the board examinations, and selects test constructors from the dental and dental hygiene education communities. Although licensure is controlled by the states, these national board examinations are relied on heavily for decisions regarding licensure. The certification examination for dental assistants is within the dominion of the American Dental Assistants' Association, through the Dental Assisting National Board Examination. Dental laboratory technologists are certified through their National Board for Certification. These associations, organized by health care professionals, set quality and performance standards for services provided by their members, thereby establishing a standard of care, discussed in Chapter 4.

Fourth, should a health professional be accused of committing some wrong, he or she will be summoned before a board of medical or dental professionals that renders decisions regarding specific infractions of the rules and specifies punishment or sanctions if necessary. This can include loss of licensure or certification. Since these boards are usually composed of individuals selected by professional organizations, they have been criticized for being too lenient with their fellow practitioners.

Fifth, associations supply information and express collective opinions; most publish monthly journals. This improves the flow of health care information to professionals and the public. In many ways this is a positive service to both the professional and public sectors; however, it does produce much uniformity regarding medical and dental treatment.

Sixth, another mechanism of control is related to the large legal departments that some of these organizations employ. Their attorneys are hired to protect the professions and often **litigate** to protect the special interests of the organization. The organizations often hire lobbyists who oversee federal and state legislation. The lobbyists directly participate in the political process to obtain passage or defeat of specific legislation that has an impact on the practice of the health care professionals for whom they lobby. Therefore, most legislation concerned with a particular health profession is shaped by that profession.

Professional medical and dental organizations contend that such power vested in their particular professions is in the public interest, as the public cannot assess the quality of health care.[2] Right or wrong, we rely very heavily on professional associations to maintain quality in the delivery of health care services. We do so despite the fact that the medical profession has a consistent record of resistance to legislation directed toward changing health care policy, delivery modes, or means of payment. The following are examples of such resistance.

The American Dental Association has opposed the rules and regulations established by the Occupational Safety and Health Administration (OSHA). OSHA was charged with reducing health hazards and implementing safety standards in the work place. In December 1991, it issued its final rule governing employers' ob-

LITIGATE

To settle a dispute in a court of law.

---

[2]*Sebastier v. State*, 504 So.2d 45 (Fla. App. 1987).

ligations regarding occupational exposure to hepatitis B virus (HBV), human immunodeficiency virus (HIV), and other blood-borne pathogens. The final standard took effect in July 1992. In December 1991, the American Dental Association sued OSHA in federal court, arguing that the standard would impose unnecessary and unjustified requirements upon dentists. The lawsuit was decided in favor of OSHA. In June 1992, when Congress was considering the 1993 budget, the ADA initiated a political campaign to cut OSHA's budget appropriations. A major budget cut would have impaired OSHA's ability to enforce implementation of the standard.

The American Medical Association has opposed workers' compensation laws, social security, Medicare and Medicaid, health maintenance organizations, and the creation of Professional Standards Review Organizations to review the work of physicians involved in federally funded programs.

Generally, the public expresses frustration with specific practices of professional organizations. The failure of the medical profession to provide quality, affordable, health care for all citizens, despite publicly touted claims of excellence and technological achievements, represents the most critical factor that has triggered the increasing presence of the federal government in the health care system.

EXECUTIVE AGENCIES OF THE FEDERAL GOVERNMENT

Laws passed by Congress are often implemented and administered by agencies and departments of the executive branch. These agencies develop rules and regulations, which are published in the *Federal Register*. These rules have the force of law. Some agencies provide services. Many oversee the distribution of federal funds, to ensure that they are utilized according to statute (e.g., funds for Medicare or the Centers for Disease Control).

Other agencies (such as the Federal Trade Commission and the Product Safety Commission) have **regulatory power.** Some are part of cabinet departments (e.g., Food and Drug Administration and Occupational Safety and Health Administration). Most health-related functions are within the Department of Health and Human Services. The Public Health Service is under the direction of this Department, which also includes the Alcohol, Drug Abuse and Mental Health Administration, the Centers for Disease Control and Prevention, the Food and Drug Administration, the Health Resources and Services Administration, the National Institutes of Health, and many others.

The Occupational Safety and Health Administration, a division of the department of labor, is of particular concern to dental office staff members, as it regulates work place safety and health; specifically it is responsible for the implementation of the standards for occupational exposure to blood-borne pathogens. These standards assist in providing a safe work environment for health care providers who are exposed to blood and other body fluids routinely. Copies of OSHA's standards and interpretations are available through the U.S. Government Printing Office. Other information is available on OSHA's web site, http://www.osha.gov.

OSHA's standards were developed with input from the Centers for Disease Control. The CDC recommends methods to prevent disease transmission. "Rec-

REGULATORY POWER

The authority to issue regulations to ensure uniform application of the law and to carry out the intent of the law. Regulations are not the same as laws; however, they influence how laws are interpreted.

ommended Infection Control Practices for Dentistry" contains specific strategies for dental health care providers. These recommendations are more specific than OSHA standards. The two agencies are constantly updating their standards and recommendations on the basis of current research.

MEDICARE AND MEDICAID

Despite the efforts of the medical profession, in 1965 Congress passed the Medicare and Medicaid amendments to the Social Security Act. For better or worse, this established the **precedent** of the federal government's involvement in the administration of health care.

Medicare is a federally administered program providing hospital insurance (part A) and supplemental medical insurance (part B) for persons 65 years and older, regardless of financial status. Disabled persons under the age of 65 who receive cash benefits from social security or railroad retirement programs and certain persons with chronic kidney disease are also eligible for Medicare benefits. Hospital insurance benefits include:

1. Inpatient hospital services for up to 90 days for an episode of an illness, plus a lifetime reserve of 60 additional days of hospital care after the initial 90 days are used
2. Care in a nursing home for up to 100 days after a period of hospitalization
3. Up to 100 home health visits after hospitalization

Supplemental insurance benefits include:

1. Physicians' and surgeons' services, certain nonroutine services of podiatrists, limited services of chiropractors, and services of independently practicing physical therapists
2. Certain medical and health services, such as diagnostic services, diagnostic x-rays, laboratory tests, and other services, including ambulance services, and some medical supplies, appliances, and equipment
3. Outpatient hospital services
4. Home health services (prior hospitalization not required) for up to 100 visits per calendar year
5. Outpatient physical and speech therapy services provided by approved therapists

There are deductibles and coinsurance amounts that are the responsibility of the beneficiary.

Medicaid provides for services rendered to the indigent. States are permitted to include medically needy, aged, blind, and disabled poor, as well as their dependent children and families. The federal government matches funds with state welfare agencies. Medicaid is administered by the states; therefore, services covered vary from state to state.

These programs were not designed to exert control over physicians, change the structure of health care, or change the distribution or quality of health care. They are administered through insurance companies. Some claim that these two programs contributed to the rising costs of health care, as they provided a means of

PRECEDENT

A court decision that serves as the basis for a subsequent case involving the same or a similar question of law.

MEDICARE

A federal program that provides medical insurance for the elderly.

MEDICAID

A program of assistance to low-income families. Funds for Medicaid are provided jointly by the federal and state governments.

passing excessive demands for payment on to insurance companies rather than to individual health consumers. The most disturbing outcome is the fact that many states are overburdened with Medicaid fraud and abuse. Congress funds Medicaid Fraud Control Units within states to recover funds and prosecute fraud and abuse.

Medicare and Medicaid Case Examples

To provide some perspective on the magnitude of the problem, let's examine some statistics from Massachusetts alone. In 1997, Massachusetts' Medicaid program administered over $3.8 billion for health care goods and services to nearly 600,000 recipients. Since 1991, Massachusetts' Medicaid Fraud Control Unit has recovered more than $27 million in criminal and civil restitution, fines, penalties, and costs. It has executed search warrants and administrative document requests, and it has obtained 295 convictions. The criminal prosecutions run the gamut from physicians to transportation companies.

- A psychiatrist was ordered to serve a one-year House of Correction sentence as a result of Medicaid fraud and larceny conviction. The defendant's license to practice medicine was also revoked. Massachusetts alleged that he stole in excess of $300,000.[3]
- A physician pleaded guilty to charges of Medicaid fraud and larceny from the state's Medicaid program, involving more than $25,000. He was sentenced to two years in the House of Correction, one year to serve and the balance to be suspended for five years, and was placed on probation for five years. He also relinquished his right to $98,000 in unpaid claims that the Medicaid program had withheld prior to his **indictment**.[4]
- A pharmacist was sentenced to serve 30 days of a six-month term in the House of Correction for filing false Medicaid claims. He was also ordered to pay $18,000 in restitution. His corporation was ordered to pay $6,500 in fines. The guilty pleas were the result of the filing of claims for services that were not rendered.[5]
- A dentist agreed to pay $123,000 in civil penalties and $62,000 in restitution to settle **allegations** of Medicaid fraud and abuse in his billing practices. He had fraudulently billed for cosmetic dental services, billed for services not covered by Medicaid, and billed for services to patients who were not yet Medicaid eligible.[6]
- A footwear distributor pleaded guilty to five counts of Medicaid provider fraud and four counts of larceny from the Medicaid program. The defendant was sentenced to a three-to-five-year suspended sentence and 10 years of supervised probation. He was ordered to pay $150,000 in restitution, and he must perform 100 hours of community service for each year he is on probation. He defrauded Medicaid by overcharging for orthopedic shoes or supplying the

INDICTMENT

A charge that must be proven at trial in order to convict an individual of a crime.

ALLEGATION

A claim or assertion in the pleading of a party to a lawsuit, specifying what he or she expects to prove.

---

[3]Commonwealth of Massachusetts, Office of the Attorney General: *Medicaid Fraud Control Unit: Significant Case Activities, 1991-1997*. This report was issued by the Massachusetts Attorney General's Office in 1997.
[4]*Medicaid Fraud Control Unit*, supra.
[5]*Medicaid Fraud Control Unit*, supra.
[6]*Medicaid Fraud Control Unit*, supra.

shoes to those who did not need them. He also overbilled Medicaid for removable arch supports, charged the program far in excess of the maximum allowable amount for orthopedic footwear, and charged for custom-made shoe inserts that were actually pre-made.[7]

- A rest home agreed to pay $40,000 in restitution to settle allegations that it violated state Medicaid regulations for long-term care facilities by billing the Medicaid program for reimbursement of services that were never rendered to residents.[8]
- The Massachusetts Medicaid Fraud Control Unit entered into 77 civil settlement agreements with transportation companies that provided taxi, ambulance, and chair-car transportation to Medicaid recipients. The total amount recovered was approximately $1,165,795. Allegations included padding mileage, billing for individual fares when two or more recipients were transported in the same taxi trip, billing for trips that were never made, and failing to obtain completed medical necessity forms for chair-car and ambulance rides.[9]

Nationwide, the General Accounting Office estimates that 15% of total expenditures for health care are attributable to fraud and abuse—nearly $100 billion in 1996 alone. Other health-related activities conducted by the federal government seem to involve less abuse than Medicare and Medicaid.

The False Claims Act

The False Claims Act[10] was originally passed in 1863, during the Civil War, to address the unscrupulous practices of the private industries providing supplies, equipment, and services to the government. For instance, a common practice was to supply sawdust rather than gunpowder. The Act permitted employees of companies that do business with the government to bring suit on behalf of the United States under the qui tam provision (qui tam means "he who brings the action for the king, as well as for himself"). This law was amended in 1986 and was used against fraud in the defense industry. An important aspect of the amendment is that it forbids employers from retaliating against employees who file such complaints. Therefore, individuals employed by any of the businesses discussed above could file suit on behalf of the government for Medicare or Medicaid fraud and have the protection of this Act. An individual filing a lawsuit under this Act must also file a memo with the government. The government has 60 days to decide whether to intervene in the suit. If the government opts out and the suit proceeds, the person may recover individually unless the court finds that the individual brought the suit for frivolous reasons or to harass the employer. Figures from the Justice Department indicate that the number of these cases is on the rise. In 1988, 50 cases were filed and recoveries totaled $2,000,000; in 1994 the number of cases increased to 221, with recoveries totaling $379,000,000. With fraud in the medical industry continuing to escalate, we are apt to see an increase in these types of lawsuits.

---

[7]*Medicaid Fraud Control Unit*, supra.
[8]*Medicaid Fraud Control Unit*, supra.
[9]*Medicaid Fraud Control Unit*, supra.
[10]31 U.S.C. §§ 3729-3733.

CABINET DEPARTMENTS

Cabinet departments whose responsibilities relate to health matters are as follows:

1. The *Department of Agriculture* is responsible for inspection of meat, poultry, and egg products, the food stamp program, the school breakfast and lunch programs, and the Supplemental Food Program for Women, Infants and Children.
2. The *Department of Defense* is responsible for medical care of active and retired members of the military and their dependents.
3. The *Department of Housing and Urban Development* provides grants for community development, which may relate to improvement of community health.
4. The *Department of Education* is responsible for programs related to rehabilitation and education of the handicapped. The department develops educational programs for drug and alcohol abuse and health and sets standards for voluntary agencies that accredit educational programs and institutions.
5. The *Department of Justice* is responsible for the control of narcotics and other drugs. It regulates the manufacture, distribution, and dispensing of drugs. Dentists and other health professionals who dispense or prescribe drugs must register with the Drug Enforcement Administration, which is part of this department.
6. The *Department of Labor* is responsible for the Occupational Safety and Health Administration. which enforces laws and regulations related to industrial health and safety. These regulations are directly applicable to dental offices.
7. The *Department of Veterans Affairs*, formerly known as the Veterans Administration, operates various hospitals, clinics, nursing homes, and residential homes for veterans of the armed forces who have service-related disabilities and who are indigent. The VA hospitals also serve as training facilities for medical and dental educational programs.

INDEPENDENT AGENCIES

There are independent agencies whose responsibilities relate to health issues. To mention a few:

1. The *Consumer Product Safety Commission* enforces safety standards and regulations related to consumer products. These products include dental products.
2. The *Environmental Protection Agency (EPA)* implements legislation relating to environmental quality control. For instance, the EPA has set guidelines for the management of infectious waste. Dental offices are directly affected, as human blood, blood products, contaminated sharps, and human tissue (including extracted teeth) are designated as infectious waste. The EPA excludes teeth taken home by children from the regulated waste definition.
3. The *Federal Trade Commission (FTC)* regulates interstate commerce, including the labeling and advertising of nonprescription drugs. It seeks to eliminate anticompetitive practices by health professionals and institutions, as well as deceptive practices or unfair methods of competition. Professional associations have been in direct opposition to various activities of the FTC and have

fought to diminish its power. For example, the FTC found professional organizations' ban on advertising to be a restraint of trade. The ban was subsequently lifted through litigation. Associations may still regulate advertising, but they may not ban it.

There are innumerable other government agencies, quasi-agencies, institutes, and services, as well as private organizations, that relate to medical and dental health. This discussion was intended to provide an introductory overview, not a detailed listing. Most of these agencies will gladly provide information regarding their activities and functions.

SUGGESTED READINGS

Centers for Disease Control: Recommended infection control practices for dentistry, *MMWR* 35:237-242, 1986.

Centers for Disease Control and Prevention: Recommended infection-control practices for dentistry, *MMWR*, vol 42, no RR-8, 1993.

Cockerham WC: *Medical sociology,* Englewood Cliffs, NJ, 1978, Prentice-Hall, Inc.

Controlling occupational exposure to bloodborne pathogens in dentistry, Washington, DC, 1992, US Department of Labor, OSHA publication 3129.

Fitzpatrick M: OSHA update, *Access* 11(2):21-27, February 1997.

Miller CH, Palenik CJ: *Infection control and management of hazardous materials for the dental health team,* ed 2, St Louis, 1998, Mosby.

Reidinger P: Fraud doctors, *American Bar Association Journal* 82:50-54, May 1996.

Wilson F, Neuhauser D: *Health Services in the United States,* Cambridge, Mass, 1985, Ballinger Publishing Co.

US Department of Labor, Occupational Safety and Health Administration: Occupational exposure to bloodborne pathogens, final rule, 29 CFR part 1910.1030, *Federal Register* 56(235):64004-64182, December 1991.

AUTHOR'S CASE STUDY COMMENTS

Reread the Case Study and Study Questions for Section III
Questions 1 through 8 are examined in the following analysis:

1. Are both Ms. Casey and Ms. Smythe in violation of the Maine dental practice act? If so, explain.

Ms. Casey and Ms. Smythe moved from a state with an open dental practice act to one that lists duties that may be performed by dental hygienists and dental assistants. Amalgam restorations are not among those listed duties; therefore, they are in violation of the Maine dental practice act. (See Appendix H.) Ms. Casey is in violation for an additional reason: she is practicing without a license, and Maine has no provision for acquiring a temporary license.

2. Should a violation be found, will their punishment be the same?

As stated at the beginning of this book, ignorance of the law is no excuse. Both Ms. Casey and Ms. Smythe had the duty to know the law of the state in which they practiced. Ms. Casey runs a greater risk, as she could have her license to practice dental hygiene revoked, or in this case perhaps she could not receive a license because of her illegal activity. The scope of their punishment would be within the discretion of the Maine Board of Dental Examiners.

3. Is Dr. Kemper in violation of the Maine dental practice act?

The illegal activity in the dental office jeopardized the licenses of the dental hygienist and the dentist. Courts can inflict penalties upon individuals who perform or delegate services that are beyond the scope of those permitted under the dental practice act of a particular jurisdiction.

4. What are the possible consequences if one is in violation of the dental practice act?

Violations vary in scope and severity, and the laws of each jurisdiction differ. Depending on the jurisdiction, one could be guilty of a misdemeanor or a felony, subject to temporary or permanent revocation of a license, fined, or imprisoned. Remember: one could be subject to one, any combination, or all of the above for one infraction.

5. What rights do Ms. Smythe, Ms. Casey, and Dr. Kemper have regarding any actions against them by the Maine Board of Dental Examiners?

Assuming that Ms. Casey will have obtained her license prior to any action by the Board, both she and Dr. Kemper will then hold professional licenses. A professional license is a property right, which under the United States Constitution cannot be revoked without due process. Due process means that prior to revocation of a license, the holder of that license has a right to notice of the charges, discovery of information against him or her, and a hearing.

AUTHOR'S CASE STUDY COMMENTS—cont'd

6. What if Dr. Kemper's office was located in Casper, Wyoming, rather than Maine; would there be any different outcome?

The outcome could be different for Ms. Casey, as placing, carving, and finishing amalgams are on the list of accepted expanded duties. After Board approval she could perform these duties legally. Unfortunately for Ms. Smythe, these duties are not listed as legal procedures for a dental assistant.

7. What would the outcome be if Dr. Kemper's office were located in your state?

Most dental hygienists and dental assistants have been faced with the decision of whether to perform dental services that extend beyond the practice acts of their particular jurisdictions. Many have done so and probably have not considered themselves to be engaging in criminal behavior. *However,* it is critical that all health professionals become familiar with the practice acts of the jurisdictions in which they provide their services. They must be prepared to discuss them with prospective employers during an interview, not after accepting employment.

8. Has Dr. Albright committed any violations?

Dr. Albright is committing a felony—Medicaid fraud. Most states have a Medicaid fraud and abuse agency. However, should your state not have such an entity, the attorney general's office is usually the appropriate contact to report such abuse. Medicaid fraud affects us all, as we pay higher premiums for health insurance, higher medical bills, and/or higher taxes to subsidize those who are illegally securing Medicaid funds.

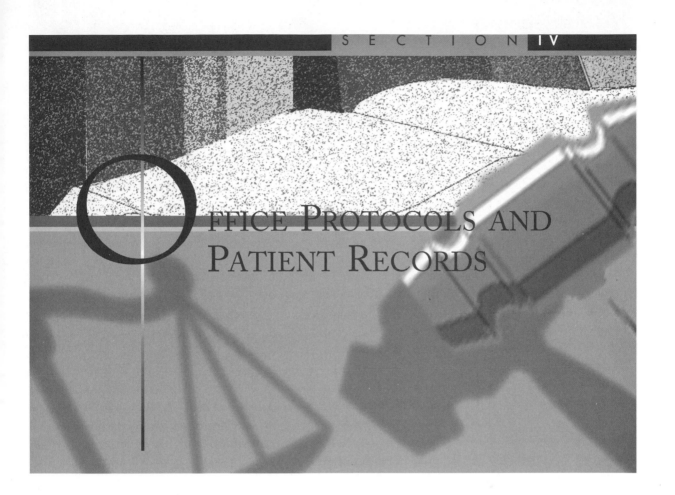

SECTION IV

OFFICE PROTOCOLS AND PATIENT RECORDS

CASE STUDY

A new patient, Susan Scott, arrived for an appointment with Dr. Hastings; she complained of a bad taste in her mouth and bleeding gums. She reported that she was a nonflosser, because dental floss is too painful to use. Upon examination, clinical findings included generalized profuse bleeding and pocketing of 4 to 6 mm. Her gingival tissue was bright red, with rolled margins and puffy papillae and generalized moderate plaque with moderate to heavy calculus on the lingual surfaces of the mandibular teeth and the buccal surfaces of the maxillary posterior teeth. No teeth were missing, with the exception of #1, #16, #17, and #32. However, there were restorations on teeth #18, #3, #14, #15, and #30 and no carious lesions. Ms. Scott had not been to a dental office for ten years.

Ms. Scott is 31 years of age. There were no positive findings in her medical history, and she was taking no medication. She reported to Dr. Hastings that she was in the process of a divorce and was a bit stressed but that, otherwise, she has always been healthy, except for a venereal disease that she received antibiotic treatment for three weeks ago.

Ms. Scott was scheduled with Dr. Hastings' dental hygienist, Ms. Gale, for four periodontal scaling appointments. After her treatment was completed, she scheduled a six-month recall examination and prophylaxis.

Figures 1 and 2 are copies of Susan Scott's records in Dr. Hastings' office.

Dr. Hastings' next patient, Mike Dru, 33 years old, was a regular patient of Dr. Hastings. Mr. Dru reported having severe pain on the left side of his mouth since last week. An examination of the patient revealed a large carious lesion in tooth #19. Finding no radiographs in Mr. Dru's records, Dr. Hastings informed Mr. Dru that a full-mouth series of radiographs must be taken for a complete diagnosis. Mr. Dru refused radiographs. He stated that radiographs were not necessary, as the doctor could see the problem. Dr. Hastings refused to treat the tooth without a radiograph and made an appointment for Mr. Dru with an oral surgeon to have tooth #19 removed. Dr. Hastings wrote prescriptions for Mr. Dru for amoxicillin and acetaminophen with codeine.

Figure 3 is a copy of Mike Dru's record in Dr. Hastings' office.

Mr. Dru canceled his appointment with the oral surgeon and went directly to the office of another dentist, Dr. Roberts. Dr. Roberts examined Mr. Dru and informed him that he recommended seeing an oral surgeon for extraction of tooth #19. In addition, Dr. Roberts informed Mr. Dru that he had periodontal disease and could suffer tooth loss if the disease were left untreated. Mr. Dru had the oral surgeon extract tooth #19 and returned to Dr. Roberts' office for treatment of his periodontal disease. Figure 4 shows Dr. Roberts' patient records for Mr. Dru, including dental hygienist Joan Wills' treatment records for Mr. Dru's periodontal therapy. Mr. Dru was told that several of his teeth had either a guarded or a poor prognosis.

Mr. Dru then made a visit to his attorney. He

Text continued on p. 141

Patient Acquaintance Form

Name *Susan Scott*   Address *151 Main St.*

City_____ State_____ Zip_____ Home Phone *878-8887*

Work Phone *878-1000* Sex (M/F̶) Marital Status *M*

Birthdate *4-25-68* Social Sec.#_____ Driv. Lic.#_____

Name of Responsible Party *self*_____

Billing Address *same*_____

Insurance (Y/N̶) Employer Name_____ Phone_____

Address_____ City_____ State_____ Zip_____

Insurance Company Name_____ Phone_____

Referred By_____

Does Your Medical History Include Any Of The Following:

1.	Rheumatic Fever	___Yes	✓No
2.	Heart Murmur	___Yes	✓No
3.	Heart condition or stroke	___Yes	✓No
4.	High blood pressure	___Yes	✓No
5.	Hepatitis or liver disease	___Yes	✓No
6.	Bleeding problems or anemias	___Yes	✓No
7.	Allergies - if yes, list:	___Yes	✓No
8.	Emphysema, Asthma, or other breathing problems	___Yes	✓No
9.	AIDS or AIDS related complex	___Yes	✓No
10.	Epilepsy or convulsion disorders	___Yes	✓No
11.	Diabetes	___Yes	✓No
12.	Drug or alcohol dependency	___Yes	✓No
13.	Kidney disease	___Yes	✓No
14.	Stomach or intestinal disorders	___Yes	✓No
15.	Cancer - if yes, list:	___Yes	✓No
16.	Mental or emotional illness	___Yes	✓No
17.	If female, are you pregnant?	___Yes	✓No
18.	Presently undergoing medical treatment? Please describe below:	___Yes	✓No

Pt. reports being diagnosed w/chlamydia 5-10-98

19.	Prosthetic joint replacement (hip, knee, etc.)	___Yes	✓No
20.	Do you experience headaches?	___Yes	✓No
21.	Clicking sounds when you open or close your mouth?	___Yes	✓No
22.	Are you fearful of dental treatment?	___Yes	✓No
23.	Are you unhappy with the appearance of your teeth?	___Yes	✓No
24.	Do you have any objection to silver-mercury fillings?	___Yes	✓No
25.	Do your gums bleed when you clean your teeth?	✓Yes	___No
26.	Are you concerned about a problem with bad breath?	✓Yes	___No
27.	Are your gums red, swollen, or tender?	✓Yes	___No

28. List your physician's name: *Dr. Wm. Smith*

29. List the name of your previous dentist:_____

30. List drugs you are presently taking:_____

31. In case of emergency, notify: *Ms. Paula Weis*

Susan Scott *6-30-98*
Patient signature   Date

FIGURE 1

Patient acquaintance form (Susan Scott).

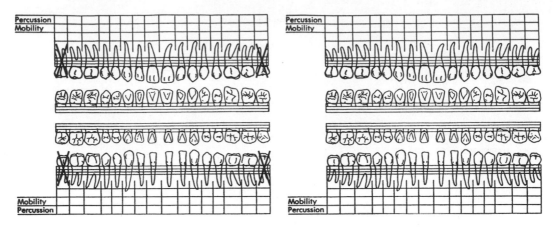

DATE	TOOTH	SERVICE	DATE	TOOTH	SERVICE
6-30-98		Pt complains of bad taste in mouth - gingival inflamation no cat			
		~~scribbled out~~			
		~~scribbled out~~			
7-5-98		quad scale MR			
7-30-98		quad scale mand R			
8-15-98		quad scale mand L			
8-30-98		quad scale max L			
10-1-98		X-rays received from Dr. Thomas FMX dated 10-8-89			
1-4-99		Pt refused to update medical hx uncooperative - doesn't care about her teeth - completed perio treatment only because she had insurance benefits pro-exam			

FIGURE 2
Patient chart with services (Susan Scott).

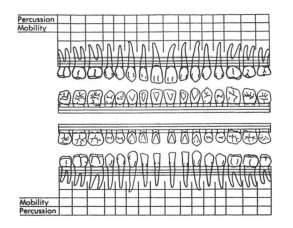

DATE	TOOTH	SERVICE	DATE	TOOTH	SERVICE
12-3-87		Exam - No tx needed			
7-5-88		Pro			
2-9-89		Pro			
10-15-91		Pro			
5-8-92		Pro			
6-6-93		Pro			
7-15-95		Pro			
8-20-97		Pro			
10-1-98		Pain #19 - pt refused			
		X-rays - referred			
		to oral surgeon			
		R amoxicillin			
		acetaminophen w/codeine			

FIGURE 3

Patient chart with services (Michael Dru).

Name __Michael Dru__   Address __321 Ayles__

City _____ State _____ Zip _____ Home Phone __854-1321__

Work Phone __890-1500__   Sex (M/F)   Marital Status __M__

Birthdate __4-25-66__   Social Sec.# __276-90-5084__   Driv. Lic.# __100854__

Name of Responsible Party __self__

Billing Address __same__

Insurance (Y/N)   Employer Name __EB Black, Inc.__   Phone __890-1500__

Address _____ City _____ State _____ Zip _____

Insurance Company Name __Atlas__   Phone _____

Referred By __Betty Dru__

Does Your Medical History Include Any Of The Following:

1. Rheumatic Fever .... ___Yes X No
2. Heart Murmur .... ___Yes X No
3. Heart condition or stroke .... ___Yes X No
4. High blood pressure .... ___Yes X No
5. Hepatitis or liver disease .... ___Yes X No
6. Bleeding problems or anemias .... ___Yes X No
7. Allergies - if yes, list: ...Penicillin.................... X Yes ___No
8. Emphysema, Asthma, or other breathing problems .... ___Yes X No
9. AIDS or AIDS related complex .... ___Yes X No
10. Epilepsy or convulsion disorders .... ___Yes X No
11. Diabetes .... ___Yes X No
12. Drug or alcohol dependency .... ___Yes X No
13. Kidney disease .... ___Yes X No
14. Stomach or intestinal disorders .... ___Yes X No
15. Cancer - if yes, list: .... ___Yes X No
16. Mental or emotional illness .... ___Yes X No
17. If female, are you pregnant? ..NA......................... ___Yes ___No
18. Presently undergoing medical treatment? Please describe below: ..... ___Yes X No

19. Prosthetic joint replacement (hip, knee, etc.) .... ___Yes X No
20. Do you experience headaches? .... X Yes ___No
21. Clicking sounds when you open or close your mouth? .... ___Yes X No
22. Are you fearful of dental treatment? .... X Yes ___No
23. Are you unhappy with the appearance of your teeth? .... X Yes ___No
24. Do you have any objection to silver-mercury fillings? ...... ___Yes X No
25. Do your gums bleed when you clean your teeth? .... X Yes ___No
26. Are you concerned about a problem with bad breath? .... X Yes ___No
27. Are your gums red, swollen, or tender? .... X Yes ___No

28. List your physician's name: __Dr. Long__

29. List the name of your previous dentist: __Dr. West__

30. List drugs you are presently taking: _____

31. In case of emergency, notify: __Fran Dru__

__Michael Dru__   __10-1-98__

Patient signature   Date

FIGURE 4

A, Patient acquaintance form.

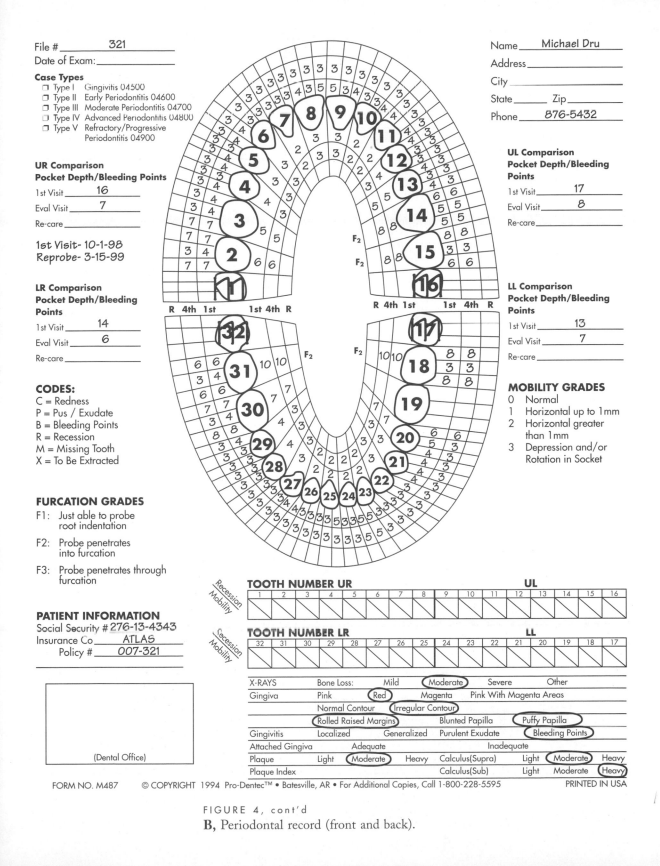

FIGURE 4, cont'd

B, Periodontal record (front and back).

File # _____321_____

Date of Exam: _____

Case Types
- ☐ Type I   Gingivitis 04500
- ☐ Type II   Early Periodontitis 04600
- ☐ Type III Moderate Periodontitis 04700
- ☐ Type IV   Advanced Periodontitis 04800
- ☐ Type V   Refractory/Progressive
             Periodontitis 04900

UR Comparison
Pocket Depth/Bleeding Points

1st Visit _____16_____

Eval Visit _____7_____

Re-care _____

1st Visit- 10-1-98
Reprobe- 3-15-99

LR Comparison
Pocket Depth/Bleeding Points

1st Visit _____14_____

Eval Visit _____6_____

Re-care _____

CODES:
C = Redness
P = Pus / Exudate
B = Bleeding Points
R = Recession
M = Missing Tooth
X = To Be Extracted

FURCATION GRADES

F1: Just able to probe
     root indentation

F2: Probe penetrates
     into furcation

F3: Probe penetrates through
     furcation

PATIENT INFORMATION
Social Security # 276-13-4343
Insurance Co _____ATLAS_____
Policy # _____007-321_____

(Dental Office)

Name _____Michael Dru_____

Address _____

City _____

State _____ Zip _____

Phone _____876-5432_____

UL Comparison
Pocket Depth/Bleeding Points

1st Visit _____17_____

Eval Visit _____8_____

Re-care _____

LL Comparison
Pocket Depth/Bleeding Points

1st Visit _____13_____

Eval Visit _____7_____

Re-care _____

MOBILITY GRADES
0   Normal
1   Horizontal up to 1mm
2   Horizontal greater
    than 1mm
3   Depression and/or
    Rotation in Socket

TOOTH NUMBER UR								UL							
1	2	3	4	5	6	7	8	9	10	11	12	13	14	15	16

Recession / Mobility

TOOTH NUMBER LR								LL							
32	31	30	29	28	27	26	25	24	23	22	21	20	19	18	17

Recession / Mobility

X-RAYS	Bone Loss:	Mild	(Moderate)	Severe	Other
Gingiva	Pink	(Red)	Magenta	Pink With Magenta Areas	
	Normal Contour	(Irregular Contour)			
	(Rolled Raised Margins)	Blunted Papilla	(Puffy Papilla)		
Gingivitis	Localized	Generalized	Purulent Exudate	(Bleeding Points)	
Attached Gingiva	Adequate		Inadequate		
Plaque	Light	(Moderate)	Heavy	Calculus(Supra)	Light (Moderate) Heavy
Plaque Index				Calculus(Sub)	Light Moderate (Heavy)

Michael Dru

	Hygienist Notes and Treatment Progress	Patient Comments
Examination Visit Date ___10-1-98___ ☑ Complete / Perio Exam ☑ X-Rays **FMX** ☑ Document all Findings ☑ Consultation ☐ Prophylaxis, if Appropriate ☑ Other **FMP**		Pt states that he is unaware of his periodontal disease -no past diagnosis Does not with to see periodontist.

Treatment #___1___ Date___11-15-98___
☑ Scaling/Root Planing
  ☑ Full Mouth *Gross Debridement*
  ☐ Quadrant–First
☑ Sub-Gingival Medication
☐ Rota-dent Instruction
☑ Adjunctive Hygiene Instruction
  ☑ Dental Floss
  ☐ Rota-Points
  ☐ Other
☐ Fluoride Therapy
☐ Rx for Home Care
☐ Other
	Microscopic exam spirochete activity ↑ 25 / field not able to floss in post - max + mand profuse bleeding irrigate w/ .12% Chlorhexidine Gluconate	

Treatment #___2___ Date___1-15-99___ ☑ Monitor Plaque Control ☐ Rota-dent Re–Instruction ☑ Scaling/Root Planing **Max + Mand Rt** ☐ Quadrant–Second ☑ Sub-Gingival Medication ☑ Fluoride Therapy ☐ Other	Plaque at gumline irrigate - w/ .12% Chlorhexidine gluconate Rec. daily fl₂ rinse - brushing inst. disp. floss holder	Pt states his displeasure with floss.
Treatment #___3___ Date___2-1-99___ ☑ Monitor Plaque Control ☐ Rota-dent Re–Instruction ☑ Scaling/Root Planing **Max + Mand Lt** ☐ Quadrant–Third ☑ Sub-Gingival Medication ☐ Fluoride Therapy ☐ Other	Interprox plaque No plaque at gumline irrigate - w/ .12% Chlorhexidine gluconate rotapoint instructions	Pt reports using fl₂ rinse daily.
Treatment #___4___ Date___2-15-99___ ☑ Monitor Plaque Control ☐ Rota-dent Re–Instruction ☑ Scaling/Root Planing **fine pale FM** ☐ Quadrant–Fourth ☑ Sub-Gingival Medication ☐ Fluoride Therapy ☐ Other	No plaque irrigate - w/ .12% Chlorhexidine gluconate reviewed homecare	
Treatment #___5___ Date___3-15-99___ ☑ Re-Probe and Assess Therapy Results ☑ Final Polish ☑ Evaluate questionable areas for possible specialist referral ☑ Appoint for Maintenance Interval ☐ Other	↓ areas of pocketing ↑ 3mm. - no plaque good brushing and rotapoint technique Pt advised of areas of pocketing ↑ 3mm	Pt states that he is satisfied w/tx results.

© COPYRIGHT 1994 Pro-Dentec™ • For Additional Copies, Call 1-800-228-5595

FIGURE 4, cont'd
B, For legend see p. 139.

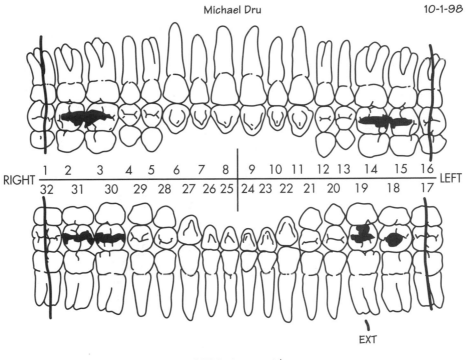

FIGURE 4, cont'd
C, Dental chart.

was very upset about his treatment in Dr. Hastings' office for the past 10 years. He claimed that no one had explained to him that he had periodontal disease or that he was in danger of any tooth loss. The attorney filed a suit for negligence on Mr. Dru's behalf against Dr. Hastings. Within the year Mr. Dru had to have teeth #14 and #15 extracted as the pockets deepened surrounding the teeth and they became mobile. He then became dissatisfied with Dr. Roberts' and Joan Wills' treatment and filed suit against both for negligence.

Mr. Jim Scott, Susan Scott's husband, entered Dr. Hastings' office and demanded his wife's records. He claimed that he needed the records to calculate their income tax. Ms. Charles remembered that Dr. Hastings had told her never to give out original records. Therefore, she told Mr. Scott to have a seat while she made a copy. She also told him that there would be a $10 charge for duplica-

tion. Twenty minutes later, Mr. Scott paid the $10 and left Dr. Hastings' office with his wife's records in hand.

That same afternoon, a local police officer entered Dr. Hastings' office and requested the records of Vera Smith. Vera had been in a fatal car accident that morning with three other individuals. In the aftermath of the accident, flames had charred everyone in the automobile. An examination of the patient's file revealed that only the information shown in Figure 5 was in the patient's record. Fearing repercussions from Mrs. Smith's family because of a lack of information to adequately identify her on the basis of her dental records, Dr. Hastings refused to turn over the record. The next day two police officers returned to Dr. Hastings' office with a subpoena for all of Dr. Hastings' patient records.

Ms. Jane Jones is a 54-year-old patient who is extremely fearful of the dental office. In the past

PROGRESS NOTES

PATIENT'S NAME _Michael Dru_

DATE		CODE
10-1-98	CC: #19 pain	
	Reviewed med/dent hx, hx of pen. allergy	
	otherwise neg. – vital signs WNL	
	soft tissue exam WNL, FMP, FMX	
	#19 carious lesion – DB cusp & DL cusp fractured	
	below gumline – ref. to Dr. Gray for ext.	
	Red, bulbous gingival tissue, generalized	
	profuse bleeding, mod. plaque, heavy	
	sub.ging. cal.	
	Patient advised of the presence of	
	periodontal disease and of the	
	possibility of loss of dentition, however,	
	patient refuses referral to periodontist.	
	Michael Dru	
	R. Roberts, DDS	
	Paula Adams, Witness	
	Written informed consent for tx in record.	
	_RR_	
11-15-98	Reviewed med hx – nc V.S. – WNL	
	gross debridement w/ ultrasonic scaler	
	profuse bleeding, tenacious sub. cal.	
	OHI – brushing & flossing technique	
	irrigate tissue	
	NV – scale max & mand R w/hA – review brush & floss	
	_j.w._	

FIGURE 4, cont'd

D, Progress notes.

DATE		CODE
1-15-99	Reviewed med hx - n.c. V.S. WNL	
	Scale max & mand R w/LA - ↓ bleeding	
	Review flossing + brushing technique	
	Plaque at gumline problem flossing post	
	disp. floss holder - irrigate tissue.	
	NV - Scale max & mand Lt. w/LA	
	review brushing and flossing	(JW)
2-1-99	Reviewed med hx -n.c. V.S. WNL	
	Scale max & mand Lt w/LA	
	↓ tissue redness -no gumline plaque	
	interprox. plaque - pt. finds flossing	
	difficult. rec. & review -rotapoints.	
	NV -fine scale -review brushing + rotapts.	(JW)
2-15-99	Reviewed med hy-n.c. V.S. WNL	
	fine scale max. & mand. disclosed -no plaque	
	reviewed brushing + rotapts. - pt has good	
	technique -sl gingival bleeding in post	
	irrigate.	(JW)
3-15-99	Reviewed med hx -n.c. V.S. WNL	
	fine scale post., polish, reprobe - ↓	
	pocketing -disclosed - no plaque, improved	
	tissue contour. Discussed need for	
	more frequent annual visits due to	
	depth of periodontal pockets -pt. agreed.	
	NV - 3 mos recall	

FIGURE 4, cont'd
D, For legend see opposite page.

AUTHORIZATION FOR RELEASE OF HEALTH INFORMATION

I, _Michael Dru_ ,

RESIDING AT _321 Ayles_ AUTHORIZE THE RELEASE

OF A COPY OF MY DENTAL RECORDS AND ANY INFORMATION RELATED TO MY

HEALTH HISTORY, DENTAL HEALTH STATUS, TREATMENT RECORD AND

RADIOGRAPHS TO:

Robert Roberts, D.D.S.
NAME

_421 W. 8th St_
ADDRESS

Michael Dru   _10-1-98_
PATIENT'S SIGNATURE   DATE

FIGURE 4, cont'd
E, Authorization for release of health information.

Dr. Hastings has always given Ms. Jones either pre-medication or nitrous oxide to provide even the simplest treatment. She had been waiting for her appointment with Dr. Hastings for 35 minutes and now was showing greater signs of agitation because of the wait and her fears. When the police entered Dr. Hastings' office, she appeared to become even more anxious. Suddenly, she experienced severe chest pain with no loss of consciousness. Ms. Charles quickly rushed to get the oxygen for Ms. Jones.

REQUEST FOR TREATMENT - INFORMED CONSENT

I hereby request that Dr. Roberts provide treatment for me for the following condition:

periodontal disease . I have been afforded the time and

opportunity to discuss this proposed treatment, the alternatives and risks with Dr. Roberts

and I understand:

1. The means of treatment will be: _a series of visits to clean teeth above and below gums, root plane -roots of teeth Provide instructions for my participation in control of plaque in my mouth._

2. The alternative means of treatment is: _periodontal surgery_

3. The advantages of proposed treatment over alternative treatment is: _non- surgical means_

4. That all treatment including the one proposed have some risks involved. The risks of importance involved in my treatment have been explained to me, and they are: _The possibility of little or no tissue response with future increased pocketing_

5. The risks of non-treatment are: _Continuation of disease with possible future tooth loss_

Michael Dru
Signature of Patient

_10-1-98_
Date

Paula Adams
Signature of Witness

Robert Roberts, DDS
Robert Roberts, D.D.S.

FIGURE 4, cont'd
F, Request for treatment/informed consent.

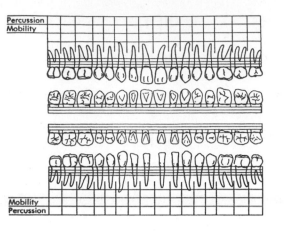

DATE	TOOTH	SERVICE	DATE	TOOTH	SERVICE
1-5-96		ex, pro			
2-15-96		pain UR asymptomatic			
3-15-96		pain UR asymptomatic			
4-1-97		ML resin #9			
7-8-97		ex, pro			
1-12-98		ex, pro			
2-12-98		TMJ pain-			
		fabricate mouthguard			
		imp for mouthguard			
3-5-98		seat mouthguard			
8-5-98		~~adjust mouthguard~~			
8-20-98		ex, pro			

FIGURE 5
Patient chart with services (Vera Smith).

RESPONSE TO CASE STUDY

Morris L. Robbins, D.D.S.

An adage that has been around dentistry for a long time is "Never treat a stranger." This applies to all aspects of a patient's care, from the medical history to the dental examination and the recording of information regarding the treatment provided.

As we look at each case, keep in mind the three issues of not knowing the patient, patient information, and the record. In the case of Ms. Scott, it appears that sufficient medical information had been received and discussed with her. The information issue is strong in this case. The treatment record shows that an incomplete oral examination occurred, with no emphasis on periodontal evaluation. No diagnosis was recorded, nor was it noted that any discussion to inform the patient had ever occurred. Note that quadrant scaling was performed by the dental hygienist (we assume, not noted on chart). To further emphasize that Dr. Hastings and Ms. Gale were treating a stranger, no x-rays were available until they were received from another practitioner after the quadrant scaling had been completed. The last entry includes the inappropriate judgment "doesn't care about her teeth" and a seriously questionable statement that the periodontal treatment was completed only because the patient had insurance benefits.

Yes, a stranger was treated in this office, and when Mr. Scott came in to demand his wife's records, they should not have been given to him without her permission. One can only speculate on the future as far as litigation is concerned, but both Dr. Hastings and Ms. Gale should be very concerned, since their services were provided to a stranger without the gathering of proper information.

The case of Michael Dru could be even more damaging for Dr. Hastings. It is clearly evident that he treated a stranger in Mr. Dru for more than ten years. It appears that periodontal disease and decay existed in his mouth and were not treated properly by Dr. Hastings. The basics of dental education had been abandoned, and treatment had proceeded without proper information gathering and recording by the dentist and information being given to the patient concerning his advancing dental disease.

Dr. Hastings was ten years too late in requesting that Mr. Dru have a full-mouth x-ray series. Even though Mr. Dru refused the x-rays on October 1, 1998, Dr. Hastings did the right thing in this incident by referral. A stark contrast exists between Dr. Hastings and Dr. Roberts in relation to strangership and information. The way in which issues of information are handled by Dr. Roberts and his hygienist is clearly head and shoulders above Dr. Hastings' practices in this regard and provides clear evidence that Dr. Roberts did not treat a stranger and also that he gave clear and succinct information to Mr. Dru. Negligence will be almost impossible to prove.

A healing arts practitioner must always know the patient thoroughly, be prepared to gather necessary information, and, when a diagnosis and treatment plan are ready, clearly inform the patient of them and answer any questions the patient may have. Documentation of these safeguards in the records will assist the practitioner in a myriad of ways.

RESPONSE TO CASE STUDY

Marilyn Cortell, R.D.H., B.S., M.S.

A simple knowledge of recordkeeping is not enough; vigilance in regard to accurate and thorough documentation is essential. It is necessary to adopt, maintain, and utilize a systematic, logical, and predictable approach to recording and maintaining all entries made in the patient's clinical records. We should be able to view effortlessly what observations were made and discussed, what services were provided, and what future treatment recommendations were made. Keeping in mind that a dental record may provide the only chronological and detailed history of a patient's treatment will make us more thorough when we record.

The following is a mnemonic developed to help dental health professionals utilize a systematic approach to recording and documenting. I have personally used this method, and it has become second nature to me. In addition, I have lectured on the topic of documentation to audiences in the dental health professions, who also have found it useful to commit the mnemonic to memory.

For the case study, all entries made in the clinical record should follow the order of this mnemonic:

Dental **H**ealth **E**xaminers **R**adiate **G**ingerly, **P**roviding services, **P**atient education, and **T**reatment plans **S**incerely.

Study this sentence until it becomes familiar; then assign meaning to the first letter of each word:

D	Date every entry
H	Health history
E	Extraoral and intraoral tissue exam
Radiate	Radiographic assessment
Gingerly	Gingival and periodontal evaluation
Providing services	State services provided
Patient education	Disease prevention recommendations
Treatment plans	State treatment plans, objectives, and alternative options
Sincerely	Sign your name

It is possible that you will feel burdened with paperwork when making entries into a patient's record. Perhaps you will feel that your schedule does not permit time to be thorough. However, when you are feeling particularly overwhelmed, keep in mind that it is your responsibility to be sure that nothing is left to interpretation or assumption. Remember: *If it isn't written, it didn't happen.*

Susan N. Scott, Patient of Dr. Hastings:
Susan Scott was thorough in reporting her chief complaint (cc) as having a "bad taste in her mouth and bleeding gums"; the dentist and the hygienist were good listeners and provided appropriate services; however, gross deficiencies in documentation and recording are evident.

Date
Provide a date for all chart entries.

Health History
Personal data on the medical history form are part of the patient's clinical record and must be complete, thorough, and signed by the patient or guardian; there should be no blank spaces. In Susan's personal information, city, state, and zip code are missing. The name of Ms. Paula Weis is listed for emergency notification, but no telephone number is given. The address and telephone number of her physician are missing. No details on the current treatment of chlamydia are given; they should include the treating doctor's name and the treatment protocol. There is no record of dialogue with the patient regarding the chief complaint, dental concerns, or any other relevant conversation.

RESPONSE TO CASE STUDY—cont'd

Examiners
Extraoral and intraoral tissue (cancer) exam and charting are not recorded; the assumption is that the exam was not performed.

Radiate
Radiographs are not up to date in Ms. Scott's record. The last films were taken at a previous dental office, nine years ago. Appropriate diagnosis and treatment planning cannot be made without a radiographic assessment.

Gingerly
Initial periodontal observations and examination were not carried out.

Providing Services
Susan had four quadrant scaling appointments, with no detail of how actual services were performed.

Patient Education
Ongoing oral hygiene education and recommendations for Susan to prevent disease should be discussed and written out.

Treatment Plans
Future treatment needs should be recorded, along with a chronology of conversations with the patient regarding treatment recommendations and treatment options, followed by a comprehensive explanation of consequences if the plan is not accepted. Using "next visit" or "N/V" to transition from one visit to the next will help to clarify what procedure is next.

Sincerely
Sign your name when all documentation has been appropriately and accurately recorded.

Example of Chart Entries for Susan Scott, Using the Mnemonic: This is an example only and rep-resents one possible method for chart documentation. Feel free to adapt and supplement it by using your own style and abbreviations.

6/30/98
√ HH: pt recently diag w chlamydia. Underwent ABx w single 1-gm dose Zithromax . cc: pt states bad taste, bleeding gums, not flossing, too painful. In process of divor, feeling stressed, otherwise usually healthy. EIOE: WNL. FMX: NCF. Ging: gen bright red, rolled marg w enlarg papillae, mod ging infl, tissue blds easily. Gen 4-6 mm pkts w BOP. Gen mod plaque w mod-heavy calculus ling low ant & buccal max mol. Provided: compl clinical and perio exam, FMX Reviewed pts home care, B/F demo, rec 2x/day w Listerine rinse

Tx plan: 4 quad SCRP, reinf HCI
N/V: begin quad SC
M Gale

7/5/98
rev HH, no ch, pt reports B/F regul. Feels "glad she decided to come for Tx" Dr H admin 2 carp lido 1-100.000 w epi infilt. SCRP max rt w ul-trasonic followed by hand scale. Tissues bled throughout. Calculus heavy & tenacious, rev HCI. N/V: max rt, begin mand rt A
M Gale

Mike Dru, Patient of Dr. Hastings:
Dr. Hastings' records for the treatment of Mike Dru are grossly deficient, lacking relevant and necessary information. Many omissions are obvious and have been exaggerated for purposes of emphasis. The absence of a complete and current medical and dental history should make it impossible to provide further treatment for Mike. Without an updated and accurate medical history, Dr. Hastings is unable to assess whether

RESPONSE TO CASE STUDY—cont'd

necessary or proposed treatment will present any degree of risk to Mike. Note omissions such as the name of the oral surgeon, which should be in the record along with the specific prescription and dosage. A follow-up call should be made to the oral surgeon's office, with date, time, and who Dr. Hastings spoke with being recorded in Mike's record.

Mike Dru, New Patient of Dr. Robert Roberts:
The records from the office of Dr. Roberts show significant improvements over the records from the office of Dr. Hastings.

Date
10-1-98

Health History
1. Mike's medical history form had "yes" answers. A further probe of these answers should be conducted and additional information recorded directly on the medical history form. The health history should be updated each visit.
2. Address is incomplete.
3. Not clinically significant, but important from a business perspective, is insurance company information.
4. Emergency information is lacking: current doctors, contact person, name, address, telephone. Informed consent, optional although important, is a means of ensuring that both patient and service provider have communicated, with a mutual understanding of future treatment recommendations and of consequences if the treatment plan is refused.

Examiners
Complete oral examination, vital signs, and charting were performed adequately and well documented.

Radiate
A complete series of radiographs were exposed. Radiographic findings were recorded in clinical chart.

Gingerly
On 10/1/98 a thorough periodontal examination was performed, along with a gingival observation. Notes were made on Mike's subsequent visits, giving providers a detailed chronology of the patient's progress and compliance.

Providing Services
Services provided are well documented, as is relevant dialogue. Note the logical, predictable sequence of each subsequent visit. We must make sure that the patient's name appears at the top of each form in the record. Specific data on administering local anesthesia, indicating type and concentration, should be included. Again, using "next visit" or "N/V" to end the entry is acceptable.

Patient Education
Ongoing communication is essential to properly educate the patient about the importance of continuing care. This patient education dialogue should be well documented and reinforced each visit.

Treatment Plans
This is the place on the chart to note future treatment recommendations, always including recall visits in addition to the patient's other dental needs.

Sincerely
Sign your name when all documentation has been appropriately and accurately completed.

RESPONSE TO CASE STUDY—cont'd

Vera Smith, Patient of Dr. Hastings:
Dr. Hasting's record of Vera Smith's treatment is obviously characterized by negligence, which clearly reinforces the significance of a well-documented clinical record. Had the mnemonic been followed, Vera Smith's record would have contained radiographs along with a thorough and comprehensive charting, which would serve as forensic identification for Ms. Smith's family.

Jane Jones, Patient of Dr. Hastings:
Given that Ms. Jones is an established patient of record and is waiting in the office for her appointment, the assumption is that all records are present and current in her file. Emergency treatment should be based on information relating to the patient's prior history.

COMMON ABBREVIATIONS

Administered	admin
Amount	amt
Antibiotic	ABx
Appearance	appear
Assessment	A
Bleeds	blds
Bleeding on probing	BOP
Brushing and flossing	B/F
Buccal	buc
Calculus	calc
Carpules	carp
Change	ch
Check	$\vee$
Chief complaint	cc
Complete	compl
Continue	cont
Demonstrated	demo
Decrease	$\downarrow$
Diagnosis	diag
Enlarged	enlar
Epinephrine	epi
Extraoral and intraoral exam	EIOE
Full-mouth radiographic series	FMX
Followed	follo
Generalized	gen
Gingiva	ging
Health history	HH
Home care instruction	HCI

Continued

COMMON ABBREVIATIONS—cont'd

Improve	imprv
Increase	↑
Infiltration	infil
Inflamed	infl
Lidocaine	lido
Lingual	ling
Lower	low
Mandible	mand
Margins	marg
Maxilla	max
Month	mnth
Molar	mol
Moderate	mod
Millimeters	mm
Next visit	N/V
No changes	no ch
No clinical finding	NCF
Oral cancer screening	OCS
Oral hygiene instruction	OHI
Papillae	pap
Patient education	pt ed
Plaque	plaq
Pockets	pkts
Provides services	pro serv
Quadrant	quad
Radiographic	radio
Recommend	rec
Re-evaluate	re-eval
Reinforce	reinf
Review	rev
Scaling, root planing	SCRP
Slight	sl
Treatment	Tx
Treatment plan	TxP
Ultrasonic	ultra
With	w
Within normal limits	WNL or wnl

CASE STUDY QUESTIONS

1. Patient Dru has initiated litigation against Dr. Hastings and Dr. Roberts. Which doctor's patient record is more likely to succeed in a court of law? Why? List strengths and weaknesses of both.

2. Does Patient Scott have any legal claims against Dr. Hastings? If so, what are they?

3. Patient Scott's treatment record indicates that she refused to update her medical history when she returned for a prophylaxis and examination. What should Dr. Hastings do?

4. Is it likely that Patient Dru will prevail in his lawsuit against Dr. Hastings? Why or why not?

5. Is it likely that Patient Dru will prevail in his lawsuit against Dr. Roberts and/or Joan Wills, the dental hygienist employed by Dr. Roberts? Why or why not?

6. What should Dr. Hastings do regarding the police officers and the subpoena for his patient records?

7. What health and/or legal issues exist regarding patient Jones?

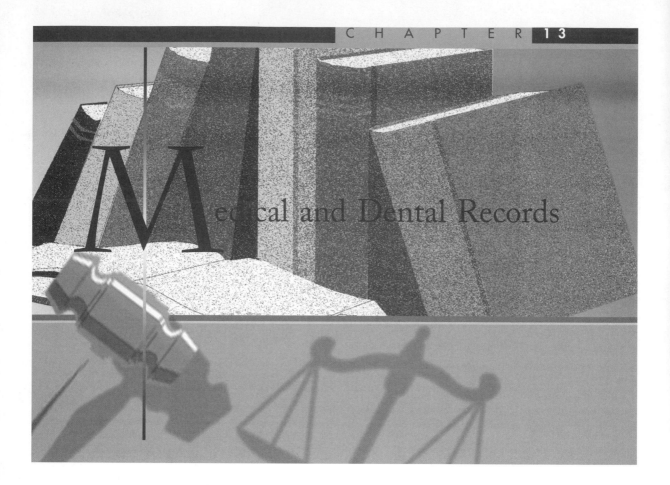

Medical and Dental Records

LEARNING OUTCOMES

After reading this chapter, you should be able to:

- Discuss critical reasons for keeping accurate patient records.
- Describe types of patient identification data essential to a patient's dental records.
- Compare and contrast accurate and inaccurate means of making entries in a dental patient's progress notes.
- Discuss how a patient's dental record may be utilized in a court of law.
- Understand the legal consequences of altering a patient's record.
- Discuss the confidentiality of patients' medical and dental records, specifying when it is essential to keep information confidential and when it is appropriate to release information contained in such records.

KEY WORDS

CONSENT FORM
CONTROLLED SUBSTANCE
DENTAL HISTORY
MALPRACTICE
MEDICAL HISTORY
PATIENT IDENTIFICATION
   DATA
PROGRESS NOTES
REFERRAL
SUBPOENA

KEEPING ACCURATE RECORDS

Failure to keep adequate patient records may constitute **malpractice** for a variety of reasons. First and foremost, the health care provider treating the patient could be missing critical information and, as a result, incorrectly treat a patient. Insufficient documentation in the patient's record may lead to a guilty verdict in a court of law even though there was no negligence on the part of a health care provider.

Most medical and dental records contain patient identification data, a medical and/or dental history, reports of tests or procedures, informed consent documents, diagnostic and therapeutic orders, and clinical observations. The bulk of entries made in the patient record are the progress notes.

PATIENT IDENTIFICATION DATA

Patient identification data include the patient's name, address, work and/or home telephone number, social security number, birth date, person to contact in case of emergency, including telephone number, physician's name and phone number, and financial information, such as insurance companies or other responsible parties. Data are updated at all recall visits or whenever changes occur for the patient. Financial agreements and insurance information are to be kept separate from the progress notes.

CONSENT FORMS

Signed **consent forms** are part of the patient's file (see Chapter 6). All states require a patient's informed consent prior to treatment. Consent may be in writing or oral. Whether written or oral, consent is to be documented in the patient's record. A patient may decide not to proceed with recommended treatment. A patient has the right to be informed of the consequences of refusing treatment. After the patient is informed and then refuses, he or she has given informed refusal. Courts now view informed refusal as a duty of the health care provider to the patient, when recommended treatment is not initiated. Treatment recommendations of the professional and the possible outcomes of noncompliance are documented in the patient's record and signed by the patient. For example: "1-13-99: Generalized advanced periodontal disease with 5-9 mm pocket depths and profuse bleeding. Patient was advised of the presence of disease and of the possibility of loss of dentition; however, patient refuses recommended treatment or referral to a periodontist." After refusal, the patient's periodontal status is evaluated at subsequent visits, appropriate treatment recommended, and information documented at each recall. Notations such as these protect the professional from claims of malpractice. They also may provide a basis for dismissal of a patient without fear of allegations of abandonment.

MEDICAL AND DENTAL HISTORY

A complete medical and dental history must be documented in the patient's record prior to treatment. The **medical history** should include information relating to allergies, potential drug sensitivities, including reactions to dental anesthesia, present medications and/or treatment, systemic diseases, such as diabetes, hepatitis, or

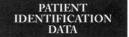

MALPRACTICE

Failure to exercise reasonable care by a professional, which results in harm to another; negligent conduct by a professional or a breach of a standard of care.

PATIENT IDENTIFICATION DATA

All data collected to provide medical and dental information about a specific patient.

CONSENT FORM

A signed document indicating a patient's agreement to receive treatment and acknowledging his or her understanding of the specific treatment or procedure recommended by a health practitioner.

MEDICAL HISTORY

A record of all past and current medical conditions and treatment received by an individual.

AIDS, cardiac conditions, history of rheumatic fever, arthritis, bleeding problems, or nervous disorders, and general health and physical appearance. The medical history must be dated and signed by the patient. This document should be reviewed with the patient verbally to ensure that the patient understands all questions. Medical histories are to be reviewed prior to all appointments and so noted in the progress notes. At each appointment the patient should be asked if he or she has seen a physician, taken new medications, or had injuries or illnesses since his or her last visit. Any changes need to be documented with a date and signature. A complete review of the medical history should be done at least once a year.

It is sometimes necessary to confer with the patient's physician to clarify issues regarding the patient's health. It is imperative that all telephone conversations be documented in the patient's record. Written communications that request information, and any responses as a result, are to be kept in the patient's record. The **dental history** should include the patient's chief complaint and information regarding past dental treatment. If it is necessary to obtain records from the patient's past dentist, permission should be requested from the patient prior to making the request and the patient should be asked to sign an authorization for the release of information in his or her past dental record.

DENTAL HISTORY

A record of all preventive, restorative, and aesthetic treatment a person has received, as well as his or her dental experiences.

REFERRAL

Sending a patient to another practitioner to seek advice about medical or dental treatment or diagnosis.

REPORTS OF TESTS OR PROCEDURES

Documentation of **referrals** to specialists for treatment or evaluation and their responses are part of the patient's permanent file. Reports from other professionals, such as oral surgeons' reports regarding biopsy findings or results of microbial testing, are also maintained in the patient's chart. All diagnostic tests performed are documented in the patient's record. If test results are within normal limits, that also is noted in the progress notes.

CLINICAL OBSERVATIONS

Documented clinical observations provide baseline data for diagnosis, treatment planning, and future treatment. Clinical observations include findings of a head and neck examination, as well as an examination of the mouth. All findings should be documented, including screening for oral cancer and other pathology, teeth present and missing, current caries and restorations, endodontic status, existing partial or full dentures, existing crowns and fixed bridges, periodontal status, and notations on occlusion and temporomandibular joint function. When the presence of lesions is noted in or around the mouth, the circumference should be measured with a probe. This information allows for a more accurate determination of actual change at a later evaluation. The general appearance of the lips, oral mucosa, gingiva, tongue, and pharynx, as well as any evidence of erosion or attrition, bruxism or clenching, or mouth breathing, should also be noted. Radiographs, diagnostic photographs, and study models are part of the patient record.

A diagnosis and a treatment plan, based on clinical findings, are to be clearly stated and in writing. The patient needs to understand cost, risks, and benefits of treatment and alternative treatment. Both the patient and the provider sign and date the treatment plan. All alterations in the treatment plan and/or the diagnosis should be recorded. Any adverse reactions are noted, as well as postoperative instructions.

In the past, conflicting tooth numbering systems and radiograph mounting systems were often responsible for treatment of the incorrect tooth; thus the existence of these various systems contributed to unnecessary dental malpractice claims. To resolve this problem, the American Dental Association adopted a policy system on tooth numbering and radiograph mounting. It states: "Teeth should be numbered 1-32 starting with the third molar (1) on the right side of the upper arch, following around the arch to the third molar (16) on the left side, and descending to the lower third molar (17) on the left side, and following that arch to the terminus of the lower jaw, the right third molar (32). Consecutive upper case letters (A-T), in the same order as described in the numbering system, should be used to identify the primary dentition. Looking at the teeth from outside the mouth, radiographs should be viewed in the same manner and so mounted."[1] The American Dental Association has developed guidelines covering many aspects of the dental office and patient treatment. Generally, the courts look to these guidelines to determine whether there has been a breach in the standard of care. If, in the court's opinion, a dental health care provider's conduct has fallen below the standard of care, as evidenced by a particular guideline not being followed, liability could be established.

A high prevalence of malpractice litigation is based on the failure to diagnose, treat adequately, or refer patients with periodontal disease. It is a legal and ethical obligation of the dental health care provider to provide adequate treatment for periodontal disease or refer the patient to a specialist. Each dental visit should include a review of the patient's periodontal assessment.

Items to be assessed clinically are:
1. Gingival bleeding
2. Attachment loss (probing depths plus gingival recession measured from the cementoenamel junction)
3. Furcation involvements
4. Tooth mobility

Items to be assessed radiographically are:
1. Absence of bone loss
2. Crestal bone loss
3. Horizontal bone loss
4. Angular bone loss

PROGRESS NOTES

Progress notes are chronological notations of actual patient treatment performed. Items include pretreatment procedures (premedication, anesthetics, etc.), any unusual circumstances or incidents, actual treatment, changes in treatment or diagnosis, oral hygiene instructions, home care recommendations and noncompliance by patient, postoperative instructions, critical telephone conversations, medications

PROGRESS NOTES

A record, kept on a continuing basis, of all treatment provided to a patient and observable conditions pertaining to his or her health.

---

[1] The ADA House of Delegates adopted the universal system of tooth numbering and radiographic mounting, to be used by all dental professionals, in 1968.

taken or prescribed, and treatment planned for the next visit. If a patient refuses to have a radiographic series, document the refusal and have the patient sign or initial the entry. If a radiograph is a necessary part of treatment and the patient refuses, it would be wise to dismiss the patient. Should the patient be dismissed, the appropriate procedures are to be followed to prevent an allegation of abandonment (see Chapter 8). The patient's compliance with prescribed premedication is always documented in the progress notes. Document the dosage of any medication given and the amount and type of anesthetics administered.

The Drug Enforcement Administration imposes federal regulations on dentists who prescribe, dispense, or administer **controlled substances;** that information must be documented in the patient's record. This documentation includes a description of the treatment performed or the diagnosis, the name and strength of the drug or drugs, the quantity of the drug or drugs, and the date prescribed, dispensed, or administered. An additional inventory and dispensing document is to be maintained for every drug that is classified as a controlled substance and kept in the office.

Each entry in the progress notes includes the date and the signature and status or title of the individual making the entry. If records are computerized, a numbering system may be utilized to identify which practitioner provided a particular service. Documenting each procedure is a must. Should you find yourself in a court of law with missing entries in your patient record, a jury may decide that the missing services were never provided. All entries are made as soon as services are provided. Some practitioners wait until the end of the day to complete the records for their patients. With such a method, it is very easy to omit critical observations or services. If time does not permit completion of each record at the close of each appointment, utilize a small tape recorder and later transcribe your oral narration into the patients' records.

Do not make entries on patient records for the next day. Obviously, it is often quite possible that the treatment planned the previous day may not actually be performed.

Handwriting should be clear, and spelling should be accurate. There can be no continuity of treatment if the notes for previous treatment are illegible. Inaccurate spelling or illegible entries reflect poorly on the competence of the provider making such an entry. If handwriting is not easily readable, one should print. If spelling is problematic, the solution is as simple as a small electronic dictionary that easily fits in a pocket during working hours. An accurate knowledge of charting abbreviations is essential. There are no standard abbreviations, but a system should be devised for each office. Determine where a list of the abbreviations utilized in your particular employment setting is located, and keep it available at all times.

Review all policies regarding patient records with regularity. The courtroom is not the place to discover that employees are each documenting patient treatment differently. This would reflect badly on the quality of treatment that patients are receiving. Properly documented, legible patient records are one of the best defenses in any litigation.

CONTROLLED SUBSTANCE

Any substance designated as a narcotic under state or federal law. The purpose of this designation is to control the distribution, use, and sale of these drugs.

All members of the dental staff may place information in the patient's progress notes. A staff member might document an observation or an entry at the request of the dentist or another staff member. Any staff member who observes or participates in treatment can make a treatment entry. All documentation in the patient's record must include the signature of the person making the entry and the signature of the dentist.

MAINTENANCE OF PATIENT RECORDS

The statute of limitations regarding the preservation of patient records varies from state to state. Records are typically retained for seven to ten years, depending upon the state's statute of limitations. Specific provisions for certain items such as radiographs are often included in the state statute. States generally have a statute that relates to minors and/or incompetent individuals. The statute may not begin to run until the minor reaches the age of majority. Regarding incompetence, the statute of limitations may not run until the incompetence is removed. Incompetence must exist at the time the cause of action arose.

Failure to maintain or store medical or dental records may be considered medical malpractice in a court of law.[2] Failure to properly maintain patient records can subject the professional to other sanctions, such as having a license revoked or being barred from participation in insurance programs (including Medicare or Medicaid).[3] More than half of the states have enacted statutes that permit patients access to their medical and/or dental records. Given the fact that the statute of limitations may be extended to a period beginning when the patient knew or should have known about his or her injury, a patient could initiate a lawsuit several years beyond the statutorily recognized time.[4] Obviously, the longer patient records are kept, the better. For example, in the event of a patient's death, the administrator or executor of an estate may take legal action against a health care provider on behalf of the estate of the deceased person.

DISCOVERY OF RECORDS

When a patient's medical condition and/or treatment is an issue in a civil lawsuit, medical or dental records pertaining to the suit may be obtained by the opposing party. There are several means by which they may be obtained:

1. The defendant can request the records from the plaintiff.
2. The defendant can make a formal discovery request for production of documents.
3. The defendant can request an authorization by the plaintiff to release medical records.
4. A **subpoena** may be issued to a third party requiring a record custodian to appear in court and bring documents listed in the subpoena.

SUBPOENA

A legal document commanding an individual to attend court under penalty for failure to appear.

---

[2]*Brown v. Hamid, M.D.*, 856 S.W.2d 51 (Mo. 1993).
[3]*Koh v. Perales*, 570 N.Y.S.2d 98 (N.Y. App. Div. 1991).
[4]*Warrington v. Pfizer*, 80 Cal. Reptr. 130 (1969).

ALTERATION OF RECORDS

A patient's medical or dental record is essential not only for treatment considerations; it provides critical information for third-party payers (insurance) and for both parties to civil litigation involving medical or dental malpractice. Providers may be tempted to alter records if the documentation reflects substandard care or if the documentation is substandard. Altering medical records is both unethical and illegal. In addition, alteration of records may be the basis for an insurance carrier to cancel a health care provider's malpractice coverage.[5] Altering or falsifying records is fraud. Punitive damages are often awarded for fraudulent behavior. In all probability, an insurance carrier would not cover damages for such behavior.

Technology has made it possible to identify an altered record. Ink analysis, handwriting analysis, light reflection, and so forth, can be used to detect any irregularity. Patient records may be corrected as long as the new entry clearly reflects that it is a correction and the original entry is still readable. A single line should be drawn through the original entry; there should be no erasing and no obliterating with pen or correction fluid. The person correcting the entry should sign or initial and date the alteration. Any erasures or obliterating of the initial entry tends to make it appear as though someone is trying to hide the content of the entry, especially in a court of law. Corrections should be written in the next space available. No spaces are to be left between entries. Leaving an extra line or lines between entries is not a good practice, as entries could be made at a later time and the record could give the appearance that entries are made in this manner with regularity. Since medical and dental records are permanent records that are never altered, ink is always used for all entries. Patient records may be typewritten or may be in the form of a computer printout that is clearly dated, signed, and kept with the rest of the patient's record. Each page in the patient's record should be headed with the patient's name.

QUALITY OF DOCUMENTATION

An important factor to keep in mind in regard to patient records is to make entries that are free of comments that would negatively characterize the patient. Frivolous or humorous remarks about the patient are not to be placed in the patient's record. Eliminate adjectives that describe the patient rather than the patient's condition. It is very easy to become discouraged when a patient behaves badly or does not comply with professional recommendations. These feelings can all too easily be transcribed into the patient record; then it could be argued that because of his or her animosity toward the patient, a practitioner provided substandard care. Rather than documenting your feelings or interpretation, clearly document the patient's behavior or provide a statement of facts describing what occurred during treatment. It is usually a safe practice to quote the patient should his or her comments have a direct bearing on his or her treatment or physical condition. Certainly document any patient refusal relating to treatment. This includes refusals for specific diagnostic tests, for treatment, or to provide specific information in a health history survey.

---

[5]*Mirkin v. Medical Mutual Liability Insurance Society of Maryland*, 572 A.2d 1126 (Md. Spec. App. 1990).

High-quality patient care depends on an accurate patient record. Any vague statements in the record that another health care provider would have a problem quantifying should be avoided. For instance, describe which symptoms the patient is currently experiencing or which symptoms are no longer a problem for the patient. It is impossible to maintain continuity of treatment between providers if a later provider has no understanding of the condition of the patient earlier or the nature of the previous treatment. For instance, if an entry in the patient's record stated that the treatment produced "good results" or the patient was "doing well," this would have no meaning to another health care provider who later treated the patient, nor would it provide specific documentation in a court of law. As mentioned earlier, medications are always documented. In addition to federal requirements, entries noting the patient's need and the patient's response are prudent for all medications administered. Also, a copy of each prescription or a notation in the progress notes regarding each prescription written is part of the patient record. In the event that a pharmacist incorrectly transcribes the prescription and the patient receives the wrong medication, a written record would negate liability.

It may be as valuable to document nontreatment as it is treatment. All patient cancellations and missed appointments need to be documented. These entries could be evidence of patient noncompliance and may be critical in response to allegations of malpractice.

CONFIDENTIALITY OF PATIENT RECORDS AND ACCESS TO PATIENT RECORDS

Patients are entitled to access to information in their medical and dental records in a reasonable time, place, and manner. Therefore, a copy of a record may not be withheld for any reason, including nonpayment of a fee for services. An appropriate duplication charge may be made, to the patient or anyone the patient authorizes in writing to receive a copy of the patient's record. Original records should never be released to anyone. This includes radiographs. Radiographs are the basis for diagnosis and are necessary to explain the basis of treatment. In a court of law, testimony regarding a radiograph is inadmissible unless the radiograph is produced.[6] The original record is the work product of the individual who created it. If information included in the record is required by anyone, that person should be provided with a copy. The only exception is in the event that a court subpoenas the original record; in that case, the practitioner should be sure to keep a copy. Whenever a copy of a patient's record is given to the patient or another authorized individual, the transaction should be noted in the patient's record.

Patient records contain confidential information between the patient and the professional. Without written authorization, this information should be released to no one except the patient. This applies to spouses, children of aging parents, siblings, parents of adult children, friends, other professionals who are consulted or to whom patients are referred, insurance companies, and other agencies. A patient could allege breach of confidentiality for the unauthorized release of his or her

---

[6]*Fletcher v. Industrial*, 255 N.E. 2d 403 (Ill. 1970).

medical or dental records to another individual. Also, an allegation of malpractice would be appropriate if another health care provider was unable to provide continuity of medical or dental treatment because the patient's record had not been made available despite the patient's authorization.

Patient records are to be kept in a place where confidentiality is maintained. File cabinets that contain patient records should be locked overnight or when no one is working in the area. If patient information is entered into a computer, safeguards (such as passwords or other controls against unauthorized entry) should prevent individuals, other than staff personnel, from gaining confidential information. Not only are the contents of patient records confidential, but all financial and account information, including insurance information, is likewise confidential. Computer screens are not to be in plain view so that patients may be privy to confidential information. In addition, a backup storage system for information entered into the computer is required. A backup of computerized patient records is completed daily, and the floppy disk or tape of the backed up information is to be taken off the premises when the office or facility is closed.

Remember, in addition to patient records, phone conversations as well as face-to-face conversations office personnel have with patients in the office are confidential. Incoming messages on answering machines may contain information that is considered confidential. Appropriate actions must be utilized to safeguard the confidentiality of these situations.

In summary, properly kept patient records are a valuable defense in a court of law; all records should be complete, objective, accurate, unaltered, and confidential.

SUGGESTED READINGS

Institute of Medicine: *Health data in the information age: use, disclosure and privacy*, 1994.
Risk management: protect yourself against malpractice, Chicago, 1991, American Dental Association, Seminar Series.
Samuels B, Wolf SM: *Medical records: getting yours*, Public Citizen's Health Research Group, 1992.

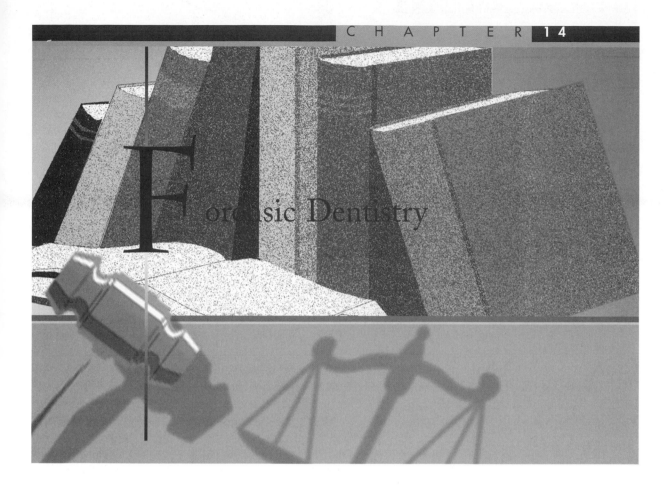

Forensic Dentistry

LEARNING OUTCOMES

After reading this chapter, you should be able to:
- Discuss how dental records may be utilized to identify physically unrecognizable deceased individuals.
- Discuss how bite mark evidence is obtained and how it is used for identification purposes.
- Discuss problems regarding the use of bite mark evidence in a court of law.
- Discuss the chain of custody for legal evidence, including the importance of maintaining the chain.

KEY WORDS

ANTEMORTEM
CHAIN OF CUSTODY
FORENSIC DENTISTRY

FRYE TEST
POSTMORTEM

FORENSIC DENTISTRY
The science of dentistry as it relates to the law. For example, utilizing the human dentition to identify a deceased individual.

ANTEMORTEM
Prior to death.

POSTMORTEM
After death.

No discussion of dental records would be complete without a discussion of **forensic dentistry.** Dental identification is based on a comparison of **antemortem** records with the charted records of **postmortem** remains. A complete dental record may be essential to the identification of deceased individuals. Throughout history, there has been a need to identify victims of mass disasters that occurred as a result of nature or the actions of humans.. The identification process would be far less successful without the assistance of forensic dentistry. One of the most recent disasters occurred on April 19, 1995, when a bomb exploded in the federal building in Oklahoma City, Oklahoma. In the midst of the turmoil, local dentists, dental faculty members, and dental students were mobilized; they assembled at the University of Oklahoma College of Dentistry to assist the medical examiner with victim identification. They gathered antemortem dental data and compared them with postmortem dental findings.

ANTEMORTEM DENTAL DATA

Where does one begin to search to obtain adequate information? In disasters such as airline crashes, there is generally a roster of passengers. In Oklahoma City many family members knew who was in the federal building that day. In such circumstances, family members should be questioned regarding a victim's current dentist and any previous dentists who may have provided treatment for the individual, including specialists such as orthodontists, oral surgeons, periodontists, endodontists, or pedodontists. For instance, cephalometrics, radiographs of root canal therapy, or study models could assist in the identification process. Family members may be able to provide information about whether a victim had been treated at a dental school or had any hospital admissions. Either situation might produce helpful records or radiographs. Prison records of former convicts may be helpful. If an individual ever had dental insurance, the insurance company may have computer-stored records pertaining to the dentition. Generally, when the dentist of a victim is located, the medical examiner or forensic dentist contacts the victim's dentist and requests the patient's records, including radiographs, photographs, study models, and so forth, for use as evidence. A state official such as a police officer is sent to take custody of the patient's records. This officer signs an affidavit documenting that he or she took the records and including a description of the records and the time, place, and date. The officer then delivers the records to the medical examiner. The medical examiner signs a statement to indicate that the evidence is in his or her custody. An investigation is performed by someone trained in forensic dentistry, who then signs an affidavit stating whether, in his or her professional opinion, the identity of the deceased matches the identity of the patient's records. The evidence is to be locked in a protected place until the investigation is completed and the records are returned to the dentist. In such situations a dentist must relinquish the patient's records, or the court has the power to subpoena all of the dental records of an uncooperative practitioner.

For an excellent example of precisely how identifications are made in the face of major disasters, see Box 14-1, which is a case report of the January 31, 1974, crash of a Pan American airliner. It should be noted that a dental team of six

BOX 14-1 FORENSIC INVESTIGATION CASE EXAMPLE

On January 31, 1974, a Pan American 707 airliner carrying 101 passengers approached Pago Pago in the Samoan Islands in a blinding rainstorm. The plane came down short of the runway and made a relatively soft landing in jungle growth. As it settled into a ravine, spilling gasoline, it exploded into flames. Ninety passengers perished immediately, with the toll ultimately rising to 96. Because adequate facilities did not exist in Samoa, 90 unidentified bodies were flown to the Los Angeles Chief Medical Examiner Coroner's Office for forensic investigation.

In the Samoan Islands airline personnel flew in a small plane from island to island, attempting to gather information, including dental data, that would be helpful in the identification process. Information gradually came in from all over the world by messenger, mail, teletype and telephone. However, a major problem was the fact that many of the victims were husky Samoans who never had the services of a dentist. Thus, there were no dental records and little medical information for many passengers. Also, the enormous distances involved made it difficult to verify, amplify or question incoming data. Additionally, some passengers were almost incinerated and only small, burned fragments were available for identification. On the positive side, the population of victims was known, because the passengers went through customs with their passports, making the passenger list verifiable.

Autopsies included estimation of age, based principally on arthritic and arteriosclerotic changes, and general evaluation of other organs. The maxilla and mandible were resected and age estimation was also included in the dental examination. A huge master information chart was constructed. For each unknown body, it was possible to enter weight, height, color of hair, color of eyes, name (when determined), information on teeth, fingerprints, property, tattoos, medical x-rays, dental x-rays, method of identification, clothing, medical and surgical autopsy findings, and age range. Thus, if one were trying to identify a 40-year-old male passenger with black hair and brown eyes, he could glance at the chart and quickly develop a list of "possibilities." But if that passenger were badly charred, conceivably he might not be on the list.

The dental phase began on February 6, 1974. During the first three days 77 oral autopsies were performed. "Full mouth" radiographs were taken on all cases using the medical examiner-coroner's recently installed dental x-ray machine. During this period, incoming dental information on passengers was entered on "antemortem dental charts." Also, a number of identifications were accomplished during this phase.

During the third day, the comparison and identification process went into full swing. Antemortem and postmortem charts were compared. When de-

From Vale GL, Noguchi T: The role of the forensic dentist in mass disasters, *Dental Clinics of North America* 21(1):132-145, January 1977.   *Continued*

BOX 14-1 FORENSIC INVESTIGATION CASE EXAMPLE—cont'd

tailed dental information appeared on the passenger's antemortem chart, tentative identification could usually be made in a matter of minutes or even seconds. This was then verified by x-ray comparison or other identifying information. The few passengers with gold restorations were quickly and easily identified. A number of identifications were considered ideal in that there were matching x-rays and numerous concordant points.

After the first three to four days, the process slowed considerably, since it was necessary to wait for more information to arrive. Thus, the dental team logged 138 man-hours during the first three days, but only 37^1/$_2$ man-hours during the next three days. Overall, the investigation involved six dentists, one dental hygienist, and six dental assistants.

As the number of cases with good antemortem records trickled to an end, the work became more challenging. When 30 "Does" remained unidentified, the dental team constructed its own "elimination chart," generally following the method described by Salley.* This saved much time in evaluating the possible matches for a given passenger.

It also became increasingly necessary to combine dental findings with other information. Thus, a close working relationship with the forensic pathologists was absolutely essential; the processes of categorization, association and exclusion were utilized increasingly.

To illustrate the process, there were six unidentified male bodies with dentures. Two were subsequently identified by fingerprints. Of the four remaining, one had only one testis. This body was identified because only one male passenger was known to have one testis and dentures.

Of the three remaining denture cases, one had a full upper denture, with natural teeth in the mandible. This body was identified because there was only one passenger in this age range known to have a full upper denture and natural lower teeth. Two denture cases now remained unidentified. Information was received that one man with dentures had an appendectomy. Autopsy findings showed one of the two remaining denture victims had had an appendectomy, so that body was considered identified and shipped to a distant city

*Salley JJ et al: Dental identification of mass disaster victims, *Journal of the American Dental Association* 66:827, 1963.

dentists, three dental assistants, and one dental hygienist performed this forensic investigation.

POSTMORTEM DENTAL FINDINGS

It is said that no two sets of teeth are identical; a possible exception may be identical twins, who also have identical fingerprints. Therefore, in the absence of other methods, the oral cavity provides distinct characteristics to make possible the iden-

BOX 14-1   FORENSIC INVESTIGATION CASE EXAMPLE—cont'd

for burial. However, word was subsequently received that another passenger also had dentures and an appendectomy. Consequently, the body that had been sent out was brought back. An old upper denture was obtained from one victim's family and found to fit the decedent very well, thus helping to verify the original identification. When tested in the body of the other denture wearer the denture did not fit.

As further verification, the dentist of the one remaining denture victim was able to give the mold number of his patient's denture teeth. Teeth were removed from the denture and cross-matched. The question remained as to why the medical history for this victim showed a removed appendix and the autopsy report listed the appendix as being present. It was concluded that, in the appendectomy, the pursestring suture had failed to contain a short inverted appendiceal stump, thus giving the appearance that the appendix was present.

Finally, there were three unidentified male bodies in the age range of the late twenties or early thirties. There were also three unidentified male passengers aged 26, 29 and 32. One of these passengers was known to have had an appendectomy. This matched the findings of one of the victims, with general support from dental findings. Of the two remaining passengers, a photograph of one showed a very massive maxilla and mandible. Of the two remaining victims, one had massive jaws, whereas the maxilla and mandible of the other were diminutive and delicate, thus permitting differentiation.

Using pubic bone aging, with dental aging, medical x-ray findings, studies of the uterus, and the process of exclusion, similarly it was possible for the forensic pathologists to establish identity of the remaining females.

Finally, after a five-week investigation that spanned the world and included nearly 239 hours of dental time, all 90 victims were identified and returned to their families. In that 51 of the victims were identified by dental means, this is believed to be one of the largest recorded disasters utilizing identification by dental evidence.

tification of a deceased individual with a reasonable degree of medical certainty. To explore how identification is possible, examine the structures of the oral cavity. Our teeth represent the most durable structure of our body. Enamel that covers the anatomical crown of the tooth is the hardest tissue found in the human body. The hardness is due to the high degree of calcification. The mineral hydroxyapatite makes up 95% of the total weight of enamel. Hydroxyapatite makes up 70% of the total weight of dentin and 45% of the total weight of bone. Teeth exposed to high heat become brittle at 400 degrees Fahrenheit and break down to ash at about 900 degrees Fahrenheit. Restorations may withstand even higher temperatures. The human dentition, therefore, may be the only remaining portion of the body to assist in positive identification.

Identification is possible because each individual has up to 32 teeth, each with five clinically visible surfaces. There are a number of identifiable variables in regard to restored or carious surfaces, teeth present or missing, occlusion and malaligned teeth, existing partial or full dentures, existing tori, variations in arch size, periodontal status, and so forth. If radiographs are available, the combinations of identifying features increase. With the assistance of radiographs, root canal fillings, periodontal bone loss, impacted teeth, dilacerated teeth, retained root tips, trabecular patterns, and other pathological conditions may be identified.

Postmortem radiographs are helpful when there are no restorations or no teeth. Bone trabecular patterns, nutrient canals, nerve foraminae, or pathologic processes may lead to identification. If a denture is available, they are now marked with the identity of the owner when they are fabricated, and positive identification may be possible. The identifying mark is generally found on the maxillary right buccal flange and the mandibular right lingual flange.[1]

Because of possible oral changes during a person's lifetime, one single area of dissimilarity does not rule out positive identification as it does with bite mark examination. Identifying a deceased individual by the dentition of the remains is an established part of forensic medicine; utilization of a bite mark to establish the identity of the perpetrator of a crime is a newer procedure.

BITE MARK EVIDENCE

There are many historic references to the utilization of a bite mark for identification purposes. The history of the use of bite marks in the United States includes debtors who came from Britain or Europe to America to work as servants. These individuals verified their agreements by biting the seal on the pact in lieu of a signature and became known as indentured servants.[2]

Today, bite mark evidence is primarily used in investigation of cases involving child abuse and sexual assaults such as forcible rape. Bite marks are also found in significant numbers in primarily two types of homicide cases: a child victim and an adult involved in sexual activity prior to death. The value of the bite mark is that it is evidence that tends to prove or disproves the alleged biter's active participation in the crime. Since it is impossible to inflict a bite mark without leaving traces of saliva, the bite mark is swabbed for traces of saliva for DNA analysis and blood typing. A photograph is taken as a means of recording the mark. If the bite left depressions in the skin, an impression can be taken with dental impression material, followed by pouring of dental stone into the impression to produce a model.[3]

There are several problems in using the bite mark for identification. The skin is

---

[1]For a more detailed discussion, see Mertz CA: Dental identification, *Dental Clinics of North America* 21(1):47-67, January 1977.
[2]Rothwell BR: Bite marks in forensic dentistry: a review of legal, scientific issues, *Journal of the American Dental Association* 126:223-232, 1995.
[3]Levine LI: Bite mark evidence, *Dental Clinics of North America* 21(1):145-158, January 1977.

not an ideal medium for precise impressions. Distortions may occur for a multitude of reasons, including edema, stretching of the skin, exposure to fluctuations in temperature or humidity, and movement of the biter or victim during biting. In addition, the dentition of the perpetrator may change as a result of restorations, extractions, caries, periodontal disease, orthodontics, and so forth.

For competent identification, one must secure impressions for models, an intraoral photograph, and a wax bite impression from the accused. Impressions of teeth of all suspects to be utilized for comparison with the bite mark are taken only with informed written consent or by court order. Models are made according to acceptable dental criteria and are labeled as evidence in the particular case. Comparisons are made between the bite mark and the wax impression made of the suspect's bite and/or the model of the suspect's dentition. A report of the final analysis is provided to both the defendant and the prosecutor. Bite mark evidence is sometimes key to the conviction or exoneration of a criminal defendant. For positive identification, the presence of four to five teeth marks is required. Bite marks are commonly those of anterior teeth, often those of premolars, and rarely those of molars. The American Board of Forensic Odontology provides guidelines for accurate bite mark analysis, including photography, impressions, and swabbing.[4]

CHAIN OF CUSTODY

All materials are labeled to maintain a clear **chain of custody** for evidentiary purposes. Unless a chain of custody is maintained, the evidence will be of no value in a court of law. The name of the deceased and the case number, a list of items that relate to the case, and the signatures of individuals taking custody and those being relieved of custody of items, with the date, time, and reason for each exchange, are to be documented. Reasons for exchange are transportation, examination, storage, and so forth. Storage areas, whether rooms, laboratories, or refrigerators, should be adequately secured. Evidence should never be unprotected, and custodians of the evidence should always be known. These procedures are sometimes breached by law enforcement personnel, thus making the evidence inadmissible in a court of law.

> **CHAIN OF CUSTODY**
> When an item of real evidence is offered in a court of law, the party presenting the evidence must account for the care of the evidence from the time it reaches his or her possession until the time it is presented in court.

ADMISSIBILITY OF BITE MARK EVIDENCE

Judges and juries often rely on the testimony of expert witnesses to explain matters related to their fields of expertise. A judge or a jury lacking expertise in a particular field would be uninformed about the subject matter of the testimony in the case before them. Because the goal of the court is to establish truth and often two expert witnesses provide conflicting testimony, the courts will scrutinize the admissibility of evidence produced by new scientific technology.

The Frye Test

When courts are called upon to determine whether to admit scientific evidence, they often rely upon a test first expressed in *Frye v. United States*.[5] *Frye* stated:

---

[4]American Board of Forensic Odontology: *Policies, procedures and guidelines*, July 1995, Colorado Springs, Colo, American Academy of Forensic Sciences.
[5]293 F. 1013 (D.C. Cir. 1923).

"While courts will go a long way in admitting expert testimony deduced from a well-recognized scientific principle or discovery, the thing from which the deduction is made must be sufficiently established to have gained general acceptance in the particular field in which it belongs." The **Frye test** was followed by many states but not all, as numerous difficulties surrounded the vagueness of the wording.

Courts applying the Frye test often arrived at different conclusions. For instance, in both *Bundy v. State of Florida*[6] and *State v. Hurd*,[7] the Frye test was applied to the utilization of witness hypnosis. In *Bundy* the court concluded that "the testimony of a witness tainted with hypnosis should be excluded in a criminal case and that hypnosis was not considered sufficiently reliable by experts in the field." The *Hurd* court found that "hypnosis is generally accepted as a reasonably reliable method of restoring a person's mind."

The Federal Rules of Evidence

The Federal Rules of Evidence (Rule 702)[8] developed a more flexible approach to the admissibility of novel scientific evidence. The rule suggests that the questions to be asked regarding the admissibility of such evidence are:

1. The soundness and reliability of the process or technique used in generating the evidence
2. The possibility that admitting the evidence would overwhelm, confuse, or mislead the jury
3. The connection between the scientific research or test to be presented and the particular disputed factual issues in the case

Again, some states have rules of evidence that parallel the Federal Rules of Evidence, and others do not. Therefore, the admissibilty of bite mark evidence has been decided on a case by case basis, with some courts relying on its authenticity and others believing that bite mark evidence is without scientific merit.

Bite Mark Case Examples

One of the first cases to utilize bite mark evidence was *People v. Johnson*.[9] Such evidence was admitted to convict the defendant of rape and aggravated battery. Four years later, in *People v. Milone*,[10] a disagreement between the experts regarding bite mark evidence prompted the court to declare that such disagreements "did not affect admissibility but influenced the weight of testimony." Basically, this left it up to the judge and the jury to decide which expert was more believable. One of the most well-known cases involving bite mark evidence was *Bundy v. State of Florida*.[11] Bundy left bite marks on several of his victims. Two dentists testified as expert witnesses. Photographs were taken of the bite marks and enlarged to actual

---

[6]471 So.2d 9 (1985).
[7]432 A.2d 86 (1981).
[8]Federal Rules of Evidence, St Paul, 1997, West Publishing Co.
[9]289 N.E.2d 722 (Ill. 1972).
[10]356 N.E.2d 1350 (1976).
[11]455 So.2d 330 (Fla. 1984).

size. Pursuant to a judge's warrant, law enforcement authorities arranged for a dental expert to take impressions and photographs of the defendant's teeth. Models were fabricated from the impressions, and a positive identification was subsequently made. The trial court found that "the science of odontology, which is based on the discovery that the characteristics of individual human dentition are highly unique, is generally recognized by scientists in the relevant fields and therefore is an acceptable foundation for the admissibility of expert opinion into evidence."

As McClure notes in her article, "Elastomeric impression materials are now available, as well as specialized photography, including infrared, ultraviolet, and narrow-band illumination. The use of videotape can help illustrate the details of bite marks."[12]

Advanced radiographic techniques and computerized electronic image enhancement equipment have aided the presentation of courtroom evidence. Technological advances such as these will bring additional evidence that is unimaginable today into the courtroom of the future.

SUGGESTED READINGS

American Society of Forensic Odontology: *Manual of forensic odontology*, Colorado Springs, Colo, 1984, American Society of Forensic Sciences.

Frese P: Denture identification, *Dental Hygienist News* 9(3):3, 1997.

Mertz CA: Dental identification, *Dental Clinics of North America* 21(1):47-67, January 1977.

Rawson RD et al: Statistical evidence for individuality of the human dentition, *Journal of Forensic Sciences* 29:254-259, 1984.

---

[12]McClure EA, Carroll D: Bite marks: a new mark of evidence? *Access, American Dental Hygienists' Association* 12(7):31-33, August 1998.

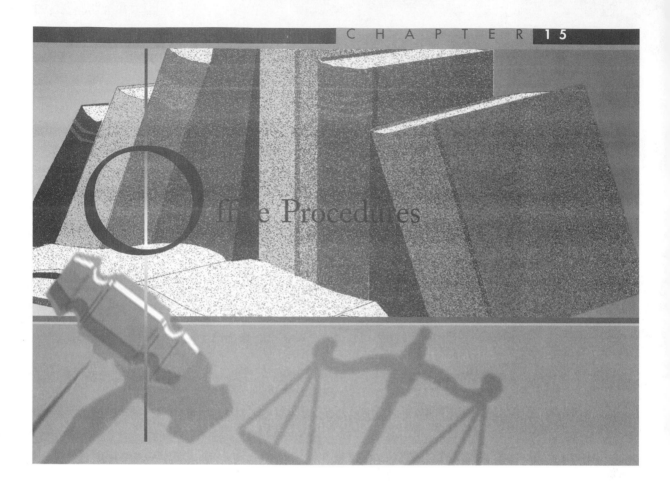

CHAPTER 15

Office Procedures

LEARNING OUTCOMES

After reading this chapter, you should be able to:
- Discuss emergency treatment in the dental setting.
- Understand the use of aseptic techniques in the dental setting.
- Discuss the possible legal consequences of improper use or poor maintenance of equipment in the dental setting.
- Discuss the possible legal consequences of lax housekeeping procedures in the dental setting.
- Identify essential techniques for ensuring quality care in regard to radiation safety.
- Discuss the dental health care professional's responsibility in the event that a minor patient presents signs of abuse or neglect.

KEY WORDS

ASEPSIS
INVITEE
STERILIZATION

SUBROGATE
WANTON

Numerous procedures that are performed daily in the dental office have the potential for either becoming the basis for a lawsuit or providing a solid defense against possible liability.

The following discussions of emergency medical treatment, asepsis and sterilization, office equipment, housekeeping, and radiographic techniques all include information relating to procedures that can be a good defense when performed correctly or a liability if performed poorly. The topic of child abuse is also included, because of the legal ramifications for dental professionals if they do not report suspected abuse. Ultimately, the goal of these discussions is to provide quality care. If patients are to receive quality care, the standard of care should not be breached. For a variety of reasons, we sometimes overlook details that require our attention if we are to provide quality care.

In addition to the materials in this chapter, see Appendix F for a Safety Mini-Audit for an office safety program, developed by Turbyne and Associates.

EMERGENCY MEDICAL TREATMENT

All emergency treatment must be within the standard of care; liability in a court of law is likely if the standard of care is not met. Emergency treatment encompasses procedures that most dental office personnel rarely need to perform. Therefore, a periodic review of these procedures is a must. Develop a written emergency plan, and review it three to four times each year. Emergency phone numbers should be placed conspicuously by the telephone; not all areas have 911 available. Review the monitoring of vital signs. All personnel need to be familiar with the locations and operation of the oxygen tank, emergency drug kit, first aid kit, fire extinguisher, and eye wash station. Drugs and medications in the emergency drug kit should be checked for expiration dates on a monthly basis. This is an area that is easily forgotten. There are companies that provide automatic replacement services for expired items in the emergency kit. OSHA requires that fire extinguishers be checked and that documentation of this procedure be placed on the attached label. All staff members should have a current CPR certification.

Prior to treatment, each patient must have a complete and current medical history, including the name and phone number of the patient's physician. The medical history would be valuable to paramedics arriving in response to any emergency.

It is essential to utilize preventive measures such as high-speed evacuation, rubber dams, and safety glasses for the patient, to avoid emergencies. Take vital signs prior to administering any form of anesthesia. This provides baseline data in the event that emergency medical treatment is required.

ASEPSIS AND STERILIZATION

Appropriate **sterilization** and **aseptic** techniques minimize the risk of liability and constitute a vital defense in certain types of cases. For example, if a patient developed a postoperative infection and sued for negligence, any sound defense would require proof of methods of sterilization utilized in the dental office. A brief overview follows.

To protect patient and dental care provider, latex, vinyl, or nitrile gloves are worn

STERILIZATION

The process of destroying all microorganisms.

ASEPSIS

The absence of microorganisms.

during the delivery of patient services. To protect the integrity of the gloves and prevent contamination, nails should be short; no rings or nail polish should be worn. Never reuse or rewash gloves; they are intended to be disposable. Washing is likely to cause cross-contamination, as it does not remove microorganisms. Washing may also weaken the integrity of the glove. Heavy-duty utility gloves are worn for cleaning the operatory and instruments. Place instruments in the ultrasonic cleaner; there should be no hand scrubbing. This avoids accidental puncturing or tearing of gloves during instrument processing. Hand washing is to be performed before and after each patient, and each time gloves are removed, with an antimicrobial soap to keep microbes on the hands at low levels. Faucets and soap dispensers should be hands free.

Face masks are worn during patient treatment to protect the patient and the clinician from splatter and inhalation of aerosols or other infectious materials. Masks should be replaced for each patient. Masks should be replaced when wet (or every 20 minutes), as they lose their ability to filter. Protective eyewear (safety glasses or prescription glasses) should be worn by patient and clinician to protect the eyes from physical damage and infectious agents. Eyewear should be decontaminated between patients. Face shields may be used as eyewear if they are chin length, curved on the sides, and made with heavy material. Masks should still be used when face shields are worn. No street clothing is to be worn during patient treatment. Watches or exposed jewelry tend to harbor organisms and should be worn only if covered. However, rings should not be worn under gloves. Protective clothing (scrubs and smocks) guards the patient and the clinician from contamination and/or infection and should not be worn outside the office. Laundering of these garments is to be done on site or provided by a professional service. Hair is to be away from the face; hair covers are available for maximum protection.

Surface barriers are used to cover surfaces that cannot be sterilized and are easily contaminated during treatment. Surface asepsis may be accomplished by using a surface cover or by disinfecting the surface after contamination and before another patient is treated in the operatory. A wide variety of plastic materials are available for covering surfaces in the dental operatory. Spray all exposed surfaces with a cleaning agent, or wipe with a wet towel or gauze. Then disinfect all surfaces with an iodofor or a sodium hypochlorite solution. Alcohols are not as acceptable. Protective clothing, eyewear, masks, and utility gloves should be worn while one is cleaning and disinfecting the dental operatory.

Sterilization should be accomplished in one of three ways:

1. Steam autoclaving for 20 to 30 minutes at 121 degrees Celsius (250 degrees Fahrenheit) or for 3 to 10 minutes at 134 degrees Celsius (273 degrees Fahrenheit)
2. Unsaturated chemical vapor for 20 minutes at 132 degrees Celsius (270 degrees Fahrenheit)
3. Dry heat for 60 to 120 minutes at 154 degrees Celsius (320 degrees Fahrenheit) (static air) or for 12 minutes at 184 degrees Celsius (375 degrees Fahrenheit) (forced air)

Occasionally, instruments that are not heat resistant require sterilization. In such cases a 2% to 3.4% solution of glutaraldehyde may be used to sterilize these items.

Instruments must be in this solution for at least 10 hours to reach sterilization. The solution should be placed in a closed container. Persons using this method should utilize protective wear.

All nondisposable instruments that are used in the mouth should be sterilized, including handpieces. Sterilization should be constantly monitored. Chemical indicators on the inside and the outside of each instrument package (that change color when reaching a specific temperature) are used to ensure that the sterilization process is functioning properly. Biologic monitoring confirms that the method of sterilization being used is actually destroying microorganisms. This method should be conducted once per week for every sterilizer in the office. There are testing services across the country that provide the tests, culturing, and notification if positive results should occur.

The office manual should contain a section that specifically lists sterilization protocols to be used. This must be available for all employees to read and refer to as necessary. The office manual should also include the proper procedure, documentation, and treatment should a dental health care provider accidentally experience an exposure, such as a needle stick or bodily contact with potentially harmful solutions. These protocols should be in compliance with CDC guidelines, OSHA regulations, and applicable state and local laws. Should an accident such a needle stick occur, confidentiality of the source of the exposure is to be maintained. It is of no value to document these protocols unless they are followed when an exposure occurs. Testing of both the provider and the source patient should be conducted. Regarding the use of appropriate office protocols and procedures, records of employee training must be maintained. Records should include date and content of training as well as names of all employees attending the training session and names and qualifications of persons providing the training.

Health officials investigate clusters of disease transmission. One area of investigation is to determine whether there is a common source for a particular disease. If the universal precautions described in this section are followed, the possibility of disease transmission from patient to health care provider, health care provider to patient, or patient to patient is drastically reduced.

Disease Transmission Case Example

The most widely reported case involving transmission of disease from health care provider to patient was initially reported by the Centers for Disease Control in 1990. It was the case of Dr. David Acer, a Florida dentist who had contracted AIDS. A patient of Dr. Acer, Kimberly Bergalis, contracted AIDS. During its investigation the CDC found four additional cases of AIDS among Dr. Acer's patients. Genetic sequencing revealed that the direction of the virus was from dentist to patient and produced no evidence of patient-to-patient transmission. Further investigation showed that six of Dr. Acer's patients who were HIV positive had DNA sequencing linking their disease to Dr. Acer.

Investigation of his office procedures resulted in the following findings:
1. Dr. Acer had very inefficient communication with his staff.
2. There was no staff training in infection control.

3. There was no written infection control protocol.
4. Staff members responsible for sterilization did not know the name of the sterilant or any of the parameters for its use.
5. Only surgical items were sterilized; instruments were sometimes just wiped with alcohol.
6. Overall, infection control was spotty.

This was far below the standard of care in 1988 and 1989, when the disease transmission took place. Training in universal precautions and other infection control protocol was commonly incorporated into the practice of dentistry by 1985. Tragically, it was not common enough to be in place in Dr. Acer's office and to save Kimberly Bergalis' life.

In the aftermath of the Acer case, the CDC made closer examination of existing studies. One study, involving 22,032 patients of 63 HIV-positive health care providers, found no evidence indicating that any patient had been infected with HIV from a health care provider. Another study showed that, among 8,973 patients of 13 seropositive health care providers, 112 individuals were infected. Twenty-seven had been infected prior to receiving treatment, and 57 had established risk factors. The other cases were under investigation as of the date of the reporting.[1]

Infection control procedures do work, but in order to work they must be utilized.

OFFICE EQUIPMENT

Each member of the staff needs to be familiar with the uses of major equipment. If injury to a patient is caused by misuse of a particular piece of equipment, in all likelihood liability will be found.

Evaluation and maintenance of all equipment should be performed with regularity. Maintenance should be monitored by a qualified individual. All maintenance, whether it is changing radiographic solutions in developing tanks or changing the tubing or gauges on the nitrous oxide sedation equipment, should be documented. Being able to show that a particular piece of equipment was recently repaired or evaluated and found to be in good working condition may be the best defense against an allegation of negligence.

HOUSEKEEPING

INVITEE

A business visitor, such as a patient in a dental office. The business owner has the duty to protect the invitee against any known dangers and against any dangers he or she could have discovered with reasonable care.

Individuals conducting business or members of the public invited to do business are considered **invitees.** Invitees can reasonably expect that the premises have been made safe for them. The owner has a duty of care to invitees and may not impose unreasonable risk of harm upon them,, even from dangers of which the owner is unaware. The owner has a duty to inspect his or her premises for hidden dangers, and to use reasonable care in making inspections. Some states use the standard of reasonable care whereby foreseeability of harm to visitors shall be the measure of liability, no matter why an individual is on the premises.[2] In either event, it is prudent for all businesses, such as dental offices, to inspect reception areas, or any areas

---

[1]AIDS Awareness, The Acer case: an interview with a CDC investigator, *Access* 6(10):6-7, December 1992.
[2]*Basso v. Miller,* 386 N.Y.S.2d 564 (1976).

where the public will be, for broken objects or furnishings. Equally important is to inspect sidewalks, parking lots, and driveways and to keep them clear of debris, snow, ice, and so forth. It is the responsibility of all dental office staff members to minimize the exposure to liability. If rendering the premises safe is not possible, the doctor-owner should be notified of the existing condition.

Damages in personal injury cases in which liability is found can be excessive. In negligence cases in which actual physical injury is found, a plaintiff can recover for damages in addition to compensation for the physical harm itself. The plaintiff can recover out-of-pocket losses such as medical expenses, lost earnings, and the cost of any labor required to perform tasks that the plaintiff can no longer do. The plaintiff may also recover for physical pain suffered from injuries and for mental distress resulting from injuries (e.g., fright and shock, humiliation, anxiety). Recovery for future damages must be part of the settlement, and this particular matter will be litigated only once. An expert witness will be necessary to ascertain future damages. Recovery or settlement for personal injuries is tax free under the Internal Revenue Code. The plaintiff is entitled to recovery even though he or she is reimbursed for losses by some third party, such as an insurance company. In many cases the person making the payments is **subrogated** to the rights of the plaintiff or has a right of reimbursement against him or her out of any judgment, and there is no double recovery. For instance, Jane Doe sues Harry Smith for $50,000 for personal injuries, $25,000 for pain and suffering, and $9,000 for damage to her automobile, as a result of an automobile accident caused by Harry's negligence. Jane's insurance company pays her $59,000, and Jane wins a court judgment against Harry for $65,000. Now the insurance company may recover the $59,000 from Jane.

In addition, if the plaintiff receives free services, such as medical services, from a friend or family member, he or she may recover the reasonable value of those services. A plaintiff has a duty to mitigate and may not recover any damages that he or she could reasonably have avoided. As noted previously, punitive damages are sometimes awarded to penalize the defendant. In negligence cases, punitive damages are usually awarded if the defendant's conduct was "reckless" or "willful and **wanton.**" Liability insurers often do not pay for punitive damages. Therefore, obligations for personal liability are potentially a financial disaster.

> **SUBROGATE**
>
> To substitute one person in place of another. The person substituted has a claim to rights of the other.

> **WANTON**
>
> Willfully cruel or malicious.

RADIOGRAPHIC TECHNIQUES

When to take radiographs and how many to take are left up to individual practitioners, but the "reasonable and prudent dentist" standard regarding radiographs would apply. For instance, the reasonable and prudent dentist would not take a full-mouth series of radiographs for every patient annually. To do so would be unethical and in all probability would be found illegal in a court of law. This practice would fall below the standard of care.

The Consumer-Patient Radiation Health and Safety Act was passed and signed into law in 1981 (and amended in 1991) to protect consumers from unnecessary radiation.[3] The act mandated minimum standards (set by each state) for accreditation of educational programs for individuals who expose radiographs and for cer-

---

[3] 42 USC 10001, Consumer-Patient Radiation Health and Safety Act of 1981, §§ 975-983.

tification of these individuals by the states. The Secretary of Health and Human Services is primarily responsible for establishing these minimum standards.

An attempt should be made to obtain any previous full-mouth series taken. Duplicate films should be sent if a patient is transferring or being referred to another dentist, to minimize the patient's exposure to radiation. Patients are concerned with the levels of radiation to which they are exposed. They often resist the taking of even diagnostically necessary films. Once these films are exposed, the last words a patient wants to hear is that a film or films need to be retaken. It does not matter why taking additional films is necessary; patients view the exposure of additional films as unnecessary radiation.

Minimizing exposure of the patient to radiation can easily protect patients. Leaded aprons with a thyroid extension are to be worn by patients while radiographs are being exposed. The beam is to be collimated to the smallest size that will produce quality radiographs. Use fast-speed film, and check the exposure values. Never take more films than necessary to view the entire dentition and supporting structures. To further minimize patients' exposure to radiation, the x-ray machine, processing procedures, and film exposure techniques should be reviewed for quality assurance. A written description of the quality assurance system is a must for all dental offices. List items that require daily, quarterly, biannual, and annual evaluation. Simple and inexpensive tests can be performed in the dental office to identify dental radiography problems. These are described in *Fundamentals of Dental Radiography*, Chapter 15, "Quality Control in the Dental Office."[4]

Exposure to ionizing radiation is cumulative; therefore, it is essential that a person regularly exposing radiographs take precautions as well. An individual exposing radiographs should never stand in the direct path of the x-ray beam and should always stand behind the tubehead (6 to 8 feet) or behind a lead-lined shield or wall. Individuals who expose radiographs or those who are regularly in the area where radiographs are being exposed should wear a monitoring device to detect any amounts of exposure. A film badge is utilized for this purpose. It is worn for a period of time (up to one month) and then sent to a monitoring company for evaluation. The company tests the amount of radiation on the badge and submits a report to the facility regarding the exposure of the individual employee. This report could be an important legal document, should there be ongoing problems with exposure of employees to radiation.

CHILD ABUSE

Child abuse is not a recent phenomenon. Throughout history parents in all cultures have subjected their children to atrocities, from infanticide to slavery, in the name of religion or economic gain. In the United States children used to work long hours of manual labor in factories and on farms, as there were no child labor laws to protect them.

States began to pass legislation in the 1930s, and the federal government in 1973 enacted The Child Abuse Treatment Act. The act stipulates that state statutes must

[4]Manson-Hing LR: *Fundamentals of dental radiography*, Philadelphia, 1985, Lea & Febiger.

require mandatory reporting of abuse and neglect of children. Abuse is a criminal act in some states and a civil wrong in others.

The most significant limitation on parents' authority to control health care decisions relating to their children is found in state child abuse and neglect statutes. In nearly every state a parent may not act to deprive a child of basic necessities of life, including food, housing, clothing, education, and medical care. When parents neglect a child, states have the authority to take custody of the child to ensure that basic needs are met.

Approximately 3,000 children die each year as a result of abuse and neglect. That figure is small when compared with the numbers of children suffering the indignities of abuse and neglect daily. As the public has become increasingly aware of the large numbers of abused children in all socioeconomic groups in the American population, new state statutes have been enacted by the legislatures of all the states. These statutes have been intended to identify abused children and intervene on their behalf.

As a result of these child protective statutes, the law requires dental hygienists in 41 states and dentists in all 50 states to report suspected cases of child abuse. During the early years of these reporting requirements, in the 1970s, health care professionals were not anxious to report suspected cases of child abuse, for fear that if an allegation were proven false, a lawsuit for slander or malicious prosecution would follow. Immunity provisions were written into state laws to protect a person making a report in good faith. The report cannot be intended to harass anyone and must be based on facts that would cause a reasonable person to suspect that a child had been abused.

Review your state statute. Office protocol should be in place for reporting cases of abuse and should be written to conform to the law of the state where the office is located. Some statutes impose penalties for failing to report suspected abuse and/or neglect cases.[5] All state statutes provide that reports must be confidential and protect those who report in good faith from subsequent legal action.

SUGGESTED READINGS

American Dental Association, Council on Dental Practice: *The dentist's responsibility in identifying and reporting child abuse and neglect*, Chicago, 1995, American Dental Association.

Bednarsh H, Eklund K: Healthcare delivery in the age of AIDS: does risk go with the territory? *Access* 8(3):8-14, March 1994.

Byrd Mann G: Improving radiographic techniques, *Dental Hygienist News* 10(2):2-6, 1997.

Centers for Disease Control and Prevention: Recommended infection control practices for dentistry, *MMWR* 41(RR-8):1-12, 1993.

Department of Labor, Occupational Safety and Health Administration: Occupational exposure to bloodborne pathogens, final rule, part 1910.1030, *Federal Register* 56(235):64004-64182, 1991.

McGiven T: The use of glutaraldehyde for disinfection and sterilization, *The Journal of Practical Hygiene* 6(5 suppl):1-5, September-October 1997.

---

[5]Mass. Gen. Laws Ann. C. 119, §§ 51E, 51F; N.M. Stat. Ann. 1978, § 32A-4-3. These are examples of state laws that impose penalties on certain professionals who do not report suspected cases of child abuse.

Meskin L: Abusive legislation, *Journal of the American Dental Association* 126(3):1080-1082, August 1995.

Miller CH: Disinfection of surfaces and equipment, *Dental Assistant* 8:21-27, 1988.

Miller CH, Palenik CJ: *Infection control and management of hazardous materials for the dental team*, ed 2, St Louis, 1998, Mosby.

Mouden LD, Bross D: Legal issues affecting dentistry's role in preventing child abuse and neglect, *Journal of the American Dental Association* 126(3):1173-1180, August 1995.

Peterson C et al: Effects of beam collimation on image quality, *Journal of Dental Hygiene* 71(2):61-70, 1997.

Sanger RG, Bross DC: *Clinical management of child abuse and neglect*, Chicago, 1984, Quintessence Publishing.

Scaramucci M., Cook S: Medical emergencies in the dental office, *The Journal of Practical Hygiene* 6(6):41-46, 1997.

AUTHOR'S CASE STUDY COMMENTS

Reread the Case Study and Study Questions for Section IV.
Questions 1 through 7 are examined in the following analysis:

1. Patient Dru has initiated litigation against Dr. Hastings and Dr. Roberts. Which doctor's patient record is more likely to succeed in a court of law? Why? List strengths and weaknesses of both.

Obviously, Dr. Roberts' records are more extensive and provide more information regarding the treatment Patient Dru actually received and, therefore, are more legally defensible than Dr. Hastings' records. Chapter 13 presents specific criteria in regard to the maintenance of patient records.

Both patient records include a dental chart with an acceptable tooth numbering system, patient identification data, medical and dental history, and progress notes. A major difference is the manner in which the progress notes were completed. A brief documentation of treatment appeared in patient Scott's record, while patient Dru's record clearly listed detailed treatment in chronological order. Patient Scott had no radiographs exposed or periodontal assessment prior to treatment. In addition, the unflattering remarks written in patient Scott's record may be considered defamatory. Her record was partially obliterated in order to make a change, rather that utilizing a single line with a signature and date.

Although Patient Dru's record is not perfect, it includes additional documentation, such as a periodontal assessment, a detailed treatment record, a signed release form for patient records, and a signed informed consent and informed refusal statement. It may have been clearer if all treatment information had been in one document rather than being divided between the progress notes and the periodontal assessment. However, the important task of documentation was far more complete than for patient Scott.

2. Does Patient Scott have any legal claims against Dr. Hastings? If so, what are they?

When Dr. Hastings' office furnished a complete copy of Ms. Scott's record to her estranged husband, there was a breach of the duty of confidentiality to the patient. Since there was information in the record that was damaging to Ms. Scott, Dr. Hastings incurred even more liability.

3. Patient Scott's treatment record indicates that she refused to update her medical history when she returned for a prophylaxis and examination. What should Dr. Hastings do?

Generally, a patient's dismissal would be in order, to protect the patient's health and reduce the risk of liability for the dental health care provider in situations in which there is no updated medical history. In this situation, Dr. Hastings should communicate with this patient to determine why she is unwilling to provide his office with vital information. It is possible that he may not know of the breach in confidentiality regarding this patient's record. Since most lawsuits are initiated because of ei-

AUTHOR'S CASE STUDY COMMENTS—cont'd

ther a lack of communication with patients or poor communication with them, a few moments of quality communication with this patient might be well worth the extra time spent.

4. Is it likely that Patient Dru will prevail in his lawsuit against Dr. Hastings? Why or why not?

Patient Dru may claim that Dr. Hastings abandoned him when he refused to treat tooth #19. Patient Dru may claim that Dr. Hastings was negligent in not diagnosing his periodontal disease and in prescribing amoxicillin when his medical history clearly stated that he had an allergy to penicillin. Regarding abandonment, since Patient Dru refused to have radiographs taken to document his oral status and in particular the status of #19, Dr. Hastings was well within his rights to dismiss the patient. In addition, Dr. Hastings provided patient Dru with emergency treatment (examination and prescriptions) and scheduled an appointment for him with the oral surgeon. Prescribing amoxicillin to patient Dru when he had an allergy to penicillin documented in the medical history certainly exposes Dr. Hastings to liability for negligence. Remember, negligence is a tort action, and all of the elements of a tort must be met (duty, breach of duty, harm or injury, and causation). As his dentist, Dr. Hastings certainly owed a duty to his patient, Mr. Dru, and negligently writing a prescription for a drug that the patient had indicated he is allergic to was a breach of that duty. We have no information about whether patient Dru experienced an allergic reaction to this drug. In fact, since he proceeded directly to Dr. Roberts' office, it appears as though he did not have the prescription filled by a druggist. If we have no harm or injury, we have no cause of action for a lawsuit. However, negligence for failure to diagnose periodontal disease is one of the major sources for lawsuits in dentistry. Patient Dru has been a patient of Dr. Hastings for the past 10 years, and there is no entry in his record to indicate that he was advised as to the condition of his mouth. Therefore, Patient Dru would be more likely to prevail in a court action based on failure to diagnose periodontal disease.

5. Is it likely that Patient Dru will prevail in his lawsuit against Dr. Roberts and/or Joan Wills, the dental hygienist employed by Dr. Roberts? Why or why not?

As discussed earlier, Dr. Roberts' records are fairly well documented. Our case study indicates that Patient Dru was informed that several of his teeth had either a guarded or a poor prognosis. Was this documented in the progress notes? No. However, the informed consent form clearly states that the patient was aware that the risk involved in treatment was the possibility of little or no tissue response, with future increased pocketing.

Regarding Joan Wills' liability, it is possible that the doctrine of respondeat superior would apply and that the dentist would be liable for the acts of the dental hygienist as his employee. In addition, in several cases in which a dental hygienist has been named in the lawsuit, the insurance companies have settled out of court despite the fact that a dental hygienist is not permitted to diagnose. In this situation, the documentation indicated that prior to treatment the patient gave his informed consent and that he was apprised of his condition before and after treatment. Such action reduces the likelihood of liability for the dental health care providers.

6. What should Dr. Hastings do regarding the police officers and the subpoena for his patient records?

Dr. Hastings has no valid grounds to refuse to surrender Vera Smith's dental record to the authorities. Dr. Hastings is faced with a subpoena for all of his patient's records, because of his noncompliance. At this stage he could decline the release of the records and make a motion to the court to quash the subpoena. Alternatively, he should contact the person issuing the subpoena (probably the district attorney or the state's attorney general) and negotiate to release only the records of Vera Smith.

Note: a defendant, in this case the dentist, has a right to file a motion to quash a subpoena. A sitting judge, for good cause shown, may negate the subpoena.

7. What health and/or legal issues exist regarding Patient Jones?

The patient's symptoms indicate hyperventilation syndrome, angina pectoris, or an acute myocardial infarction. Her medical history should be checked to assist in diagnosis. In such situations it is critical to have an accurate, updated medical history for the patient. It is also critical that an emergency plan of action be in place, with all personnel familiar with their roles in such an emergency. The patient should be seated in an upright position to relieve pressure on the heart. Upon an examination of patient Jones' medical history, it is discovered that she is extremely anxious during each visit to the dental office and that hyperventilation syndrome has occurred on three other occasions. The patient needs carbon dioxide to slow her respiration rate. She should breathe into a paper bag, cupped hands, a face mask, or a headrest cover. It is important that all office personnel be certain of what emergency treatment to administer. If Ms. Charles actually administered oxygen to patient Jones, her condition would deteriorate rather than improve.

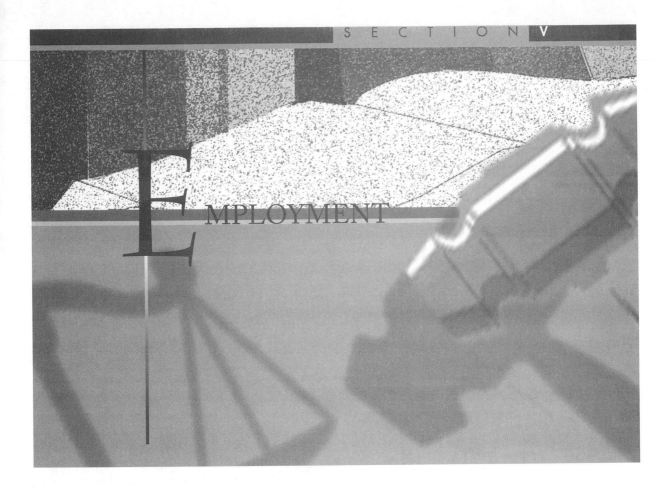

SECTION V

EMPLOYMENT

SECTION OUTLINE

CASE STUDY

As discussed in a previous case study, Ms. Clara Jenret was employed by Dr. Kenneth Hastings for eighteen years. Her employment was surprisingly terminated by Dr. Hastings. Now she is searching for new employment. Her only employment has been as a dental assistant, and she has no other employable skills. As she browsed through the classified section of the newspaper, she noticed three job opportunities for dental assistants.

One read:

We are looking for a bright, articulate, and enthusiastic female dental assistant with the ability to handle a fast-paced yet challenging group dental practice. We need an experienced self-starter who is a team player. Please send resume and photo to: Oakbrook Dental, 100 Main St., Wilmington, DE. No phone calls please.

The second read:

Need dental assistant to be a girl Friday for a solo practitioner. Must be married, as no benefits are provided with this position. Must be flexible and occasionally able to work long hours. If interested, please call 1-800-321-7654.

The third read:

Come join our friendly environment. We have a state-of-the-art dental practice and need a full-time dental assistant to join our team. Must be a nonsmoker, nondrinker, with no history of drug abuse or a criminal record. If you fit the bill, please stop by. Our office is at 2001 Market Place.

Ms. Jenret prepared her resume and sent a copy to Oakbrook Dental. She then placed a call to the author of the second advertisement and made an appointment for an interview for the following day. She was then off to 2001 Market Place, as she felt that she certainly fit the bill for this particular advertisement.

Drs. Bert Brown and William Douglas were the owners of the dental practice located at 2001 Market Place. As soon as Ms. Jenret told the staff member who she was and why she was in the office, she was asked to complete an application form. When she had completed the application form, the person at the desk thanked her for completing the form and informed her that they would be in touch with her should they wish to interview someone with her particular qualifications.

The application form that Ms. Jenret completed is shown in Figure 1.

The following day Ms. Jenret anxiously prepared for her interview with Dr. Ralph Anderson. She arrived at his office at 10:00 A.M., precisely on time. The office was a bit dingy, and when she saw the two operatories, she knew that Dr. Anderson's office did not meet OSHA standards. There were belt-driven handpieces in both operatories and no heat sterilization; the only x-ray unit had a short, pointed cone. Dr. Anderson offered Ms. Jenret a seat in his private office, and he began asking her questions regarding her dental assisting experience. He seemed impressed that she had so many years of experience and stated that he was delighted to in-

APPLICATION FOR EMPLOYMENT   Today's Date_____

Name: Last_____First_____Middle_____

Date of Birth_____Marital Status_____

Current Address: Street and Number_____

City_____State_____Zip_____

Day Phone Number_____Evening Phone Number_____

Social Security Number_____Have you applied here before?_____

Do you have previous dental office experience?_____

If yes, give dates and names of employers_____

Date Available for Work_____Hours Available per Week_____

Does your medical history include any of the following:

Heart condition_____High Blood Pressure_____Hepatitis_____AIDS_____

Epilepsy_____Drug or alcohol dependency_____Emotional illness?_____

Are you pregnant?_____List any drugs you are presently taking_____

Have you ever been arrested?___If yes, explain_____

Please furnish three professional and 3 personal references on the back of this form including: name, occupation, relationship to you, address and phone number.

I understand that any offer of employment with Drs. Brown and Douglas will be contingent upon my successful completion of any post offer preemployment physical examination that they might require. I also understand and agree that I may be required to undergo and successfully pass a screening for alcohol and/ or drugs during the hiring process or if employed, as required by Drs. Brown and Douglas.

Signature_____

FIGURE 1

terview someone who had experience using the type of equipment he utilized in his office. He also informed her that she could expect a very high rate of pay, as he did not utilize the new "high-tech" equipment and he knew how to save money in many other facets of practicing dentistry. Dr. Anderson informed Ms. Jenret that he was also able to pay her a high salary because there were no benefits with the job. He paid no insurance of any type for his employees. Dr. Anderson asked Ms. Jenret if she belonged to a specific church and, if so, whether she was active in any church activities. He explained that his practice was open every day and since it was so small, he could not have her take time off for religious holidays. At this point, Ms. Jenret, realizing that this was not the job opportunity of her dreams, politely stated that she was late for another appointment, and left.

The following week Oakbrook Dental telephoned Ms. Jenret and asked if an interview could be arranged for the following Monday. Ms. Jenret gladly met with Dr. John Dennis, the owner of the practice. The practice employed three dentists, eight dental assistants, four dental hygienists, four dental receptionists, and one office manager.

The office was beautifully decorated, and all of the equipment was new. In terms of the facility, nothing seemed to be lacking. At the conclusion of the interview, Dr. Dennis informed Ms. Jenret that she had met all of the employees, except the office manager, who was his son-in-law. He was on a much-needed vacation with his family. He then offered Ms. Jenret the job. She accepted.

After several months on the job, Ms. Jenret was sure that this job was just what she had been looking for. She considered herself very fortunate to be employed in this office, and she did not understand why others in the office had told her that there had been thirty employees who had resigned during the past year.

While having lunch with another Oakbrook employee, Ms. Taylor, Ms. Jenret discovered that Ms. Taylor and the office manager were having an affair.

Ms. Taylor hysterically told her that she had been told that if she refused the office manager's advances, she would be fired. Over the course of the next few weeks, several other employees confided in Ms. Jenret that they too had been propositioned by the office manager. One stated that she had agreed to have sex with him only because he offered her a higher salary with a new job title if she would agree. The office manager was thirty-seven years old; therefore, Ms. Jenret felt safe and thankful that she was "old enough to be his mother."

One day Dr. Dennis requested that Ms. Jenret see him in his office. Dr. Dennis asked her if she liked her job, and she replied affirmatively. He then asked if she would like to keep her job. She answered affirmatively. Dr. Dennis told her that there would be an out-of-state dental convention next month and that he would like her to join him for the week. She replied that she would have to check her calendar and would let him know by the end of the week. Ms. Jenret went home that evening with a dilemma that she had never before contemplated. Fearing that if she lost this job, she would not be able to find another at her age, Ms. Jenret spoke with Dr. Dennis the following day and agreed to attend the meeting with him.

When they arrived at the hotel where the meeting was being conducted, Dr. Dennis registered as Dr. and Mrs. John Dennis. The accommodations were lavish, and the food they consumed was always in extravagant restaurants. However, she went home feeling guilty for having had sex with her employer. She avoided him as much as possible and declined several invitations for luncheon dates with him. Dr. Dennis suddenly became annoyed with her work, finding fault with procedures she had performed for many years. After several weeks of this behavior on his part, he informed Ms. Jenret that he was putting her on notice and that if she did not improve her skills within three weeks, he would be forced to end her employment with Oakbrook Dental.

RESPONSE TO CASE STUDY   Christina Corbin Price, R.D.H., B.S.

The fact that Ms. Clara Jenret was surprisingly terminated by Dr. Hastings without any warnings raises a red flag. If an employer fires an employee for an arbitrary or unjustified reason, the employee can claim that the covenant of good faith has been breached and the contract violated. The "employee at will contract" has been modified in court through a series of relatively recent common law rulings that restrict the right of employers to fire workers. Many of these courts have held that an implied contract exists between the employer and the employee. If the employee is fired outside of the terms of the implied contract, he or she may succeed in a breach of contract action. The rules may vary from state to state. Wise employers will discharge employees only for good cause and will obtain documentation to support their positions. Employees should also be familiar with and follow company policy.

The first classified advertisement, looking for a "female dental assistant" and asking for a photo, violates Title VII of the Civil Rights Act of 1964, which prohibits certain types of discrimination by employers. Protected classes include those defined by race, sex, color, religion, national origin, and pregnancy. Employment discrimination based on any of these criteria is strictly prohibited.

In the second advertisement, asking for a "girl Friday" once again is discrimination. Discrimination law regarding the phrase "must be married" varies from state to state. Whether an employee should be "occasionally able to work long hours" depends on how the employee is compensated. Compensation should be spelled out when an employee is hired—that is, whether he or she will be salaried or paid hourly.

In the third advertisement, the words "no history of drug abuse" constitute a violation of the Americans with Disabilities Act, which does not allow an employer to ask an applicant about past drug abuse or alcoholism. However, an employer can restrict certain acts of an employee, such as smoking or drinking in the workplace or when the employee is representing the employer. Can an employer prohibit an employee from drinking on his or her personal time? An employer cannot govern an employee's personal time or habits outside the scope of work. An employee has a general right to privacy. When asking about a criminal record, an employer can ask if an individual has a criminal record conviction. An applicant may have a criminal record if he or she has been arrested and then found not guilty of the crime. Therefore, it is important for an employer to know the difference when writing classified advertisements or developing job application forms. Rewritten legally, the advertisement would read "We are a nonsmoking environment" or "Applicants with job-related criminal convictions need not apply."

The first application that Ms. Jenret fills out asks for much information that an employer cannot ask about. The first is date of birth. Within the labor laws, an employer only needs to know if an applicant is eighteen years of age. Inquiring about the marital status of an applicant could be discrimination, depending on the state. The medical history section asking about physical and mental health or past drug or alcohol dependency violates the Americans with Disabilities Act. Can Drs. Brown and Douglas make an applicant take a pre-employment physical or a drug or alcohol test? An applicant must be hired on his or her credentials alone, and then if problems arise with testing, the employee may be terminated. An employer has the right to test and to conduct further testing, provided a set policy is in place.

It appears, in Ms. Jenret's interview with Dr. Anderson, that he is asking about her religious beliefs and therefore discriminating against her. Regardless of the size of his practice, he must

RESPONSE TO CASE STUDY—cont'd

interview and hire in a nondiscriminatory manner. Employers must make reasonable accommodation for the religious requirements of their employees.

Ms. Jenret's interview with Dr. Dennis seemed to have gone rather smoothly. Ms. Jenret was hired, as an employee at will since no written contract was mentioned. A written contract would specify the number of hours per week required, the rate of pay, the day of the week on which employees are paid, benefits provided, such as vacations, holidays, sick time, insurance (health, disability, dental), retirement plan, educational allowance, and uniform allowance, and other facts that the employer and the employee agree upon.

During Ms. Jenret's employment at Dr. Dennis' office, she has learned that the office manager is sexually harassing one of her co-workers, Ms. Taylor. She then learns that the same office manager is harassing other employees. This type of sexual harassment is quid pro quo, whereby sexual favors are demanded in return for hiring, promoting, or granting other employment benefits to a person. In sexual harassment cases the employer may be liable, even though an employee did the harassing. If the culpable employee is in a supervisory position, the employer will usually be held liable for the behavior. If a lower-level employee is responsible for the harassment, the employer will be held liable only if he or she knew or should have known about the harassment and failed to take corrective action. Clearly, in the end Ms. Jenret became a victim of sexual harassment.

RESPONSE TO CASE STUDY   Jonathan Shapiro, Esq.

From overt gender, marital status, and disability discrimination in the classified advertisements, to numerous unlawful pre-employment inquiries in the employment application and job interviews, to drug and alcohol testing that violates the laws of many states, to sexual harassment and retaliation in the work place, the case study for Chapters 16, 17, and 18 is a virtual cornucopia of basic employment law issues to be identified and analyzed. Every reader of this case study should spot at least 20 significant problems or potential problems to analyze and address. I would counsel all dental hygienists that no employee has to put up with unlawful discriminatory conduct such as that of the employers in the case study. If your employer engages in conduct similar to that of the dental practices in the case study, you should go to work for a different practice (or seek legal counsel regarding your rights under federal and state law).

CASE STUDY QUESTIONS

1. May the advertisers who submitted the advertisements for a dental assistant to the classified section of the newspaper find themselves with any legal problems? If so, what are the problems?

2. Did Dr. Brown and Dr. Douglas violate any laws? If so, explain.
3. Did Dr. Anderson violate any laws? If so, explain.

4. Did the office manager at Oakbrook Dental violate any laws? If so, what are his defenses?

5. Does Ms. Taylor have a claim against Oakbrook Dental?

6. Did Dr. Dennis violate the law? If so, what are they and what are his defenses?

7. Does Ms. Jenret have a claim against Oakbrook Dental?

8. Do any other employees have a claim against Oakbrook Dental?

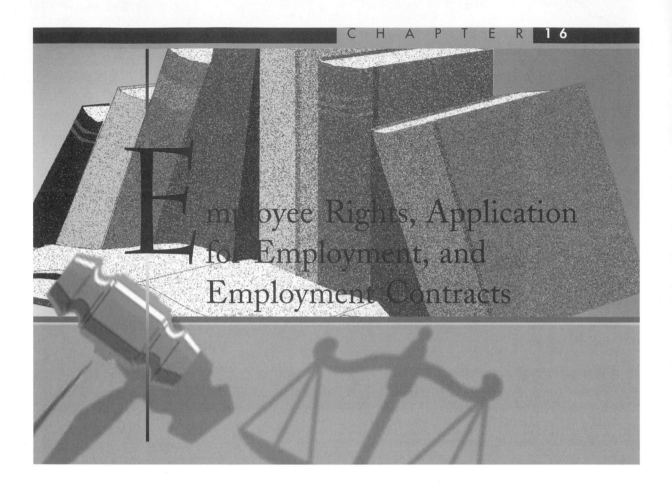

CHAPTER 16

Employee Rights, Application for Employment, and Employment Contracts

After reading this chapter, you should be able to:

- Describe employee rights that are protected by state or federal statutes.
- Identify the components of an employment contract.
- Discuss legal protections available to individuals who are discriminated against in the work place, including discrimination based on race, color, religious beliefs, gender, national origin, physical disability, or age.
- Identify permissible and impermissible questions that may be asked of an applicant during an interview for employment.
- List items that a job applicant should be evaluating during the interview process.

- Write a personal resume.
- List legal obligations that an employer has to his or her employees.
- Discuss what legal obligations an employer has to a leased employee versus the legal obligations of the temporary employment agency.
- List suggestions for preventing allegations of negligent hiring.
- Discuss legal issues relating to termination of employment.
- Describe the Employment Retirement Income Security Act (ERISA).
- Discuss employee rights regarding disability claims, unemployment compensation, and family and medical leave.

KEY WORDS

BONUS	INDEPENDENT CONTRACTOR	UNEMPLOYMENT
COVER LETTER	LEASED EMPLOYEE	COMPENSATION
ERGONOMICS	REFERENCES	UNSCHEDULED BENEFITS
FAMILY LEAVE	SCHEDULED BENEFITS	WORKERS' COMPENSATION

Employment law is a collection of state and federal statutes and case law that continues to enlarge as an increasing number of employees assert their legal rights in the employment arena. There are many state and federal statutes and regulations relating to all aspects of employment; however, they often do not apply to all businesses. Many statutes apply to businesses with a specific number of employees. This effectively exempts small businesses such as dental offices from these laws.

Having written policies and agreements that define the rights, responsibilities, and benefits of those in the employment relationship is essential to a mutually satisfying employment experience. Courts rely on employment documents such as policy and personnel manuals as part of the agreement between employer and employee.[1] Therefore, in the event of termination of employment, it can be critical that hiring agreements were initially reduced to clearly written contracts and to have clearly written policy manuals that define the expectations regarding job performance and rights and responsibilities. If manuals do not exist, it is essential that a well-defined employment contract be negotiated. If policy manuals do exist, read them and ask questions regarding any gray areas prior to accepting a position. The time to negotiate the terms of one's employment is prior to employment. It is much more difficult to attempt to negotiate for increased salary or benefits after initial employment. All negotiated agreements should be in writing.

RECRUITING AND DISCRIMINATION

A prevalent method of locating a position is through the classified section of a newspaper. Often advertisements include statements indicating that the employer is an "equal opportunity employer." This means that all qualified applicants will receive consideration for employment without regard to race, color, national origin, religion, sex, or disability. An advertisement to recruit employees should state the job title and job qualifications (e.g., the minimum education, skills, and/or experience required). All qualifications stated in an advertisement should be job related. An advertisement should not express a preference based on protected status, such as race, color, religious beliefs, gender, national origin, physical disability, or age, unless such a preference is a bona fide occupational qualification. Many state and local laws also prohibit discrimination based on sexual orientation or marital status. A majority of members of the dental assisting and dental hygiene professions are female. That does not give an employer license to selectively advertise for a female applicant, which could lead to a claim of sexual discrimination.[2] The Age Dis-

---

[1]*Lukodki v. Sandia Indian Management Co.*, 748 P2d 507 (N.M. 1988).
[2]EEOC, Policy Guide on Sex-Referent Language in Job Advertising, 405 Fair Employment Practices Manual 6847.

crimination in Employment Act stipulates that it is unlawful for employers to indicate a preference based on age in any advertisement to recruit employees. No statements referring to age that would discourage those over forty years of age from applying for a position are permissible.[3] An employer must not offer or pay a lower salary to women than to men for the same responsibilities. The skills, education, and experience required to perform duties of the position should be determined prior to recruitment, so that qualified applicants are not excluded.

RELIGIOUS DISCRIMINATION

The First Amendment to the United States Constitution states: "Congress shall make no law respecting an establishment of religion, or prohibiting the free exercise thereof." Our Constitution clearly states that one's beliefs are of no concern to government and that no one should be deprived of "civil rights" because of his or her religious beliefs. Therefore, our freedom to think is protected. Closely related to our freedom of thought is our right to privacy, or right to be left alone, a concept that is clearly important in the delivery of health care. Until the 1940s, there was very little litigation relating to what is referred to as the "establishment clause" and "free exercise clause" of the First Amendment. In *United States v. Ballard*,[4] the Supreme Court articulated its position that under the First Amendment, the question of the truth of a party's religious beliefs is barred from going to a jury, because of the subjective nature of such proof. "Men may believe what they cannot prove," so the truth or reasonableness of a belief cannot be questioned by a court. It would appear that this decision would enable anyone to view any act as discriminatory that would determine one's suitability for employment on the basis of one's subjective religious beliefs. However, *Sherbert v. Verner*,[5] a case from the South Carolina Unemployment Compensation Commission, held that a member of the Seventh-Day Adventist faith was ineligible for benefits because she was unwilling to accept jobs requiring work on Saturdays (her day of worship). The Supreme Court held that the state's action imposed an unconstitutional burden on the free exercise of religion. Also, belief in God may not be used as an essential qualification for office (or employment). When Maryland denied a commission as a notary public to a qualified applicant because he refused to declare his belief in the existence of God (as required by the Maryland Constitution for those who seek to qualify for "any office of profit or trust"), the Court held that such a religious test for public office places a burden on the applicant's freedom of belief and religion. In 1987, in *Hobbie v. Unemployment Appeals Commission of Florida*,[6] the Court reiterated that the free exercise of religion is denied when state policy forces a claimant to abandon religious beliefs and practices in order to retain employment or to adhere to religious precepts and practices in order not to forfeit compensatory benefits. In 1967, the

---

[3] 29 C.F.R. § 1625.4(a).
[4] *United States v. Ballard*, 322 U.S. 78 (1944).
[5] *Sherbert v. Verner*, 374 U.S. 398 (1963).
[6] *Hobbie v. Unemployment Appeals Commission of Florida*, 107 S.Ct. 1046 (1987).

Equal Employment Opportunity Commission (EEOC) promulgated a regulation making it mandatory that an employer make reasonable accommodations for the religious needs of employees when such accommodations can be made without undue hardship on the conduct of the employer's business.

The First Amendment bars government from making any law "prohibiting the free exercise" of religion. The free exercise clause applies not only to the federal government but also to the states, via the Fourteenth Amendment. The Fourteenth Amendment provides that no state shall "deny to any person within its jurisdiction the equal protection of the laws." The many laws prohibiting discrimination based on religious beliefs are designed to protect the individual's right of free speech. Religious beliefs and expression are forms of speech and, as such, are protected by the free speech clause of the First Amendment. In addition to the EEOC, the Federal Labor Relations Board, governmental regulations, and several United States Supreme Court decisions, most states have established human rights commissions that review complaints of discrimination based on religion. Generally, each state's attorney general has jurisdiction in this area, as well as the federal government.[7]

NOTICE REQUIREMENTS

Several federal and state statutes require employers to post specific notices advising applicants and employees of their legal rights. These postings are sometimes not applicable to the dental office setting, as the requirements do not apply unless the total number of employed personnel exceeds a certain number. The number varies with each statute. The failure to post required notices may have consequences such as money penalties or possible tolling of the statutes of limitations.

Additional postings are often required under state laws. For instance, workers' compensation, fair employment practices, maternity leave, regulations for minor employees, fire code information, state discrimination statutes, and so forth, are areas in which states have specific requirements.

THE HIRING PROCESS

Numerous state and federal laws speak to the type of information that must be included in or excluded from employment applications. Generally, contacting the unemployment office of a particular state is the best manner in which to gain information regarding the employment laws relating to the application process.

There are countless books, brochures, computer software, and other documents explaining how to write a resume and the interview process. These next few sections relating to the hiring process represent only an overview and address only specific considerations relating to the law and the dental setting.

---

[7]For additional information see Barker LJ, Barker TW: *Civil liberties and the Constitution*, ed 6, Englewood Cliffs, NJ, 1990, Prentice Hall, and Stone G, Seidman L, Sunstein C, Tushnet M: *Constitutional Law*, Boston, 1990, Little, Brown & Co.

General Elements of an Employment Application

Employment applications should be utilized to gain information to assess whether an applicant is qualified for a particular position. There is a presumption that the answers to any questions asked are being considered in the hiring process. Therefore, the burden of proof is on the employer to show that no discrimination has occurred, should a claim of discrimination be alleged by an applicant.

It is impermissible for questions to appear on an employment application that screen out applicants on the basis of their race, color, national origin, age, sex, religion, or disability. Many state statutes and rules and regulations of the Equal Employment Opportunity Commission prohibit potential employers from acquiring certain information during the application or interview process. These rules apply to application forms, job interviews, and background or reference checks. For example[8]:

1. The prospective employer may not ask questions in an attempt to determine an applicant's age. A potential employer may ascertain only if the applicant is eighteen years old or older, to determine whether the applicant is of legal age for employment.

2. The Immigration Reform and Control Act prohibits discrimination against an applicant on the basis of national origin or citizenship. A potential employer may ask whether an applicant can provide proof of work authorization. Questions about language abilities that relate to the position to be filled may be asked. A potential employer may not ask the birthplace of an applicant, or of the applicant's parents, spouse, or close relatives. An applicant cannot be required to submit a birth certificate, a naturalization record, or a baptismal record, or be asked to provide a maiden name.

3. No questions about issues that affect women more often than men (e.g., pregnancy, child rearing, family status) may be asked.

4. No questions regarding religious denomination or affiliations, church membership, or observed religious holidays are permissible.

5. Questions regarding arrests are unlawful under many state laws. Questions about convictions are permissible, but criminal convictions should not be a bar to employment unless it can be shown that the reason is job related. Any questions in this regard must include a statement that a conviction is not a bar to employment. If a potential employee is applying for a bank teller's position, it would be permissible to ask if he or she had ever been convicted of embezzlement.

6. Under the Americans with Disabilities Act, an employer may not ask about the existence, nature, or severity of a disability or conduct a medical examination until after an employment offer has been made. An employer may ask an applicant about his or her ability to perform certain job-related functions. The EEOC has listed permissible and impermissible questions utilized dur-

---

[8]For more specific information see Technical Assistance Manual on the Employment Provisions (Title I) of the Americans with Disabilities Act, EEOC, January 1992, and Leibowitz A, editor: *Drafting employment documents in Massachusetts*, Boston, 1997, Massachusetts Continuing Legal Education Books.

ing the hiring process. For example, impermissible questions would include the following:

- Do you have a disability that would interfere with your ability to perform this job?
- How many days were you sick last year?
- Have you ever filed for workers' compensation?
- Have you ever been injured on the job?
- How much alcohol do you drink each week?
- Have you ever been treated for alcoholism?
- Have you ever been treated for mental health problems?
- What prescription drugs are you currently taking?

Permissible questions under ADA are as follows:

- Can you perform the functions of this job with or without reasonable accommodation?
- Can you meet the attendance requirements of this job?
- How many days did you take leave last year?
- Do you have the required licenses to perform this job?

7. It is impermissible to request an applicant's photograph prior to hiring. No inquiries should be made regarding an applicant's weight or height.
8. It is impermissible to ask an applicant to provide information regarding marital status, children, or Mr., Miss, or Mrs., or to make any inquiry regarding gender or ability to reproduce.

The following information may be legally included in an application for employment:

- Name, address, and telephone number
- Education: high school and college; may include names and addresses of schools, years attended, degrees, and majors
- Any additional training, licenses, certification, awards
- Employment: may include names, addresses, and telephone numbers of each employer, dates of employment, job titles, responsibilities, reasons for leaving, and names of supervisors
- Position: may include the one being applied for and others that the applicant would like to be considered for
- Ability to work overtime
- Date when applicant could start should he or she be offered the job

Interviews

Before beginning an interview, an applicant should make a list of questions focusing on the office and/or business, duties of the job, and benefits of the job. However, don't be so concerned about your questions that you do not listen to the responses of the person conducting the interview. Do not discuss sex, religion, politics, or personal finances; stay focused on office or personnel policy and the requirements of the job.

When interviewing, request a job description of the position for which you are applying. A good job description is a detailed analysis of the job. It lists specific responsibilities, describing how each duty is to be performed and identifying the required or expected results. A job description lists minimum qualifications that the individual performing the job must have, including education and/or knowledge, experience, and specific skills. It should be detailed and accurate. If there are gray areas or items that are not clearly understandable, ask questions. The description should be reviewed and updated regularly. Ask when the job description was created. It may no longer be applicable to the position for which you are applying.

Examples of suggested questions for an applicant to ask during the interview are:

1. What are the specific duties and responsibilities of the position?
2. What is the average tenure of your employees?
3. Are there any changes you would like to see in the manner preventive services are offered to your patients?
4. What are the unique features of your office?
5. What is your policy for updating instruments and/or equipment?
6. May I review a copy of your infection control policy?
7. May I review a copy of your radiographic policy?
8. How are your employees evaluated, including process and criteria?
9. Who is responsible for scheduling patients?
10. How many patients per day are seen by the doctor? By the hygienist?
11. May I have a copy of a typical daily schedule?
12. What are the benefits provided with this position?
    Continuing education _____
    License or certification costs _____
    Professional dues _____
    Retirement or pension plan _____
    Health insurance _____
    Life insurance _____
    Dental benefits _____
    Profit sharing _____
    Paid holidays _____
    Other _____
13. What are the days and hours for this position?
14. May I review a copy of your office Policy and Procedures Manual?
15. What salary can you offer me?

If there is an opportunity to meet with other staff members, ask:

1. What do you like about your employment in this office?
2. What do you dislike about your employment in this office?
3. What changes would you like to see in relation to your position?

If you are moving or considering a move to a new area, you should ask:

1. What is the cost of living in the area (specifically, housing costs, taxes, insurance rates, utility rates)?
2. What hospitals, doctors, and dentists (including specialists) are in the area?
3. What is the total population?
4. What types of schools are in the area?
5. What recreational facilities are available?
6. What cultural activities are available?

Ergonomic Considerations[9]

After several years of practice, many dental health providers suffer from back, neck, and shoulder pain, carpal tunnel syndrome, and tendinitis. Since not all providers experience these disorders, the underlying causes, no doubt, vary from individual to individual. Most of the literature points to **ergonomic** issues related to patient care. Poor posture, poor body positioning, and a disregard for principles of movement contribute to these health problems. The approach to eliminating these contributing factors is twofold. First, retrain the individual who has developed poor habits relating to posture, positioning, and body movement. Second, reevaluate the ergonomics of the dental operatory to allow for optimum body posture, positioning, and movement.

It is therefore essential that every interview for potential employment include an evaluation of the equipment and instruments that you will be spending many hours per week utilizing. Poorly designed work environments often contribute to increased disability claims to workers' compensation insurance. If possible, sit in the stool you would be utilizing and test the equipment as time and circumstances will allow. A few general criteria by which to evaluate the operatory equipment are as follows. For the dental hygienist, the stool should be adjustable to accommodate your body. It should have a backrest with lumbar support that is adjustable both vertically (height) and horizontally (forward and backward). The depth of the seat cushion should accommodate leg length, with a two-inch space between the calf and the front of the seat. The seat height should adjust so that the operator may sit so that the legs are in a tripod position with the seat and there is no constriction of the back of the legs. Although arm supports are rarely present on operator stools, they are helpful because they reduce the static load on muscles of the arms and shoulders. The stool must have five casters for stability and be operated on a surface that maximizes mobility.

The patient's chair must be adjustable so that the patient may be positioned in a supine position that allows an imaginary line from patient's nose to the feet to be parallel to the floor. The delivery system should be positioned to the right of the patient (for right-handed operators), close to the operator so that instruments are accessible with no reaching beyond the arc created by sweeping the forearm while the upper arm is held at the operator's side. There should be no resistance from retractable or coiled cords on the dental unit. The dental light needs to furnish sufficient light and focus to prevent eyestrain that could result in poor posture. The handpiece must be lightweight and well balanced. An ultrasonic scaler should be available and should be placed on the unit to eliminate unnecessary reaching. Countertops must not be too high or too low for the operator to use appropriate body positioning while completing documentation in the patient's record.

For the dental assistant, the stool should be adjustable to accommodate his or her body. The feet should comfortably rest on the adjustable metal ring or foot platform at the base of the stool, with the thighs parallel to the floor. The stool's

ERGONOMICS

The scientific study of human work, specifically as it relates to the use of technology for the purpose of creating a healthy work environment.

[9]Excerpts from evaluation criteria, Davison, Price & Associates, Dental Ergonomics, P.O. Box 1559, Windham, ME 04062, 1998.

body support must wrap around the left side and front of the assistant, just under the rib cage, for support when the assistant is leaning toward the patient. The stool should be adjustable so that elbow level is 4 to 6 inches above the patient's mouth and the assistant's left thigh is parallel to the patient's chair. The stool should be positioned so that the front edge of the seat is even with the patient's mouth. The tray setup should be on a mobile cart over the lap.

Cover Letters and Resumes

COVER LETTER

A letter of introduction usually accompanying a resume or an application for employment.

The **cover letter** is simply a letter of application that accompanies your resume. It is a three- to four-paragraph letter that, first, specifically states what position you are applying for and where you obtained information about the opening. Next, provide the employer with an overview of your qualifications and how you believe they will enhance his or her business. Finally, request an interview and describe how the employer may arrange one with you. For instance, provide a telephone number and the hours you may be reached to arrange an interview. Do not address cover letters "To Whom It May Concern." Always send your letter to a named individual.

A simple concise, one-page resume should accompany the letter of application. Information on a resume should be the same as on an application:

1. Personal information: name, address, telephone number
2. Education
3. Professional or work experience
4. Professional affiliations or activities
5. Certifications, licenses, awards, and so forth

REFERENCES

Recommendations, written or oral, attesting to the competencies of an applicant for employment.

References should be sent only on request, and be sure to ask permission of individuals whose names you are submitting as references.

The rules that apply with interviews also apply with resumes and letters of application. An employer may not request information regarding age, marital status, sex, race, religion, height, weight, or disabilities. Questions regarding a husband's or wife's occupation or salary, number of children, plans to have children, personal finances, political interests, or religious beliefs are impermissible. Do not provide answers to impermissible questions in your resume or letter of application.

EMPLOYERS' LEGAL OBLIGATIONS TO EMPLOYEES

In general, during the employer-employee relationship there are fundamental responsibilities that an employer must assume. As mentioned earlier, an employer may not discriminate against an employee on the basis of race, color, sex, religion, age, national origin, or disability status.

Employee Retirement Income Security Act of 1974

An employer must comply with the Employee Retirement Income Security Act (ERISA) regarding retirement or other benefits available to employees. No specific retirement benefit is required; however, if one is offered, there is a requirement that specific information be reported to the employee. A pension plan is an employee benefit often included in a benefit plan in a small business such as a dental practice. It includes any plan that offers retirement income or results in deferral of income beyond termination of covered employment. Every plan must be documented, and the plan administrator must provide a summary of the plan to each participant and each beneficiary entitled to benefits. An individual must be given a summary of the plan within ninety days after the plan is established, when the individual becomes a participant, or when a beneficiary starts receiving benefits. On a participant's written request, the plan administrator must provide a statement of the participant's accrued benefits and vested percentage. A statement is required at least every twelve months. If the plan is materially modified, a summary of modifications must be distributed.

The required contents of the summary of the plan are as follows[10,11]:

- The name of the plan
- The name and address of the plan sponsor
- The employer identification number of the plan sponsor and the plan number
- The type of pension plan and the type of plan administrator
- The name, address, and telephone number of the plan administrator
- The name and address of a person specified to receive process in any litigation involving the plan
- The name, title, and business address of each trustee
- The eligibility requirements for participation and benefits
- The pension plan's normal retirement age, a description of any conditions on the receipt of benefits, and a summary of the plan's benefits
- A description of spousal protections
- A clear identification of any circumstances that may result in ineligibility, denial, loss, forfeiture, or suspension of any benefit that a participant or beneficiary would otherwise reasonably expect to receive
- A statement of whether benefits are insured and a summary of coverage
- An explanation of the plan's rules for counting service for eligibility, vesting, and benefits purposes
- The sources of plan contributions
- A listing of any funding vehicles and the identity of the insurers, trustees, etc.
- The date the plan year ends
- The plan's claims review procedures
- A statement of participants' ERISA rights

Any full-time employee over twenty-one years of age who has worked for the same employer for one year must be allowed to participate in the pension plan if one exists. For part-time employees, if they have worked for at least one thousand hours during the year, they must be allowed to participate to some extent in the plan. Plan benefits are not available until the employee is vested. The vesting period is the period of time an employee must work for the employer in order to receive full benefits. Vesting periods vary with plans, but seven years is the maximum under the law. ERISA requires continued coverage of employees for a period of time after their employment terminates.

---

[10]ERISA, § 102(b), and DOL Reg. § 2520.102.3.
[11]*Drafting employment documents in Massachusetts*, supra.

Workers' Compensation

Workers' compensation is an insurance program regulated by each state's insurance commission. Generally, an employer must purchase workers' compensation insurance through an insurance company. Some states permit businesses to provide this coverage through self-insured programs. Workers' compensation compensates employees should they become seriously ill or injured in the work place or as a result of conditions in the work place.

There are numerous disability claims among dental professionals. Most claims are due to ergonomic risk factors involved in repetitive tasks performed by dental hygienists, dental assistants, and dentists on a regular basis. Injuries to the neck, shoulder, arms, back, and wrists are very common and are collectively called cumulative trauma disorders, or CTDs. These disorders include damage to or inflammation of the muscles, tendinitis (inflamation of the tendons of the wrist, elbow, or shoulder), and carpal tunnel syndrome (a pinched nerve in the wrist that causes pain and/or numbness or paralysis in the hand). Claims made to workers' compensation systems are often the end result of these injuries.

Workers' compensation systems vary from state to state. Generally, every employer with at least one employee must provide coverage. A person is covered by workers' compensation as soon as he or she is hired. There are no waiting periods. Injuries that result from failure to use safety equipment, involve alcohol or drug use, or are self-inflicted are excluded from coverage in most states.

Workers' compensation provides income and medical expenses to individuals who become ill or are injured on the job. It is the sole remedy for injuries arising from the job. In other words, an employee could not collect workers' compensation benefits and then later sue the employer for the same injury. It is the employer's responsibility to pay for this coverage. The coverage is usually provided through a state fund, private insurance, or an employer's self-insured program.

Benefits available should an injury occur include medical benefits (hospital, physician, nursing, and rehabilitation services) and disability benefits. There are two types of disability benefits.

Type I, **unscheduled benefits,** is compensation for reduced earning capacity of an injured employee. Each state requires a waiting period of three to seven days. If, after the waiting period, the injured employee is unable to return to the job, he or she may qualify for disability compensation. Workers' compensation systems generally identify four types of disabilities: Temporary total, temporary partial, permanent total, and permanent partial. If an employee receives an injury, he or she is entitled to benefits for temporary disability until he or she is able to resume regular activities of the job. If an employee is unable to return to the job in full capacity, temporary benefits cease at the end of a specified recuperation period. To qualify for permanent benefits, an injured employee must qualify under his or her state's system. Unscheduled benefits are based on wages and are calculated at one half to two thirds of the employee's average weekly pay.

Type 2, **scheduled benefits,** is provided by states for specific physical injuries, such as the loss of an eye, an arm, or a leg. Scheduled benefits pay an injured employee a certain sum for each injury for a specified number of weeks. The wages lost by the employee are not a factor in scheduled benefits.

Workers' compensation claims are investigated aggressively by the state or the insurance company paying the benefits. Filing a false claim with workers' compensation is classified as fraud in all states, and such behavior can result in heavy fines as well as incarceration.

In most states, a worker's claim to receive workers' compensation for work-related injuries cannot be waived. Therefore, this is not a negotiable item in any employment negotiation. When employed in a small dental office, a person should check with the state office of workers' compensation to determine whether he or she is covered.

Unemployment Compensation

The Federal Unemployment Tax Act establishes guidelines for state unemployment plans. States control eligibility requirements and benefits. Therefore, the amount of weekly **unemployment compensation** benefit that a terminated employee can receive varies from state to state. This number is based on salary at termination. Employers are required to pay into their states' unemployment insurance systems. Generally, if an employee has worked for a specified amount of time and his or her job is terminated, that person is eligible for unemployment benefits for up to twenty-six weeks while he or she is seeking a new position. Job searches usually must be documented, and many states require a specified number of interviews or contacts each week. If you should leave the state in which you were receiving benefits to find employment, you may still be able to collect benefits from the state you left, through the unemployment office of the new state. Former employees are eligible if they were laid off or had a significant reduction in work hours and were not fired for cause or misconduct. Leaving a job to go to school may disqualify you from benefits; however, some states consider benefits to students on a case-by-case basis. You may be ineligible for benefits if your employer was a family member. An employee who has protected status (because of age, race, religion, sex, ethnicity, national origin, disability status, pregnancy, and so forth), and is fired because of that status, will be eligible for unemployment benefits. If an employee leaves employment because of an employer's illegal activity in the work place, he or she would be eligible for unemployment benefits. Unemployment benefits are taxed at the same rate as regular income. However, these taxes are not withheld from the unemployment funds one receives. To avoid an unpleasant experience with tax authorities, do not forget to set funds aside to pay taxes.

> **UNEMPLOYMENT COMPENSATION**
>
> A state insurance program that provides benefits to persons who are terminated from employment. Former employees are generally not eligible if they left their jobs without good cause or they were fired for serious misconduct.

Internal Revenue Code (and Similar State and Local Tax Laws)

Employers must withhold federal, state, and other applicable income taxes from an employee's pay. The employer must report and remit taxes as required by state law and the Internal Revenue Service. Federal taxes are explained in Circular E, Employers' Tax Guide. The amount withheld is based on:

Filing status (single, married, or head of household)
Number of dependents
Amount of gross salary

In the event that an employee owes unpaid taxes, the federal, most state, and some local taxing authorities may seize his or her wages. The amount an employee may keep depends upon the number of his or her dependents and the size of the standard deduction to which the employee is entitled.

Federal Insurance Contributions Act and Federal Unemployment Tax Act

Employers must withhold from employee's pay and remit social security contributions under the Federal Insurance Contributions Act (FICA) and remit contributions to the federal unemployment tax fund under the Federal Unemployment Tax Act (FUTA). Social security contributions include the employee's share and the employer's share. Unemployment taxes are the responsibility of the employer and are not withheld from an employee's wages. As previously mentioned, contributions to state unemployment funds are also the responsibility of the employer.

Fair Labor Standards Act

Under the federal Fair Labor Standards Act (FLSA),[12] an employer must pay a minimum hourly wage, provide overtime pay, pay in a timely manner, and keep accurate payroll records. A business is covered by this act if there is $500,000 or more in total annual sales or if the work involves interstate commerce. To meet the interstate commerce condition, courts have held that an employee is covered if he or she sends mail or makes telephone calls to or receives mail or telephone calls from other states on behalf of the employer. Under these circumstances most dental offices would be subject to this law.

Family and Medical Leave Act

FAMILY LEAVE

Unpaid absence from employment for the birth, adoption, or care of a child or for the care of a spouse, a parent, or oneself. The federal Family and Medical Leave Act requires businesses of 50 or more employees to provide 12 weeks of unpaid leave for eligible employees. Any paid leave benefits from an employer would be in addition to FMLA requirements.

The Family and Medical Leave Act (FMLA) allows eligible employees to take up to twelve weeks of unpaid leave for family emergencies, such as illnesses, or for the birth of a child. An employee's job is protected during this **family leave** period. The United States Department of Labor (DOL) oversees and enforces the Act. If a violation is not resolved, the DOL may bring court action to compel compliance. Private court action may be brought by employees whose employers violate the law. Employers are subject to the Act if they employ 50 or more employees working 20 or more weeks in the current or previous calendar year and are engaged in commerce. An employee must have worked at least twelve months and at least 1,250 hours during those twelve months to be eligible. The employee must also work in a location where at least 50 employees live in a 75-mile radius.

Pregnancy Discrimination Act

Under the Pregnancy Discrimination Act an employer may not:
- Refuse to hire
- Refuse to promote
- Fire

---

[12]29 U.S.C. § 201 et seq.

an employee because of pregnancy or related medical conditions. An employee has the right to be reinstated at the same level of seniority and with the same retirement benefits following childbirth or pregnancy. An employee may not be asked to take maternity leave at an arbitrary time. In addition, an employer may not fire or refuse to hire a woman who has chosen to have an abortion.

Americans with Disabilities Act

The Americans with Disabilities Act (ADA) is one of the more recent laws. This law establishes policy and procedures regarding opportunities provided to disabled individuals in the work place. The Equal Employment Opportunity Commission initiated this legislation to protect the rights of disabled individuals and to assist in their integration into the work force. The Act has been in effect since July of 1992.

A person is considered disabled when he or she:
1. Has a physical or mental impairment that substantially limits one or more major life activities *or*
2. Has a record of such impairment or is regarded as having such an impairment

Major life activities include walking, speaking, breathing, performing manual tasks, seeing, hearing, learning, taking care of oneself, working, sitting, standing, lifting, and reading. The impairment must substantially limit one of the major life activities for protection under the ADA. In addition to having a qualifying impairment to receive ADA protection, the individual must be qualified to do the particular job in question. Homosexuality, bisexuality, illegal drug use, and sexual or behavioral disorders are not considered disabilities by the ADA.

Employers must attempt to reasonably accommodate disabled employees, unless doing so creates an "undue hardship." Reasonable accommodation includes: handicap ramps, modifying work schedules, telephone amplifiers, reassignment to a vacant position, work stations that accommodate wheelchairs, and job restructuring.

Age Discrimination in Employment Act of 1967

The Age Discrimination in Employment Act (ADEA) bars all state agencies, local governments, the federal government, and all private employers with 20 or more employees from discriminating against individuals over 40 years of age. An employer may not refuse to hire, train, or promote, fire, or force retirement on a person over the age of 40 solely because of that person's age.

Occupational Safety and Health Act

There are many federal laws relating to employment with which an employer must maintain compliance to protect the employee. One of the most important federal laws affecting the daily lives of those of us who are employed in the dental setting is the Occupational Safety and Health Act (OSHA). OSHA was enacted to protect workers from physical hazards in the work place. The Act addresses the handling of hazardous substances and mandates infection control procedures for dentistry. The Occupational Safety and Health Administration has the authority to establish the mandatory occupational safety and health standards for all dental practices as well as other business establishments.

LEASED EMPLOYEES

LEASED EMPLOYEE

An employee who is provided by a temporary-employee leasing service. An employer pays the leasing service a fee to hire one of its employees for short-term employment.

Leased employees are employees of a temporary employment service or agency. They are assigned to work for a client of the service or agency as temporary workers for a specific period of time. The employment agreement is between the leasing service or agency and the leased employee. Therefore, the service or agency is solely responsible for the employee's wages, withholding federal and state income taxes, paying social security taxes, and providing unemployment insurance and workers' compensation insurance and other obligations of an employer.

There are many agencies throughout the United States that lease dental office personnel such as dental receptionists, dental assistants, and dental hygienists. Their clients are most often dentists who rely on temporary employees when there is a staff vacancy or when their employees are on sick leave, vacation, or maternity leave. Leased dental employees may be utilized in settings other than the dental office, such as dental education programs, research projects, public health settings, and nursing homes.

Under certain circumstances, the leasing agency and the client may be regarded as joint employers of the employee. The greater the degree of supervision and control exercised by the client and the longer the leasing arrangement, the greater the likelihood that the leased employee would be regarded as an employee of both agency and client. A court of law may assign liability to one or both for acts of the employee. This can include acts of discrimination by the leased employee against others.[13]

In determining if a leased employee meets a common law definition of "employee" status, courts will examine:

1. Whether the leased employee is performing exactly the same work as others who are employed by the client *and*
2. Whether the employee is being treated by the client essentially in the same manner it treats its own employees *and*
3. Whether the leasing agreement goes on for an extended or indefinite period of time

If all of these elements are found, a leased employee can be considered a common law employee and is thereby entitled to the same benefits as other employees employed by the client of the service or agency.[14] If leasing agreements are carefully articulated, most leased employees do not become eligible for benefits they were given no expectation of receiving.[15]

---

[13]*People of the State of New York v. Holiday Inn, Inc.*, 62 FEP Cases (BNA) 826 (1993).
[14]*Bronk v. Mountain States Tel & Tel; Inc.*, 943 F.Supp. 1317 (Dist. Colo. 1996).
[15]*Abraham v. Exxon Corp.*, 85 F.3d 1126 (5th Cir. 1996).

NEGLIGENT HIRING

An employer must lawfully gather information regarding potential employees. An applicant's privacy is a critical consideration in the employer's manner of collection and the type of information relating to potential employees. However, an employer has a duty to obtain factual information regarding the competence of his or her employees. An employer has a duty to protect customers, clients, visitors, members of the general public, and employees from injuries caused by employees who the employer knew or should have known posed a risk or harm to others.[16] Should someone become injured or have his or her property damaged or stolen by an employee whose background was not carefully checked, the employer can be sued in a court of law for negligent hiring. State statutes govern negligent hiring cases and examine whether an employer adequately investigated the fitness of a prospective employee. Likewise, should an employer retain an employee who is performing below the standard of care and someone is injured as a result, the employer can be sued for the negligent retention for failing to supervise or failing to fire the employee. Most state statutes governing negligent hiring stipulate that an employer must adequately investigate the fitness of a prospective employee. Therefore, contacting an applicant's previous employers and personal references may provide a good defense against allegations of negligent hiring. Employers should keep a written record of any investigation into the background of a potential employee.

The doctrine of negligent hiring may make an employer liable for the wrongful or criminal acts of an employee. An employer may be found liable even if the act or acts occur outside of the scope of employment. The initial contact between the employee and the plaintiff must have occurred during the employee's employment with that particular employer. Therefore, the employee's harmful acts need not take place during working hours.[17]

Employees have sued former employers under a variety of legal theories for providing unfavorable references. Negligent misrepresentation, infliction of emotional distress, defamation, and intentional interference with business relations are all allegations that may be the basis of these lawsuits. As a result, former employers often provide information only regarding position, length of employment, and salary. On the other side of the coin, a former employer could be held liable for failure to warn a prospective employer regarding an employee's past. *Conway v. Smerling*[18] held that: "an employer has a 'privilege,' if not a duty, to speak the truth even if the disclosure of the facts might negatively affect the subject's job prospects." Some states protect employee references under public policy. Communications that are reasonably necessary to further a legitimate business interest have a conditional privilege. The privilege may be lost if the communication is made with actual malice or recklessly.[19]

---

[16]*Restatement of torts, second*, § 283, St Paul, 1977, American Law Institute.
[17]*Doe v. Blanford*, 525 N.E.2d 403 (1988).
[18]*Conway v. Smerling*, 635 N.E.2d 268 (Mass. 1994).
[19]*Bratt v. Int'l Business Mach. Corp.*, 467 N.E.2d 126 (Mass. 1984).

There are steps employers can take to protect against employer liability and to protect the privacy rights of the employee. When asking prospective employees to list references, be sure to obtain written consent to contact present and former employers. Reference requests from former employers should be in writing and should include a copy of the applicant's consent form indicating permission for the former employer to disclose requested personal information. Request that the former employer validate dates, titles, duties, and other related information. When providing information requested by a prospective employer, a former employer should provide only information that a former employee knows is in his or her personnel file. If the request is by telephone, verify the caller's identity. This may be accomplished by returning the call. Do not provide information regarding the reason an employee is no longer employed in a particular employment setting, unless you have firsthand information. Responses to requests for a reference should be in writing. If that is not possible, keep a written account of oral communication. Do not report opinions in response to reference requests; state only facts that can be substantiated.

CREDIT CHECKS

In most cases a credit check by a prospective employer is an intrusion into an individual's private life. However, credit checks can be justified when they are relevant to employment. For instance, it would be justifiable to conduct a credit check for individuals who apply for positions that would require management of finances. The EEOC looks closely at this procedure should there be any resulting allegations of discrimination, as requiring good credit may be a subtle means of barring minority groups from employment. State laws also address the use of credit information during employee selection.

The federal Fair Credit Reporting Act regulates consumer credit reporting agencies and the use of consumer credit reports for employment purposes.[20] Under the Act, a consumer credit report consists of any written, oral, or other communication of any information by a consumer credit reporting agency that bears on an individual's creditworthiness, credit standing, or credit capacity, which is then used as a factor in evaluating an applicant for employment, promotion, reassignment, or retention.[21] A consumer credit report may be made available only to a prospective employer who intends to use the information for employment purposes with the written permission of the job applicant to whom it relates. The party requesting a credit report must certify the purpose for which the information will be used and state that the information will not be used for any other purpose. As with other types of credit reporting, should a potential employee be denied employment wholly or in part because of the information contained in the consumer credit report, the employer must notify the applicant and furnish the name and address of the consumer credit reporting agency making the report.[22]

---

[20]15 USC §§ 1681-1681(t).
[21]15 USC §§ 1681(d) and (h).
[22]15 USC §§ 1681 m(a).

CRIMINAL RECORDS CHECKS

State laws differ regarding access to criminal offender record information. Some states permit certain information to be released concerning prior convictions of an applicant for employment. Generally, states seal juvenile records; therefore, they are not available to a prospective employer or anyone else. Some states do not permit inquiries regarding minor offenses or misdemeanors that go back more than five years if no subsequent convictions are on record. Generally, private employers cannot obtain federal criminal history information.[23] A number of federal courts have held, under Title VII of the Civil Rights Act of 1964 as amended,[24] that because minority group members are substantially more likely than whites to be arrested relative to their respective proportion in the population, basing employment decisions upon arrest records is likely to have a disparate impact upon minority group members.[25]

IMMIGRATION STATUS CHECKS

Under the Immigration Reform and Control Act (IRCA),[26] all new employees, including citizens, must fill out Immigration and Naturalization Service Form 1-9, Employment Eligibility Verification, which requests biographical information and requires applicants to certify under penalty of perjury that they are citizens or aliens entitled to work in the United States. Applicants must submit documents verifying their identity and status, and the employer must verify and maintain the documents for three years or for one year after the employee has left the job, whichever is longer. Employers having three or more employees are barred from discrimination in the hiring process on the basis of an individual's national origin or citizenship.

MEDICAL INFORMATION

Both federal and state laws limit the medical information that employers can request from prospective employees. Under the Americans with Disabilities Act an employer may not require an applicant to take a medical examination, to respond to medical inquiries, or to provide information about workers' compensation claims before the employer makes a job offer. A job offer may be contingent upon an applicant passing a medical exam. If such an exam is required, it must be required of all entering employees who are performing the same job. An employer would be in violation of the ADA if medical exams were required only for individuals with disabilities or for persons who are believed to be disabled.

Such an examination "may not disqualify an individual with a disability who is currently able to perform essential job functions because of speculation that the disability may cause a risk of future injury." Should an employer withdraw a con-

---

[23]29 C.F.R. § 20.1.
[24]42 U.S.C. §§ 2000e et seq.
[25]*Gregory v. Litton Sys., Inc.*, 472 F.2d 631 (9th Cir.1972).
[26]8 U.S.C. §§1324A-1324C.

ditional job offer made to a disabled person as a result of a post-offer medical examination, he or she must be able to show that[27]:

1. The reasons were job related and consistent with business necessity or that the person was excluded to avoid a direct threat to health and safety.
2. No reasonable accommodation could be made or such an accommodation would cause undue hardship.

DRUG TESTING

The laws relating to drug testing vary from state to state. However, courts may approve of drug testing if all of the following are true:

1. The method of testing is reliable and respectful of the applicant's privacy.
2. The applicant is informed that the drug test may be a condition of employment.
3. There is a strong basis for drug testing because of the nature of the work.

Courts will analyze pre-employment drug testing under a balancing test. The test balances the employer's legitimate needs of business against the applicant's right to privacy. If the testing is upheld in a court of law under the balancing test, it is usually because the prospective employee knows that drug testing is a condition of employment and therefore has a reduced expectation of privacy. Some state laws require that the employer give applicants a written policy statement that is separate from the application and informs applicants of the employer's drug testing procedures. The type of drug testing must be accurate, or an employer can be charged with discrimination, defamation, or breach of privacy. In *Doe v. Roe*[28] the plaintiff claimed that his urine specimen tested positive for narcotics because of his consumption of a health food bread containing poppy seeds, and not because of opiate use. His urine was subjected to two different testing methods (both resulted in positive findings). The plaintiff asserted that there was a third testing method that could have effectively distinguished opiate use from consumption of food. The court held that the employer "must come forward with evidence establishing that its testing method accurately distinguishes between opiate users and consumers of lawful foodstuffs or medications,"[29] or risk liability for unlawful discrimination based on the assertion that the employee is a drug user.

SKILLS TESTING

The Americans with Disabilities Act may be violated if skills testing by an employer does not measure actual skills and abilities necessary to perform the job for which a person is applying. Title VII and the Americans with Disabilities Act may be violated by employment practices that disproportionately deprive applicants who are members of protected groups of equal employment opportunities. A dis-

---

[27]Technical Assistance Manual on the Employment Provisions (Title I) of the Americans with Disabilities Act, supra.
[28]*Doe v. Roe*, 553 N.Y.S. 2d 365 (1990).
[29]*Doe v. Roe*, supra.

parate impact on members of protected groups may be established by showing the following:

1. The existence of a specific employment practice (skill test)
2. A disparate impact related to membership in a protected group (an adverse effect on members of a protected group as compared with the effect on members of the majority)
3. A direct relationship between the testing procedure and the impact (or failure to hire)[30]

The Civil Rights Act[31] provides that an unlawful employment practice based on disparate impact is established under Title VII if at least one of the following is true:

1. A complaining party demonstrates that a respondent (employer) uses a particular employment practice that causes a disparate impact on the basis of race, color, religion, sex, or national origin and the respondent (employer) fails to demonstrate that the challenged practice is job related for the position in question and consistent with business necessity.
2. The complaining party makes a demonstration with respect to an alternative employment practice and the respondent (employer) refuses to adopt such alternative employment practice.

Therefore, an employer must correlate any preemployment skills testing with actual skills that are required for the job as well as show that testing is consistent with business necessity.

POLYGRAPH TESTING

The federal Employee Polygraph Protection Act[32] bans the use of lie detector testing by an employer, with a few exceptions. State law may set its own exceptions and be more restrictive than federal law. Therefore, should your employer request that you submit to a polygraph test, check both federal and state law regarding your rights.

EMPLOYMENT AGREEMENTS

Generally, employees have no job security and employment is an "at will" relationship. An employer can fire an employee at any time for any reason, as long as it is not an illegal reason (based on the employee's membership in a protected class—age, sex, race, etc.). The employee is also free to resign at any time. For these reasons, it is best to negotiate a contract that provides the security of a fixed term of employment and clearly identifies the benefits connected with such employment.

In general, an employment agreement should include a job description, method of compensation, agreements to protect property rights, confidentiality and non-

---

[30]*Griggs v. Duke Power Co.*, 401 U.S. 424 (1971).
[31]Title 42 U.S.C. § 2000e-2(k)(1)(A).
[32]29 U.S.C. §§ 2001-2009.

competition covenants, minimum term of employment, fringe benefits, and severance arrangements. Specifically the terms of an employment contract are as follows:

1. Names of employer and employee
2. Description of the job, (indicating whether the job is part time or full time)
3. Length of term. The contract may state that the agreement continues until it is terminated. It is important to agree to and document the grounds for termination.
4. Salary. The contract should always state a salary. It may state whether the raises are left to the discretion of the employer or may establish annual increases. Any **bonus** programs or other incentive compensation, such as profit sharing plans, should also be documented.
5. Benefit programs. As a result of ERISA and other laws, a potential employee cannot negotiate for additional insurance plan benefits beyond those the employer is providing other employees. A prospective employee may be able to negotiate for additional monetary compensation rather than added benefits. Fringe benefits such as paid vacations, holidays, sick leave, personal days, automobiles, office space, travel expenses, continuing education expenses, professional subscriptions and dues, and liability coverage may be negotiated.
6. Proprietary rights. Generally, inventions, products, writings, and other things of value developed by an employee within the scope of employment belong to the employer. There are exceptions. Absent an agreement with the employer, only the employee who actually invents a product can apply for a patent on that product. An employer may use proprietary rights provisions to obtain rights to products or inventions produced by the employee for a certain period of time after he or she leaves employment, on the theory that it can reasonably be assumed that if an employee produces such a product shortly after termination, it must in part have been made possible by work done or facilities available during employment. An employee may need to establish ownership of products that he or she developed prior to employment. Dental products are sometimes developed by dental assistants and dental hygienists. Rights to those products should be documented prior to their development. Often, there is a tendency for dental hygienists to feel that the patients they provide services for are their patients. Patient records and patient lists are exclusive property of the dentist who owns the dental practice. Treat them accordingly.
7. Confidentiality. Each employee has a duty to keep confidential the secrets of the employer that have material business value, which include lists of patients of record in any dental office and financial information. A written agreement gives an employer the opportunity to document exactly what information he or she deems confidential and the employee the opportunity to receive that information and acknowledge it.
8. Termination. A provision allowing termination without cause gives the employer the right to dismiss an employee at any time, without any specific reason other than dissatisfaction with the employee's performance on the job. If such a provision is in a contract, a court would determine that the employment relationship is "at will" and either party may end the employment rela-

BONUS

An amount paid in addition to salary or other employment benefits.

tionship without recourse. A provision allowing termination for cause is often a part of an employment contract. Here, an employee will not be terminated except for cause, such as willful failure to perform duties, gross negligence, or chronic absenteeism or lateness. An employer may want the contractual right to terminate the employee even if there is no cause; the contract may include provision that would allow such termination if the employer pays severance to the employee. An employee cannot be required to stay on the job and has the right to terminate employment at any time and for any reason. However, a contract may contain a provision for increased severance pay if the employee terminates for cause—for instance, if the employer breaches the employment contract.

EVALUATION

An employee should request an annual or semiannual evaluation that is discussed with the employer and documented in writing. If an employee who is fired claims that he or she was fired for an illegal reason, such as discrimination, a history of well-documented positive evaluations is his or her best evidence of such illegal action. Employees have successfully sued employers who used poor evaluation procedures for "negligent evaluation," which is the failure of an employer to review employees' work fully and honestly and to warn employees that they face discipline or discharge for failure to improve. The job description should be the basis of evaluation, as the focus is on how well the employee performs the duties of the job. The evaluation is centered on job performance and not personality.

CONFIDENTIALITY

Personnel files should be kept under lock. They should be available only to people within the business who have a legitimate business need for access to an employee's file. State laws vary, but many give employees and former employees access to their own files. In some instances, the employee will not be privy to certain items, such as letters of reference, that may violate the privacy of other individuals. Beyond these exceptions, personnel files are available to no one unless a subpoena is issued for such files.

TERMINATION OF EMPLOYMENT

An employee is not entitled to severance pay unless there is a contract between the employer and the employee that requires the payment of money and/or benefits upon termination by either party. It is best to negotiate severance pay prior to employment when negotiating an employment contract. Benefits to be paid upon termination also should be described, as specifically as possible, with dates and types of benefits outlined. Of particular importance are health insurance and COBRA rights (see Chapter 18), including when notification of continuing coverage occurs, who pays the premiums, and for how long. Other benefits may include life insurance, 401(k) plans, and short- or long-term disability, and there may be compensation for loss of pension benefits as a result of early departure.

Figure 16-1 is meant to show the options that may be negotiated in an employment contract. If, upon termination, an employee does not need certain benefits,

THIS AGREEMENT made and entered into this_____day of October, 1999, between VELMORE DENTAL ASSOCIATES, PA, hereinafter referred to as Employer, and SARAH Q. NICHOLAS, hereinafter referred to as Employee.

IN CONSIDERATION of the covenants and mutual benefits herein, it is agreed to as follows:

TERM: Terms of this agreement shall begin on January 2, 2000 and shall terminate on January 1, 2004, unless otherwise stipulated in this agreement.

COMPENSATION: Employer shall pay to Employee during the period of the term a salary or $56,000 a year, payable in equal installments every two (2) weeks.

BONUSES: Employer may enter into supplemental agreements in writing with the Employee for the payment of bonuses upon such terms as Employer shall deem to be in its business interest, and shall be determined in accordance with the Office Policy Manual which is hereby incorporated by reference and made a part of this agreement. Employee acknowledges receipt of a copy of the Office Policy Manual.

WORKING HOURS: Employee shall work 37-1/2 hours per week, office hours being from 8:30 a.m. until 5:00 p.m. All employees are entitled to two 10 minute breaks each working day, the first between 9:00 a.m. and Noon; the second between 2:00 p.m. and 5:00 p.m.; and a lunch break of 1 hour.

VACATIONS: Employee shall be entitled each year to two (2) weeks of paid vacation or personal time after six months of employment.

SICK LEAVE: Employees are entitled to eight (8) days sick leave in one fiscal year. Any employee on sick leave for more than eight (8) days must furnish a doctor's statement stipulating need for absence.

BENEFITS: Employees are directed to refer to the Office Policy Manual.

UNIFORM ALLOWANCE: Employee shall have a uniform allowance of $250.00 per year, to begin after the first six (6) months of employment.

FIGURE 16-1
Employment agreement.

TERMINATION: Breach of office policy, insubordination or chronic absenteeism or lateness are grounds for immediate dismissal. The Employer may terminate this agreement at any time upon thirty (30) days written notice to Employee or payment in lieu thereof. Employee may terminate this agreement at any time upon thirty (30) days written notice to Employer.

Should this agreement terminate for any reason other than for cause, then Employer agrees to continue to pay Employee's salary for such period as Employee shall remain unemployed. Said salary shall continue to be prorated and payable biweekly for a period not to exceed three (3) months. During this salary continuation period, Employer will continue to provide Employee all medical and dental benefits in effect as of the effective date hereof, at no charge to Employee. During this salary continuation period, Employer will continue to make contributions to Employee's 401(k) plan account, and to deduct contributions from Employee's salary as payment therefor, at the same rate as presently. After the expiration of said three month period, Employee shall be entitled to and shall be given timely notice of her right to continued medical and dental coverage under the Consolidated Omnibus Budget Reconciliation Act of 1986 (COBRA).

Immediately upon the expiration of this three-month period, Employer will pay Employee for all vacation time accrued up to that date. During this period, Employee may advise third parties that her status is presently that of an employee on a leave of absence. Employer agrees not to contest any claim that Employee may make for unemployment benefits after the expiration of this three month period unless Employee is fired for gross misconduct.

OPTION TO RENEW: If mutually agreed upon, this agreement shall be renewed for a period of one year upon the same terms except that the compensation to Employee shall be negotiable. Upon mutual agreement as to compensation for the additional period, a memorandum stating Employee's salary shall be attached and made a part of this agreement for the new period.

TRIAL PERIOD: The first three months shall be a trial period of employment, terminable at will by either party. In such event, the salary continuation period as outlined herein, shall not apply.

DUTIES: The Employee shall perform duties as a Dental Hygienist as required under her job classification in the Office Policy Manual.

FIGURE 16-1, cont'd
Employment agreement.
Continued

INCENTIVE SALARY INCREASE: A salary increase, as discussed in the yearly interview, will be reviewed annually.

PROPRIETARY RIGHTS: Employee agrees that any and all presently existing business of the Employer and any business developed by Employee or any other employee of the Employer including without limitation all patient's records, patient's lists, agreements and any other incident of any business developed, earned or carried on by Employee for Employer is and shall be the exclusive property of Employer.

IN WITNESS WHEREOF, the parties have signed this agreement on the date first above written.

VELMORE DENTAL ASSOCIATES, PA

By:_____
Dr. Bert Brown, President (Employer)

_____
Sarah Q. Nicholas (Employee)

FIGURE 16-1, cont'd
Employment agreement.

such as health insurance, he or she should consider a waiver of them in exchange for more money in the overall settlement. If there is a pension plan, be sure to check for the possibility of a lump-sum distribution and check rollover and withholding rules. If life insurance is provided, review a copy of the life insurance policy. Check to see if there are any conversion rights for the employee.

Other Considerations Upon Termination

Prior to employment, an employee should review how termination affects an employee's rights in regard to all benefits. More specifically, review what occurs upon termination with respect to savings plans, bonuses, accrued vacation, and accrued sick leave. Review the personnel or office manual for discussion of these items. Also, review federal and state laws as they apply to employment benefits.

INDEPENDENT CONTRACTORS

INDEPENDENT CONTRACTOR

An individual with special skills whom an employer hires sporadically, such as a consultant.

Businesses often hire **independent contractors** rather than employees to perform some of their work. The major difference between the two classifications is that an independent contractor, rather than an employer, has control over the outcome of the work product and the means of accomplishing the end product. The Internal Revenue Service investigates small businesses that it believes hire independent contractors to avoid withholding payroll taxes and providing other employee benefits. If an employee is mistakenly classified as an independent contractor, there can be serious legal problems and tax consequences. Should a potential employer suggest that you accept a position as an independent contractor, consult an attorney prior to agreeing to do so.

CONCLUSION

In the realm of employment as well as in other aspects of our lives, it is extremely important what our Constitution, legislatures, and judges say and do, as they determine how we conduct ourselves within and outside of the employment setting. What has been discussed in this chapter is a very small portion of a very large collection of statutes, rules, regulations, and case law relating to employment.

SUGGESTED READINGS

The following are publications available from the U.S. Government Printing Office, Washington, D.C.:

The Americans with Disabilities Act: Questions and Answers, Equal Employment Opportunity Commission and U.S. Department of Justice, Civil Rights Division, May 1997.

Baxter, N: Resumes, application forms, cover letters and interviews, *Occupational Outlook Quarterly*, Spring 1987, U.S. Department of Labor, Bureau of Labor Statistics.

How to File a Claim for Your Benefits, Pension and Welfare Benefits Administration, Division of Public Affairs, 1991.

OSHA: Employee Workplace Rights, U.S. Department of Labor, Occupational Safety and health Administration, 1997.

Social Security: Basic Facts, Social Security Administration, Publication No 05-10080, March 1998.

Social Security: What Every Woman Should Know, Social Security Administration, Publication No 05-10127, July 1997.

What You Should Know About Your Pension Rights, U.S. Department of Labor, Pension and Welfare Benefits Administration, 1995.

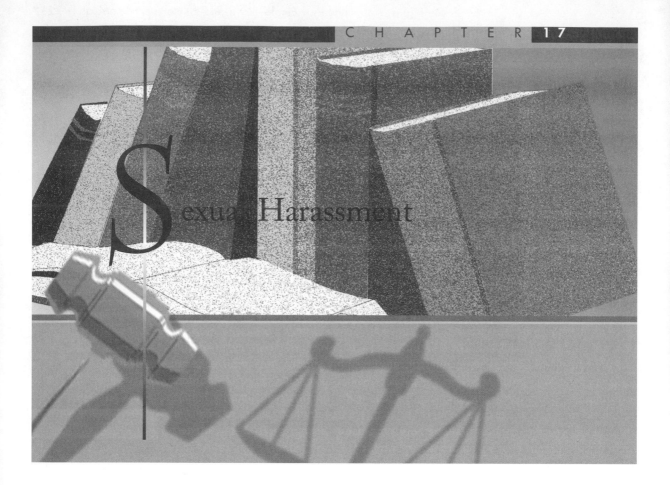

CHAPTER **17**

Sexual Harassment

LEARNING OUTCOMES

After reading this chapter, you should be able to:
- Recognize sexual harassment.
- Differentiate quid pro quo sexual harassment from hostile work environment sexual harassment.
- Discuss the responsibilities of employers when sexual harassment is occurring in the work place.
- Discuss the latest Supreme Court decision relating to same-sex sexual harassment.
- Discuss what action may be taken when a person believes that he or she is being sexually harassed in the work place.

KEY WORDS

BELLICOSE
CONSENSUAL
HARASSMENT
HUMAN RIGHTS STATUTE

PROTECTED GROUP
QUID PRO QUO
STATE FAIR EMPLOYMENT
STATUTE

What is sexual **harassment?** This is not a common question we ask ourselves, or others for that matter. Generally, we do know what it is when an incident happens to us, a family member, or a friend. Sexual harassment on the job can be of particular concern as much time is spent in the work place. Simply saying "no" or making a request to the offending person to stop the offensive behavior may fall on deaf ears. Tension between co-workers contributes to an environment that none of us wish to endure. If the boss is the underlying offender, matters are even worse. If our only source of economic security is at stake, there often seem to be no answers and there are few individuals who want to discuss the matter with us (except an attorney who is paid to listen). In this chapter we will explore what avenues are available to individuals who believe they are experiencing sexual harassment.

HARASSMENT
Words and/or actions designed to provoke another person.

ORIGINS OF SEX DISCRIMINATION LAW

Before 1980, there were no state or federal laws prohibiting sexual harassment in the work place. The original draft of the Civil Rights Act of 1964 did not include sex discrimination or age discrimination, and there was no intent to do so. Opponents of the civil rights legislation attached an amendment to the bill that included prohibiting sex discrimination, in addition to the prohibition of discrimination based on race, color, religion, or national origin. Age discrimination was prohibited by the Age Discrimination in Employment Act of 1967. The congressmen who opposed the Civil Rights Act believed that officially prohibiting sex discrimination would be so distasteful to their colleagues that the bill would fail to pass. They were wrong. However, no serious thought was given to that particular part of the legislation for several years. Originally, the Equal Employment Opportunity Commission took no action regarding sex discrimination and did not do so until women's organizations began to exert political pressure for protection in the work place.

Since sex discrimination was added to Title VII at the last minute on the floor of the House of Representatives and the bill quickly passed as amended, there was no legislative history to serve as a guide in interpreting the Act's prohibition against discrimination based on sex. Neither the courts nor the federal commission whose duty it was to write guidelines and regulations applicable to prohibiting sex discrimination in the work place had the usual guidance of the *Congressional Record* in making decisions and interpreting the law. The *Congressional Record* is the document that is generally used to interpret the intent of legislation.

DEFINING SEXUAL HARASSMENT

As mentioned in earlier chapters, Title VII of the Civil Rights Act of 1964 prohibits discrimination on the basis of sex in employment situations.[1] In 1980 the Equal Employment Opportunity Commission issued guidelines specifying that sexual harassment is a form of sex discrimination. Although these guidelines have no authority to control court decisions, they constitute a body of experience and informed judgment to which courts and parties to a lawsuit may look for guidance.[2]

---

[1]U.S.C. § 2000e-2(a)(1).
[2]*Griggs v. Duke Power Co.*, 401 U.S. 424 (1971).

The first U.S. Supreme Court decision to establish sexual harassment as a form of sex discrimination was *Meritor Savings Bank v. Vinson.*[3] Vinson was a bank employee whose supervisor constantly propositioned her, fondled her in front of other employees, followed her into the restroom, and forced her to have sex with him, among other acts. Two types of sexual harassment were identified in *Meritor*, quid pro quo sexual harassment and hostile work environment sexual harassment. Only employers can be held liable under either theory of sexual harassment. A supervisor or manager who has authority to hire and fire is also considered an employer, or more specifically an agent of the employer whose actions are deemed the actions of the employer by the authority the employer has given that supervisor or manager. A co-worker is not an employer's agent with the power to supervise and cannot be held liable under Title VII.[4] To hold an employer responsible for sexual harassment by a co-worker, one must prove that the employer knew about the harassment and did nothing to attempt to terminate the behavior.

Quid Pro Quo Sexual Harassment

Quid pro quo sexual harassment occurs when an employee is confronted with sexual demands to keep benefits, gain promotion, prevent demotion, or keep the job. In *Lipsett v. University of Puerto Rico*,[5] the court found quid pro quo sexual harassment when a "supervisor conditions the granting of an economic or other job benefit upon the receipt of sexual favors from a subordinate, or punishes that subordinate for refusing to comply." The plaintiff bears the burden of establishing a prima facie case of discrimination,[6] and a plaintiff claiming quid pro quo sexual harassment must meet a five-part test.[7] The plaintiff must show that:

1. The plaintiff-employee is in a protected group.
2. The sexual advances were unwelcome.
3. The harassment was sexually motivated.
4. The employee's reaction to the supervisor's advances affected a tangible aspect of his or her employment.
5. Respondeat superior liability has been established.

Protected Group

In defining who is in a **"protected group,"** Title VII protects both men and women from sexual harassment.[8] In a 1991 decision the court found in favor of two male employees against a company that allowed its male supervisor to force the men into various sexual activities with his secretary, with the threat of firing them if they refused.[9]

[3]477 U.S. 57 (1986).
[4]*Zabkowicz v. West Bend Co.*, 789 F.2d 540 (1986).
[5]864 F.2d 881 (1988).
[6]*Shumway v. United Parcel Service*, 118 F.3d 60 (1997).
[7]*Chamberlin v. 101 Realty, Inc.*, 915 F.2d 777 (1990).
[8]Henson v. *City of Dundee*, 682 F.2d 897 (1982).
[9]*Showalter v. Allison Reed Group, Inc.*, 767 F.Supp. 1205 (1991).

Unwelcome Sexual Advances

The question of unwelcomeness concerns whether sexual advances were uninvited and offensive or unwanted from the standpoint of the employee. In *Swentek v. U.S. Air, Inc.,*[10] the plaintiff's use of foul language or sexual innuendo in a **consensual** setting did not cause her legal protections against unwelcome harassment to be waived. A factor in determining whether sexual advances were unwelcome is the availability of an employer's sexual harassment policy and a viable grievance procedure. Failure to have a policy or a realistic mechanism for complaints would negate any claims on the part of the employer that advances were welcome because the employee failed to register a complaint.

CONSENSUAL
Characterized by mutual agreement of two parties.

The Supreme Court held in *Meritor*[11] that a plaintiff's sexually provocative speech or dress is relevant in determining whether he or she found particular sexual advances unwelcome.

Sexually Motivated Conduct

In many cases there is little question that the harassment of the plaintiff was sexually motivated. Hostile acts toward a woman or a man simply because of his or her sex is conduct that is sexually motivated. The court has found that "threatening, **bellicose,** demeaning, hostile or offensive conduct by a supervisor in the workplace because of the sex of the victim" was enough for a plaintiff to initiate litigation for sexual harassment.[12]

BELLICOSE
Belligerent or quarrelsome.

Tangible Aspects of the Job

Harassment must affect the plaintiff's compensation or the terms, conditions, or privileges of employment. Salary, benefits, promotions, hours of work, and so forth, are examples of compensation and terms, conditions, or privileges of employment.

Respondeat Superior

The doctrine of respondeat superior assigns liability to employers for acts of employees who are functioning within the scope of their employment. Employers are held strictly liable in cases of quid pro quo sexual harassment. *Meritor*[13] stated: "Where a supervisor exercises the authority actually delegated to him by his employer, by making or threatening to make decisions affecting the employment status of his subordinates, such actions are properly imputed to the employer whose delegation of authority empowered the supervisor to undertake them."

Hostile Work Environment Sexual Harassment

Hostile work environment sexual harassment occurs when "verbal or physical conduct of a sexual nature has the purpose or effect of creating an intimidating, hostile,

---

[10]830 F.2d 552 (1987).
[11]*Meritor,* supra.
[12]*Bell v. Crackin Good Bakers, Inc.,* 777 F2d 1497 (1985).
[13]*Meritor,* supra.

or offensive work environment."[14] In *Jordan v. Hodel*,[15] the Supreme Court concluded that to establish sexual harassment based on a hostile work environment, the plaintiff must show:

1. That he or she was subjected to sexual advances, requests for sexual favors, or other verbal or physical conduct of a sexual nature.
2. That the conduct was unwelcome.
3. That the conduct was sufficiently severe or pervasive to alter the conditions of the victim's employment and create an abusive working environment.

The court will determine whether a hostile work environment existed by examining both the subjective perception of the plaintiff and the standpoint of a reasonable person. The court will ask whether this particular plaintiff found the work environment hostile and also whether a reasonable person would find this particular work environment hostile. The offensive behavior must be sufficiently severe or pervasive to alter the conditions of employment and create an abusive working environment. The unwelcome conduct must be repeated and continuous rather than consist of isolated and occasional acts. "When the workplace is permeated with discriminatory intimidation, ridicule and insult that is sufficiently severe or pervasive to alter the conditions of the victim's employment and create an abusive working environment, Title VII is violated."[16]

DUTIES AND RESPONSIBILITIES OF EMPLOYERS

An employer is under a legal duty to take action to prevent or stop sexual harassment. An employer will be held responsible for sexual harassment if that employer or supervisor knew or should have known of the sexual harassment. Therefore, absence of notice does not necessarily protect an employer from liability for sexual harassment of an employee by a supervisor. An employer is liable for torts committed against one employee by another, regardless of whether they are committed in furtherance of the employer's business, that the employer could have prevented by reasonable care in hiring, supervising, or firing the offender.

In a 1988 case, three women who were members of a Iowa construction crew endured their male co-workers mooning them, fondling their body parts after cornering them between trucks, urinating in their water bottles, and constantly making lewd sexual comments to them. The women complained of the verbal abuse and the unwelcome physical touching to their supervisor. When both continued, they were forced to quit their jobs. They then brought court action against their former employer. The court found that the hostile and abusive working environment had resulted in the women's constructive discharge. Constructive discharge can occur when the sexual harassment is so unbearable that the employee is forced to resign, and the court considers this an illegal firing. In this case the court ordered the company to pay the women back pay, damages for emotional distress, and attorneys' fees.[17]

---

[14]29 C.F.R. § 1604.1 1(a).
[15]109 S. Ct. 786 (1991).
[16]*Harris v. Forklift Sys. Inc.*, 510 U.S. 17 (1993).
[17]*Hall v. Gus Construction Co., Inc.*, 842 F.2d 1010 (1988).

Employers may be liable not only for acts of other employees but also for acts of others, such as clients or patients. Should a patient make unwelcome sexual advances, request sexual favors, tell sexually explicit, demeaning jokes, comment inappropriately on your physical attributes, or perform other unwelcome acts or speak unwelcome words, ask the patient to stop the inappropriate behavior. If that does not put an end to the behavior, notify your employer or supervisor and have him or her intervene. It is the employer's duty to terminate the inappropriate behavior.

Employers attempt to use as a defense the fact that a plaintiff's sex-related conduct was voluntary or that the plaintiff was not forced to participate against his or her will. This defense was attempted in *Thorenson v. Penthouse Int'l, Ltd.*[18] Thorenson was a model who was coerced into having sex with several individuals affiliated with the company. The courts have held that the question is whether the sexual advances were unwelcome, not whether the individual's participation in sexual intercourse was voluntary.

Retaliation

Employers frequently retaliate against individuals who report sexual harassment by firing or otherwise penalizing them. Acts of retaliation are as illegal as sexual harassment, and the consequences of retaliation are the same as if the injuries had resulted from the sexual harassment.[19] For a plaintiff to demonstrate a claim of retaliation under Title VII, he or she must show that:

1. The plaintiff was engaged in an activity protected under Title VII.
2. The employer was aware of the plaintiff's participation in the protected activity.
3. The employer took adverse action against the plaintiff on the basis of his or her activity.
4. A causal connection existed between the plaintiff's protected activity and the adverse action taken by the employer.[20]

SAME-SEX SEXUAL HARASSMENT

In 1988, *Goluszek v. H.P. Smith*[21] held that claims for same-sex sexual harassment were not actionable unless the plaintiff could prove that the harasser was homosexual and thus presumably motivated by sexual desire. Therefore, when Joseph Oncale brought a lawsuit against his employer, Sundowner Offshore Services, Inc., in the United States District Court that alleged discrimination in the work place because of his sex, the District Court granted summary judgment for the employer, contending that the employee had no cause of action. Oncale took his case to the United States Supreme Court.[22] Oncale was employed as a roustabout on an eight-man oil platform crew. He alleged that he had been forcibly subjected to humiliating sex-related actions against him by some male co-workers in the presence of the rest of the crew on several occasions, that a male co-worker had physically as-

[18]563 N.Y.S. 968 (1990).
[19]*Monge* v. *Superior Court*, 176 Cal. App. 3d 503 (1986).
[20]*Cosgrove v. Sears, Roebuck & Co.*, 9 F.3d 1033 (1993).
[21]697 F. Supp. 1452 (1988).
[22]*Oncale v. Sundowner Offshore Services, Inc.*, 118 S. Ct. 998 (1998).

saulted him in a sexual manner and had threatened him with rape, and that after complaints to supervisory personnel had produced no remedial action, he quit his job in the fear that he would be forced to have sex.

The Supreme Court held that the intent of civil rights legislation was to strike at the entire spectrum of disparate treatment of men and women in employment and that harassing conduct need not be motivated by sexual desire to support an inference of employment discrimination on the basis of sex. The Court evaluated the work environment on the basis of conduct that a reasonable person in the plaintiff's position would find severely hostile or abusive, and found for the plaintiff. *Oncale* held that nothing in Title VII necessarily bars a claim of discrimination on the basis of sex merely because the plaintiff and the defendant (or the person acting on behalf of the defendant) are the same sex.

LEGAL ACTION FOR SEXUAL HARASSMENT

Title VII protects employees from discrimination and harassment. The Equal Employment Opportunity Commission investigates all claims of sexual harassment brought under Title VII. If an employee's sole goal is to stop the harassment, he or she can file a complaint with the EEOC. The employee can do so and keep his or her identity confidential by having someone file the claim on his or her behalf (e.g., an attorney, an agency, or a women's organization). The Commission has subpoena power and therefore has access to company records, as well as testimony of company personnel, to assist in an investigation. Remember that only employers can be held liable for sexual harassment under Title VII.

Title VII defines an employer as "a person engaged in an industry affecting commerce who has fifteen or more employees for each working day in each of twenty or more calendar weeks in the current or preceding calendar year, and any agent of such a person."[23] Because of the requirement of fifteen or more employees, Title VII is not applicable to most dental offices.

An individual who believes that he or she has been sexually harassed in the work place should report the harassment immediately and follow the employer's sexual harassment policy. If this step does not provide relief from the unwelcome situation, an individual may then wish to file a claim with the EEOC. If the employer is qualified under Title VII, the EEOC would first attempt to negotiate with the employer to assert the employee's rights. If the employer's behavior is egregious, the EEOC may file suit against the employer or issue a right-to-sue letter, in which case the individual would file a lawsuit to enforce his or her civil rights. The court can order the employer to: pay attorneys' fees, rehire a fired employee, provide back pay and/or benefits, grant a promotion, or award money damages if there has been a loss related to the sexual harassment. An order for injunctive relief may be issued by the court to prevent the employer from engaging in sexual harassment or to direct the employer to change company policies relating to sexual harassment. The court may stipulate one or any combination of these remedies when a plaintiff has suffered sexual harassment. The statute of limitations for filing a claim with the

[23]42 U. S. C. § 2000e(b).

EEOC depends upon the state of the employee's residence. Some states allow 180 days and others 300 days from the date on which the sexual harassment occurred. It is important to be advised of the correct period, as claims will not be acted upon if the limitations period has passed.

In determining where a claim should be filed, it is important to keep in mind that many state statutes do not permit money damages for personal injuries caused by sexual harassment. The Civil Rights Act permits $50,000 to $300,000 in damages (depending on the number of persons employed by the employer) for compensatory and punitive damages. Many states allow higher money damages than the federal statute. To file a lawsuit under federal law, one must file a claim with the EEOC. Many states require a like procedure. The EEOC will take a case to court on a claimant's behalf or issue a right-to-sue letter, which is required prior to the claimant's taking the case to court.

STATE FAIR EMPLOYMENT STATUTES

State **fair employment** or **human rights statutes** were written after the federal legislation. Almost every state has passed such statutes. However, there is no uniform applicable standard, and the content of these statutes varies widely from state to state. The federal law applies only to businesses with fifteen or more employees. If an employee works in a dental office with only five other employees, the federal law would provide no protection. The employee would have to look to his or her particular state statute for assistance. Some of the states, such as Illinois, South Carolina, Texas, Utah, Maryland, Arizona, Florida, Nebraska, Nevada, and Oklahoma, mirror the federal law and exclude employers of fewer than fifteen employees from their fair employment laws. Louisiana excludes employers with fewer than sixteen employees. Georgia's law applies only to state employees, and Alabama has no statute prohibiting sexual harassment in the work place. Some states, such as Indiana, California, Rhode Island, Idaho, and Connecticut, exclude employers who employ three to six employees, and others have no such exclusion. Many state agencies function in the same manner as the EEOC. Check to see what protection, if any, you are afforded under your state's fair employment statutes.

FILING A LAWSUIT BASED ON TORT LAW

If sexual harassment has caused serious injuries, you may want to consider filing a suit under tort law in state court. Torts vary from state to state. Many harassment claims will fit into suits for damages resulting from assault and battery, intentional infliction of emotional distress, interference with a contract, defamation, or wrongful discharge. (See Chapter 5 for discussion of intentional torts.)

A lawsuit for tort is not part of a court action under Title VII, nor would it be connected to state fair employment or human rights statutes. It is a private lawsuit, with the primary focus on collecting money damages from the perpetrator of the sexual harassment. In such cases the court cannot protect your job; therefore, you may want to file a lawsuit for tort if you are no longer interested in working for the particular employer who is the defendant to the lawsuit. If you are employed by a business with fewer than fifteen employees and neither Title VII nor your state

STATE FAIR EMPLOYMENT STATUTE

A state law that prohibits discrimination in the work place.

HUMAN RIGHTS STATUTE

A state law prohibiting discrimination, such as the Rhode Island Equal Opportunity and Affirmative Action Act (see Appendix G).

statute provides protection for your work setting, filing a tort action may be the only possible remedy. Since the statute of limitations is greater for tort actions, filing such an action may be appropriate if the statute of limitations has passed for state and federal sexual harassment claims.

Often local governments (cities and counties) have their own sexual harassment laws, which may offer better remedies than those of state or federal government. If you are seriously considering filing a claim for sexual harassment, discuss the matter with representatives of the EEOC, your state reporting agency, and your attorney to determine what action is best in your particular situation. Make your decision to go forward with a lawsuit only after you are fully informed and have had ample time to consider all of the ramifications. Lawsuits are time consuming and costly and often create considerable ill will among all individuals involved. The final outcome does not always produce the results intended.

SUGGESTED READINGS

Many organizations provide literature, videos, training, lawyer referrals, and many other services related to sexual harassment. The following are a few that will provide assistance.

American Civil Liberties Union
The ACLU has an office in each state.
Check the Internet to locate your state's office.
Internet: http://aclu.org

Institute for Women and Work
Cornell University
15 E. 26th Street, 4th Floor
New York, NY 10010

U.S. Department of Labor, Women's Bureau
200 Constitution Ave., NW
Washington, DC 20210

Women's Legal Defense Fund
1875 Connecticut Ave., NW, Suite 710
Washington, DC 20009

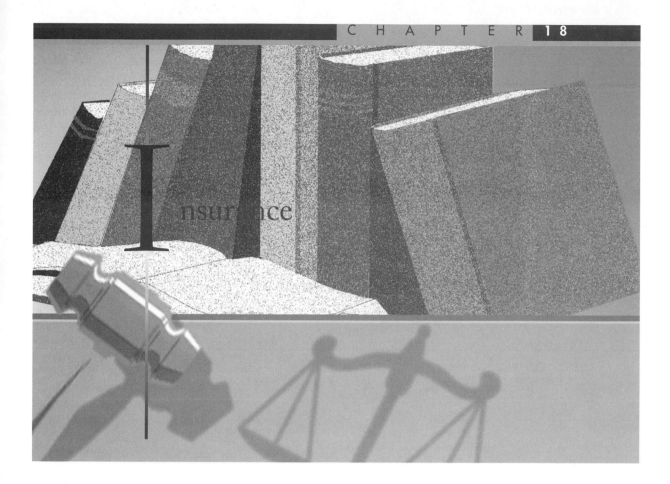

CHAPTER 18

Insurance

LEARNING OUTCOMES

After reading this chapter, you should be able to:

- Discuss the differences among the types of private health insurance (indemnity or reimbursement plans, health maintenance organizations, and preferred provider organizations).
- Describe medical savings accounts.
- Discuss employee rights protected by the Consolidated Omnibus Reconciliation Act.
- Discuss the need for disability insurance.
- Discuss term life, whole life, and universal life insurance policies and the differences between them.
- Discuss the need for malpractice insurance.
- Describe how federal insurance regulations affect the work place.

KEY WORDS

DISABILITY
HEALTH MAINTENANCE
  ORGANIZATION (HMO)
INDEMNITY PLAN
INSURANCE

MALPRACTICE
PREFERRED PROVIDER
  ORGANIZATION (PPO)
REIMBURSEMENT PLAN

Insurance is a legal form of gambling. Just as there are many forms of gambling—poker, lottery, slot machines, betting on sporting events—so, too, are there many forms of insurance: life, accident, health, liability, collision, and homeowner's, to name a few. When you buy health insurance, you, as the insured, are betting that you will contract an illness or have an accident, and the insurer is betting that you won't or that if you do, the premiums you pay will exceed your needs. Similarly, an individual's winnings from gambling rarely exceed the total amount of money spent on gambling. Actually, **insurance** is "a contract whereby, for a stipulated consideration, one party undertakes to compensate the other for loss on a specified subject by specified perils."[1]

> **INSURANCE**
>
> A written contract (policy) whereby an insured pays a stipulated sum (premium) to an insurer, who agrees to compensate the insured for losses relating to the subject matter of the policy.

Often employers provide various types of insurance as a benefits package that is offered to all employees. Some employers offer cafeteria plans. In such a plan, an employee can choose from a menu of benefits. An employer might provide a specific monthly allowance for these benefits, and any amount over the allowance would be the financial responsibility of the employee and most often would be treated as a payroll deduction. Any unused amount would be added to the employee's pay. Some types of insurance are required by law, and it is the responsibility of the employer to cover the financial costs (e.g., workers' compensation insurance). Many types that are not required, such as health and dental insurance, term life insurance, and pension plans, are tax deductible for employers. This chapter is designed to provide an overview of the common types of insurance that employers make available to their employees.

Private insurance is regulated by individual states. States charter insurance companies and license insurance agents. States oversee the financial status of insurers. There are minimum requirements for financial reserves and allowable investments. States require annual statements and conduct periodic examinations of insurers. Most states require that policy forms be filed and approved prior to utilization. The state insurance commission investigates consumer complaints. States can mandate that certain services be covered. They also can mandate that specific practitioners be paid for their services (if the same services are provided by a physician). For example, a state may mandate that insurance coverage applies to a nurse practitioner who provides services traditionally provided by a physician. If an insurance policy does not cover a specific mandated service, the policy may be reformed to reflect the coverage.[2]

HEALTH INSURANCE

One hundred eighty-six million Americans were covered by some form of private health insurance in 1995 (40.5 million were not). That same year, private health insurance paid $276.8 billion for health care. The 1995 per capita expenditure for health care was $3,621, and the total national expenditure for health care was $988.5 billion.[3]

---

[1]*Black's Law Dictionary*, ed 5, St Paul, 1979, West Publishing Co.
[2]*Di Pascal v. New York Life Ins. Co.*, 749 F.2d 255 (1985).
[3]Health Insurance Association of America: *Source book of health insurance data*, Washington, DC, 1997-1998.

Many employers provide health insurance, as the expense of obtaining an individual policy is often prohibitive, whether one person is being insured or an entire family. An employer is not legally required to provide health insurance to employees, and many small businesses do not offer health insurance as a fringe benefit. Group plans that are available to employers reduce the cost, whether the employer pays all of the premium, a portion of the premium, or none of the premium.

Health care plans vary. Generally, a plan is either an **indemnity,** or **reimbursement, plan** or a managed care plan, such as a **health maintenance organization (HMO),** a **preferred provider organization (PPO),** or a point-of-service plan. Indemnity or reimbursement plans either pay the health care facility or the physician directly or reimburse the policyholder for his or her out-of-pocket expenses for procedures covered by the policy. Often there is a deductible that the insured must pay on an annual basis before the insurer will cover any expenses. The deductible is usually $100 to $300 for individuals and $500 for families. The higher the deductible, the lower the cost of the plan. Generally, there is also a co-payment; therefore, the individual covered would be required to pay a portion of the fee (usually 20%). The insurance coverage is usually limited to a maximum amount over the lifetime of the insured. Many times individuals have expectations regarding insurance reimbursements that exceed the amount actually paid by the insurance company. Most insurance companies pay the "usual, customary, and reasonable fee" (UCR) for medical expenses, including supplies and services, incurred as a result of an injury, sickness, or pregnancy while the insured is covered under the plan. Medical services that are considered experimental, investigative, developmental, or educational are usually not considered necessary medical expenses.. The reimbursement is frequently an amount that is lower than the actual fee charged for the services an individual received.

Examine a typical situation. Assume that an individual required minor, outpatient surgery that is performed in the physician's office. The physician's fee for the service is $670. The insurance policy covering this patient has a $200 deductible and a co-payment of 20%. The usual and customary fee for the procedure is $580. To date the patient has not used this policy and now submits a claim (the physician's statement for $670) to the insurance company. The patient is aware of the co-payment ($134) and the deductible ($200), and therefore expects the insurance to pay a benefit of $336. However, a different result occurs. The usual and customary fee is $580, with the $134 co-payment and the $200 deductible. The actual benefit received is now $146 for this $670 procedure. Quite a different result! In addition, if the particular service performed was not one specified in the policy and no coverage was available, this person could find himself or herself with $670 in out-of-pocket medical expenses.

An HMO is an entity (usually made up of doctors and hospitals) that provides health care services to patients who are enrolled members, for a fixed monthly per capita fee. An HMO is both a provider and an insurer of medical services. HMOs are regulated by both state and federal statutes. Covered employees must use the HMO services, unless an emergency occurs and the HMO grants permission to utilize other emergency care.

INDEMNITY PLAN (or REIMBURSEMENT PLAN)

A contract that secures a person against unanticipated loss—for instance, an insurance plan that pays health care providers and health care facilities for services rendered or pays the patient directly for out-of-pocket medical expenses for procedures that are covered under the plan.

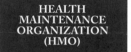

HEALTH MAINTENANCE ORGANIZATION (HMO)

An organization providing health care services for enrolled members, who pay a fixed monthly fee.

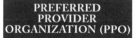

PREFERRED PROVIDER ORGANIZATION (PPO)

An organization of health care providers (doctors, hospitals, dentists, etc.). Members of a PPO discount their fees for services to subscribers.

A PPO is a network of health care providers who agree to provide services for specified fees. PPO subscribers are not limited to using health care providers or facilities with plan contracts. However, utilization of nonpreferred providers can mean higher deductibles and/or co-payments. PPOs are often administered by an insurance company, which services the claims process. A POS plan is similar to a PPO, except that a primary care physician coordinates referrals. PPOs and POSs have more flexibility on referrals outside of the plan, and a patient is partially reimbursed if he or she sees a nonparticipating provider. In a 1997 survey, the average cost per employee for an indemnity, or reimbursement, plan was $6,033. The cost of coverage under managed care was $5,325 for PPOs, $5,572 for POSs, and $5,157 for HMOs.[4]

Medical Savings Accounts

It is often financially difficult for small businesses to provide employees with health care coverage. In 1996, the Health Insurance Portability and Accountability Act was signed into law. This act created Medical Savings Accounts (MSA). These accounts are designed to be utilized by employers with 50 or fewer employees or by self-employed individuals. MSAs are intended to pay out-of-pocket medical expenses, such as for office visits, prescription drugs, eyeglasses, and dental care. To receive favorable federal tax treatment, an MSA must be used in conjunction with a qualified, high-deductible, catastrophic health plan. Selected insurance companies offer such plans. Once an individual has a catastrophic health plan, he or she may make tax-free contributions each year to his or her MSA (to 65% of the deductible for an individual and 75% for families). Medical expenses not covered under the medical plan may be reimbursed with pre-tax dollars from the employee's MSA funds. IRS regulations apply. Publication 502, Medical and Dental Expenses, explains the regulations. Unused MSA funds can be rolled over into subsequent years. Funds not used earn tax-free income. If these funds are used for nonmedical items, they are subject to taxes and a penalty. However, at age 65 one can withdraw the balance of the account for nonmedical use and without a penalty. The deductible for the catastrophic plan must be $1,500 to $2,250 for individuals and $3,000 to $4,500 for families. Co-payments are not to exceed $3,000 for individuals and $5,500 for families. These amounts are to be indexed for inflation after January 1, 1999.

Consolidated Omnibus Reconciliation Act of 1985

Since most health insurance is provided by employers, the federal government enacted the Consolidated Omnibus Reconciliation Act of 1985 (COBRA) in an effort to protect the availability of health care to individuals and families. Under COBRA, employers with group health plans must offer employees the opportunity to continue their health insurance benefits at their own expense if the employees would otherwise lose such coverage after termination of employment or reduction in hours. Termination must not be for gross misconduct. In addition, covered

[4]*Source book of health insurance data,* supra.

spouses or dependents who would lose coverage either for the above reasons or because of the employee's death, divorce, or legal separation, the employee's becoming entitled to Medicare benefits, a change in dependent status, or the employer's becoming bankrupt may elect continuation of coverage.

All covered employees and their spouses must receive a written notice of their COBRA rights at the time coverage begins under a group health plan and at the time of termination of employment. If an employee marries or remarries after receiving initial notice, a notice must be given to the new spouse. Failure to meet notice requirements leaves an employer liable for uninsured medical expenses incurred by the employee or the employee's dependent.

COBRA covers group health plans maintained by employers with 20 or more employees in the prior year. COBRA beneficiaries are eligible to pay for group coverage during a maximum of 18 months. A specific plan may establish longer periods of coverage beyond those required by COBRA.

DISABILITY INSURANCE

A **disability** is an impairment that keeps an individual from working for a prolonged period of time. Should you gamble on becoming disabled? The National Underwriters' Corporation finds that the risk of a permanent disability (one lasting for more than 90 days or for a prolonged and indefinite time) during a normal working lifetime is greater than the probability of death during that time. It is estimated that one in three people between the ages of 35 and 65 will suffer long-term disability (more than 90 days) during his or her working life. This type of insurance is often overlooked and is an important protection for the dental health provider, who is at high risk for work-related injuries. If you depend on your earned income, you need disability protection. Disability insurance should cover the difference between your monthly expenses and other sources of income you would have while you were disabled. If an employer pays the premium for employee coverage for disability insurance, the amount of the premium is tax deductible for the employer. If an employee receives payments under an employer paid policy, the employee will owe income tax on the payments.

> **DISABILITY**
>
> A condition that incapacitates an individual in some manner; an impairment that renders a person unable to work for an extended period of time.

The definition of disability under the social security law[5] is different from that used in most private disability insurance policies. A denial of a claim by social security will not necessarily result in a denial by a private insurance carrier. The private insurance carrier may assist in an appeal of the social security denial, as social security disability payments are an offset under the private policy. Be familiar with the specific plan and how "disability" is defined.

LIFE INSURANCE

Life insurance is widely used as a protection against heavy financial burdens created by the premature death of the primary wage earner. Life insurance also offers tax incentives that assist in funding retirement or other goals. Life insurance is a commonly offered benefit in the form of employer-sponsored group plans and indi-

---

[5] 42 U.S.C. § 423(d)(1)(A).

vidual policies. Employer-sponsored group plans include group term life insurance, wholesale life insurance, and salary savings life insurance. An employer can deduct the premiums paid for each employee for up to $50,000 of group term life insurance. Employees do not pay taxes on premiums an employer pays on their behalf for group term life insurance.

Individual policies are issued to individuals, who may designate specific beneficiaries. Benefits are available in various amounts to meet individual needs. Types include term life, whole life, and universal life policies. Term life insurance provides protection for a specific period of time. If during this specified period of time the policyholder dies, the face amount of the policy is paid to the beneficiary. If death does not occur, no payment is made. Term insurance is best when the need for protection does not exist for a lengthy period of time, the need is temporary, or lowering costs is essential. Whole life insurance protects a family for the lifetime of the insured. An individual can pay for a whole life policy in a lump sum, by making payments for a limited period of time (e.g., 10 to 30 years), or by making payments that are spread out over a lifetime. Whole life insurance provides permanent benefits, and the policy accumulates a cash value as the premiums paid are compounded with interest. The policy may be surrendered in part or whole, in which case the cash value is paid to the policyholder. Universal life insurance is whole life insurance that allows flexibility in the amount of protection, the length of coverage, and the size and frequency of premiums throughout the insured's lifetime. The cash value of the policy can increased by the policyholder's paying extra premiums or adding funds. As with whole life insurance, the cash value earns interest on a tax-deferred basis.

With whole life or universal life insurance, the cash value can be withdrawn or borrowed against, according to the contract, and the policy remains in force. Death benefits from all types of life insurance are income tax free to the beneficiary.

MALPRACTICE INSURANCE

MALPRACTICE

Failure of a professional to exercise reasonable care, which results in harm to another; negligent conduct by professional individuals or a breach of a standard of care.

An individual **malpractice** insurance policy is, generally, not a benefit that an employer purchases for an employee. Employees are usually informed that the doctor's malpractice insurance covers employees and that, therefore, they should not concern themselves with additional coverage. This is not legally sound advice. Should a patient sue you as a dental health care provider, he or she would probably also sue the doctor. There could be many conflicts of interest involved in defending you against such a suit. The insurance company would look after its interest first and the dentist's second; you would be third in line. (Malpractice insurance policies often have a subrogation clause, which would mean that if the company paid a claim on behalf of the employer/dentist and you, as an employee, were at fault, the insurance company would then be able to sue you for the amount paid.) A policy that would pay for all court costs, all settlements and court judgments, and all legal defense costs, with a $1,000,000 cap per incident and a $3,000,000 cap per year, would cost a dental hygienist or a dental assistant less than $100 per year, which would be a small price to pay considering the growing number of lawsuits against health professionals.

FEDERAL INSURANCE REGULATION

As mentioned earlier, no federal law requires an employer to provide health insurance as an employment benefit. However, federal requirements apply should an employer's choice of benefits include health insurance. Title VII of the 1964 Civil Rights Act prohibits discrimination in the work place with regard to "compensation, terms, conditions or privileges of employment" on the basis of an individual's sex, race, color, religious beliefs, national origin, age, or physical disability. The Pregnancy Discrimination Act of 1978 defines sex discrimination to include treatment of pregnancy, childbirth, or related medical conditions differently from other medical conditions under fringe benefit programs. If an employer offers a choice of several health plans, maternity and related benefits must be offered under all plans. Maternity-related medical conditions must be treated in the same as any other medical condition with respect to reimbursement (including maximum payments), deductibles, co-payments, coinsurance, out-of-pocket maximums, and preexisting condition limitations. In addition, dependent female spouses of employees must be treated the same as female employees.[6]

---

[6]*Newport News Shipbuilding & Dry Dock v. EEOC,* 103 S. Ct. 2622 (1983).

AUTHOR'S CASE STUDY COMMENTS

Reread Case Study and Study Questions for Section V.
Questions 1 through 8 are examined in the following analysis:

1. May the advertisers who submitted the advertisements for a dental assistant to the classified section of the newspaper find themselves with any legal problems? If so, what are the problems?

All advertisers may run into legal problems. Title VII protects individuals from being discriminated against in the work place on the basis of their race, color, national origin, age, religion, sex, or disability. All qualified applicants should receive equal consideration. All qualifications stated in an advertisement should be job related. In the first advertisement, Oakbrook Dental requested a photo. Most of the time a photo would reveal an individual's sex, race, color, and perhaps disability. The advertisement also specifically stated that Oakbrook was looking for a female, a criterion that is not job related. Oakbrook would have a difficult time defending its requests in a court of law. The second advertisement requests a "girl Friday," who must be married. Both criteria are illegal. Although most job benefits, such as health insurance, retirement plans, and uniform allowances, are not mandatory, there are several areas that are mandatory. For instance, an employer must pay into a worker's compensation fund and pay an unemployment insurance tax. An employer may not refuse to reinstate an employee because of pregnancy or childbirth. In addition, there are many benefits that must be offered to all employees if some have them. It seems that this doctor has no other employees. The third advertisement requests a nonsmoker and nondrinker with no history of drug abuse and no criminal record. There would be a need to show a job-related reason for all of these requests. An inquiry about a history of drug abuse would not be a legal request if the person were rehabilitated and there were no convictions on record.

2. Did Dr. Brown and Dr. Douglas violate any laws? If so, explain.

Dr. Brown and Dr. Douglas committed violations in their employment application. An applicant may not be asked for birth date, marital status, or record of arrests, and he or she may not be asked any of the questions relating to medical history. There can be no discrimination regarding individuals with disabilities or women who are pregnant. Dr. Brown and Dr. Douglas are within their legal rights to include the last two sentences of the application. Take note that the job must be offered to the applicant prior to any testing. Also, the testing would need to be job related.

3. Did Dr. Anderson violate any laws? If so, explain.

Dr. Anderson is in violation of OSHA standards, which should be a major consideration in any applicant's decision to accept a job. Dr. Anderson requested information relating to Ms. Jenret's religion, a clearly illegal criterion upon which to hire an individual.

AUTHOR'S CASE STUDY COMMENTS—cont'd

4. Did the office manager at Oakbrook Dental violate any laws? If so, what are his defenses?

Sexual harassment in the work place is illegal. This includes behavior such as obscene gestures and comments, unwelcome sexual remarks, sexual touching, and promises of promotion or a job for sex. By law if a manager engages in these types of behavior, the employer is responsible for the manager's acts, even if the employer did not know of the behavior. If the behavior is by a co-worker, the employer is responsible if the harassing behavior was reported to the employer and nothing was done to stop the sexual harassment. The office manager will no doubt claim that the sex was consensual as his defense. This will not provide a good defense. The courts have held that if there is intimidation, sex is not consensual. The office manager has committed sexual harassment.

5. Does Ms. Taylor have a claim against Oakbrook Dental?

As stated in the previous question, in regard to sexual harassment, illegal acts performed by a manager are attributable to the employer. The office manager engaged in quid pro quo harassment with Ms. Taylor; Oakbrook is, therefore, liable for the acts of its manager, even if Dr. Dennis, the owner, knew nothing of the manager's activities.

6. Did Dr. Dennis violate any laws? If so what are they and what are his defenses?

Dr. Dennis is also guilty of quid pro quo sexual harassment. He asked Ms. Jenret if she wanted to keep her job prior to propositioning her. His defense will also no doubt be that the sex was consensual. Again, this will not stand as a defense, as intimidation was part of the offer. Dr. Dennis has violated Title VII of the Civil Rights Act.

7. Does Ms. Jenret have a claim against Oakbrook Dental?

Ms. Jenret and Ms. Taylor have claims against Oakbrook Dental. Dr. Dennis' complaints regarding Ms. Jenret's job performance are obviously retaliation resulting from her rejection of his continued advances. Oakbrook employs more than fifteen people; therefore, the federal law would apply. Both women should visit their attorneys and ascertain whether their remedies are better under federal law or state law. If Oakbrook were found responsible for sexual harassment in the work place, Ms. Jenret and Ms. Taylor would be entitled to receive moneys for lost wages, emotional and physical damages, attorneys' fees, and punitive damages, and job reinstatement. Job reinstatement is not always the request of a plaintiff, for obvious reasons. Under the federal Civil Rights Act an employer who employs 15 to 100 people may be liable for up to $50,000 for compensatory and punitive damages. The $50,000 does not include back wages or out-of-pocket expenses such as medical bills. In this case, if Ms. Taylor files a sexual harassment lawsuit against Oakbrook under the Civil

AUTHOR'S CASE STUDY COMMENTS—cont'd

Rights Act and a jury awards her $25,000 for her medical expenses, $5,000 for back wages, $150,000 for pain and suffering, and $100,000 in punitive damages, the judge will reduce the award to an amount allowable under the law. Ms. Taylor will receive the $25,000 for medical expenses and the $5,000 for back wages, but the other $250,000 will be reduced to $50,000. Therefore, the maximum she could receive is $80,000.

It is important that both women obtain legal advice as soon as possible, as a case must be brought within six months of the last occurrence of harassment, which may be at the time of the termination of employment.

8. Do any other employees have a claim against Oakbrook Dental?

In this situation the office manager was apparently making sexual advances toward multiple employees. Sexual harassment claims can arise when sexual advances are made to two or more employees with differing results. Here, the manager gave a promotion (higher salary and a title) to a woman because she had sex with him. If he denied a promotion to another employee because she would not have sex with him, she too has experienced unwelcome sexual conduct that is classified as sexual harassment. The employee would have a sexual harassment claim based upon the improper denial of her promotion by a person in authority in a quid pro quo situation. Ms. Taylor would also have a claim if the sexual advances were unwelcome and she submitted only out of fear of losing the promotion or job. If the manager has a consensual affair with one employee and gives her promotions, raises, and so forth, in preference to another employee, he is sexually abusing both employees. While the manager is searching for the employee who will agree to his sexual requests, he is harassing the employees who refuse his advances.

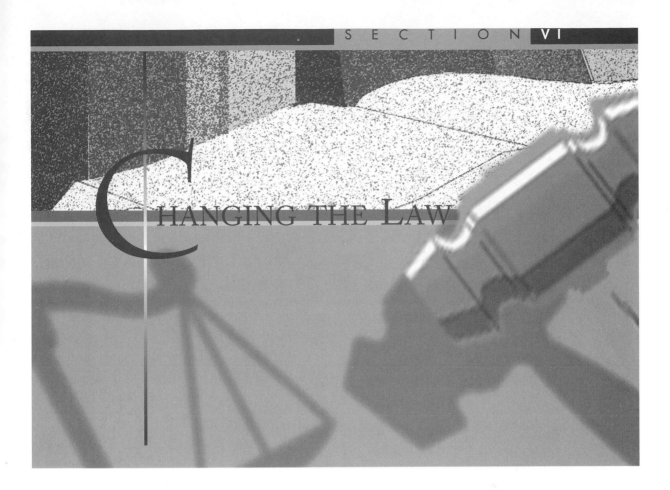

CHANGING THE LAW

SECTION OUTLINE

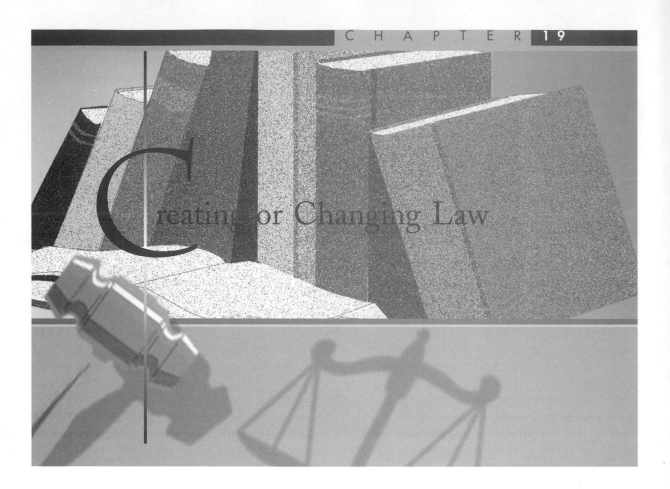

CHAPTER 19

Creating or Changing Law

LEARNING OUTCOMES

After reading this chapter, you should be able to:

- Assist in changing or creating law.
- Identify the steps that legislation must pass through before becoming a law.
- Discuss how the court system assists in changing laws.
- List future issues that need to be considered by dental professionals as new laws are created and outdated laws are revised.

KEY WORDS

ADJUDICATE
BILL
CHAMBER

LITIGATION
LOBBYIST

At this point you have read a substantial amount of material regarding the law, how it affects health care and dental care, and, more specifically, how it affects the dental professions. You have read of how certain ethical issues become involved in **litigation** and are **adjudicated** through the judicial system. Also, ethical issues are raised in federal and state legislatures, and statutes are enacted as a result. You have seen how case law and statutes provide guidelines for our professional actions. Many of these guidelines are helpful and provide a sound basis for decisions we need to make regarding our professional conduct. But what if a statute or case law appears terribly wrong to us? Change may be the solution, and perhaps change will be inevitable. As a dental health care professional, you have an obligation to your patients, your colleagues, and yourselves to assist in these changes. It is the only means by which all perspectives will be considered.

FEDERAL LEGISLATION

There is no federal right to health care under the United States Constitution. Although the federal government has no duty to provide health care, the federal government is involved in meeting the health care needs of the population by funding benefit programs that assist people who lack health care insurance or other means of paying for health care. Therefore, the federal government is directly involved in the health of the nation through the passage of statutes by Congress. Likewise, the states are involved through the passage of laws by their legislatures. The introduction of a **bill,** often referred to as a resolution, in the U.S. Senate or the U.S. House of Representatives, is done by a member of Congress. Legislation may be drafted by private organizations or by the President (Executive Branch) and introduced by a member of Congress. A proposed bill is assigned a number (e.g., HR-157 or S-296, which would mean the 157th bill introduced in the House during the session and the 296th bill introduced in the Senate). It is then sent to the appropriate committee for review, study, and public hearings. If the resolution is approved by the committee, it is then reported favorably to the full House or Senate, where it is placed on the docket (calendar) for floor action. There is no requirement that a House or Senate committee act on all bills referred to it. There is no time limit within which it must report out a bill. If a bill passes in the House or the Senate, it is forwarded to the other **chamber** for similar action. If there are differences between the resolutions passed by both chambers, the bill is sent to a conference committee. The conference committee is composed of senior members of both House and Senate committees. Once the conference committee arrives at an agreement, a conference report is voted on by both chambers. If both chambers approve, the bill is then forwarded to the President for his signature, indicating approval. If the President refuses to sign, he has by his refusal vetoed the legislation. A two-thirds vote of Congress would be required to override the veto and enact the bill into law. Once the President signs the legislation, it becomes law. Many bills are introduced at each session of Congress, but relatively few become law. Once a bill becomes law, it is assigned a number indicating the particular Congress that passed it. For instance, Public Law 93-247 indicates that this law is the 247th law passed by the 93rd Congress. Public Law 93-247 is the Child Abuse Prevention and Treatment Act.

LITIGATION
A lawsuit; court proceedings to determine legal issues regarding the rights and responsibilities between parties.

ADJUDICATE
To make a final determination of issues through court action.

BILL
A federal or state proposed law that is introduced in a legislative body for approval. Should a bill pass in the legislative body and be signed by the appropriate executive officer, it becomes a law.

CHAMBER
Normally state legislative bodies have two chambers, as does the federal legislature. The United States Congress is made up of the Senate and the House of Representatives. Nebraska is an exception; its legislative body is referred to as unicameral, as it consists of only one chamber.

Subsequently, laws are published in what is known as "Statutes at Large" and finally are incorporated into the United States Code. Laws are usually referred to by their formal names, such as the Family and Medical Leave Act or the Age Discrimination in Employment Act. Quite frequently, a law eventually becomes known by the names of its chief congressional sponsors. For example, although PL 79-725 is formally known as "An Act to amend the Public Health Service, to authorize grants to states for surveying their hospitals and public health centers and for planning construction of additional facilities," it is generally referred to as the Hill-Burton Act, after its sponsors, Senators Lester Hill and Harold Burton. This legislation, enacted in 1945, provided federal financing for the construction and expansion of hospitals and other health care facilities. The statute requires that the state provide adequate hospitals for all individuals within the state and provide services for those who are unable to pay for those services. Thus, facilities that applied for and received federal funding acquired two legal obligations by doing so. First, the "community service obligation" represents the duty to make all reasonably affordable services available to all persons in the geographical area. Second, the "uncompensated care obligation" requires that a reasonable amount of services be provided to the indigent. These duties continue indefinitely. Most hospitals and health-related institutions receive federal financial assistance through the Hill-Burton Act and the Medicare and Medicaid programs. Therefore, Congress may change laws or the agencies that administer a specific law, may change the regulations, and in either situation dramatically affect public policy as it relates to health care, just as the Hill-Burton Act expanded the availability of health care.

After a law has been passed, it must then be submitted to the Appropriations Committee of Congress; the Committee will then vote to approve or disapprove funding for the new law. Therefore, a bill may be passed by both the House and the Senate and be signed by the President, but never be enforced should the Appropriations Committee refuse to fund the legislation.

STATE LEGISLATION

On the state level, bills are introduced in the legislature basically in the same manner as on the federal level, although the exact procedures for enacting laws in each state vary. In addition, many states have provisions whereby a petition to enact a certain law may be presented to the legislature. Generally, such a petition would have to contain signatures of registered voters equal to 10% of the number of people who voted in the last gubernatorial election. For example, if 520,000 people voted in the last election for governor, then the petitions must contain 52,000 signatures of registered voters. The signatures on these petitions are then verified by the Secretary of State. Once the petitions meet the statutory requirement, the proposed bill must appear on the ballot for the next state election, to be voted on by the electorate (referendum).

LOBBYIST

An individual who is hired by various organizations to induce legislators to vote for or against specific bills pending before the legislature.

Private organizations and special interest groups petition legislators to sponsor numerous state and federal resolutions. In this regard, **lobbyists** play a major role in urging legislators to initiate legislation. Most large professional organizations, such as the American Medical Association, the American Dental Hygienists' Association, and the American Association of Dental Schools, hire lobbyists. A lobbyist is a person who is skilled in presenting a client's views to legislators and those of legislators to the client. A lobbyist is an accessible and knowledgeable resource to legislators on issues involving a particular profession. Lobbyists are often attorneys or former legislators. A former legislator knows the process and the people, and can be an excellent choice as a lobbyist. An attorney will often have developed an area of expertise (e.g., health care) and will concentrate on issues related to that specific area.

REGULATIONS

Quite often, the language of the laws enacted is very general and broad in scope. The specific details of the various laws enacted remain to be spelled out in regulations (often referred to as "rules and regulations"). At the federal level, this function is performed by the various administrative agencies of the Executive Branch. For instance, the Department of Health and Human Services promulgates regulations for the Hill-Burton Act.

Once the process of establishing rules and regulations is complete, federal laws are published in the *Federal Register* and are effective thirty days after publication. They are then incorporated into the Code of Federal Regulations and have the force of law.

CHANGING THE LAW

Our lives are affected daily by the laws, rules and regulations, guidelines, and so forth, adopted by Congress, state legislatures, and federal, state, and local administrative agencies. It is only natural that we feel compelled to exert control over these institutions, which influence our political, economic, and social lives. Our form of government permits and encourages us to challenge laws and regulations that we deem unfair. Some people are reluctant to attempt to change laws or regulations out of fear of offending employers, family, or friends. Large numbers of health care professionals are faced with choosing to assert their rights or to accept the status quo. Many believe that changes in laws or regulations that affect the manner in which they perform their jobs should be left to the political experts. But who are the experts? Members of health professions are the experts in their respective fields.

There are basic issues that affect all health professionals. We regularly research, discuss, and write about employment trends, access to health care, safety in the work place, and economic fairness. However, there exists an insurmountable imbalance of power and economic resources that prevents adequate representation in the decision-making process in regard to fundamental issues in our professional lives. As professional organizations become larger, they increase their political activity by sponsoring training programs, legislative campaigns, fund raising, and research activities, forming political action committees (PACs), and hiring lobbyists.

LITIGATION

We have read how civil litigation is utilized to settle disputes between two individuals or entities and how criminal litigation is used to protect the rights of an individual or to establish an individual's guilt beyond a reasonable doubt. Litigation is also utilized to change laws or interpretations of laws. Individuals wishing to make changes in the legal system file lawsuits as 'test cases' to accomplish such ends. Often, if a desired result is not achieved by court action, the individual or entity attempting to effect a different outcome will turn to the legislature.

CHANGES RELATING TO DENTAL HYGIENE

The American Dental Hygienists' Association has a Governmental Affairs Division to carry out directives of the membership to make specific changes in the status quo. It often becomes necessary to create relationships with appropriate state or federal agencies to facilitate working within the legislative process. Should the desired legislation be focused within a specific state or states, it would be important to communicate the underlying reasons for the recommended changes to the governor or governors. Remember, it is the governor who has the final approval once a bill has passed in any state legislature, unless a legislature overrides a governor's veto. In the 1970s dental hygienists resolved that their legislative goal was to amend various dental practice acts to allow dental hygienists to administer local anesthesia. At the time only a few states permitted administration of local anesthesia as an expanded function for dental hygienists. Many of these initiatives were successful, and now it is legal in approximately half of the states for a dental hygienist to administer local anesthesia. Today the emphasis is on dental hygiene self-regulation. Changing the state dental practice acts to permit dental hygienists to regulate their licensure and education and to have an effect on issues relating to scope of practice would give them rights similar to ones that hundreds of other professionals, such as nurses, physical therapists, dietitians, cosmetologists, and real estate brokers, presently enjoy. Currently, the state dental boards are composed of dentists; there is very little representation by dental hygienists and little or no representation by dental assistants.

CHANGES RELATING TO DENTAL ASSISTING

The critical issues for dental assistants are education and credentialing. Unlike dental hygienists, dental assistants have self-regulation of their education and certification process. However, in the majority of state dental practice acts, there is no requirement that a dental assistant be educated, certified, or licensed. A major barrier to changes in the rules and regulations of state dental practice acts in regard to education and/or certification that faces the American Dental Assisting Association is largely a situation of supply and demand. There are 27,000 certified dental assistants throughout the United States. However, this does not even come close to supplying the number needed for the existing positions available. Therefore, the majority of dental assistants receive on-the-job training in lieu of a professional education. Obviously, one critical issue is pay. It stands to reason that those with the greater educational level should receive higher pay. Dental assistants have two very persuasive arguments in their favor that support education and credentialing. First, a qualified dental assistant can increase a dentist's productivity dramatically. Studies indicate that one full-time dental assistant can enable a dentist to provide up to 63% more dental treatment. Second, hiring a qualified dental assistant can reduce the costs associated with the hiring and training process that occurs each time an unqualified individual is hired and remains an employee for only a short period of time. The challenges are numerous. There are laws to be amended, educational programs to be initiated, and procedures to be developed to enable qualified dental assistants who were trained on-the-job to obtain appropriate credentials.

CHANGES RELATING TO ALL DENTAL PROFESSIONALS

As dental professionals, we can naturally expect many changes in the manner in which we accomplish our various roles within the dental office. Two topics require our immediate attention, as they relate to issues presently identified as risks to the dental health care provider. The first is the growing number of dental health care providers (and patients) with latex allergies. These allergies are generally associated with three responses to the latex: contact dermatitis (rash, itching, cracking, chapping, scaling, or weeping skin): contact urticaria (hives); and itchy, red eyes, fits of sneezing, runny or stuffy nose, itching of the nose or palate, and shortness of breath, wheezing, chest tightness, or difficulty breathing, resulting from inhalation of latex aerosols. It is estimated that 17% to 37% of dental health care providers are affected, and the incidence seems to be growing. Box 19-1

BOX 19-1   DENTAL OFFICE PRODUCTS THAT CONTAIN LATEX
Ambu-bag, stethoscope Blood pressure cuff and tubing Pulse-oximeter finger monitors Laderal pocket masks, airways Anesthetic, injectable medication plunger diaphragms Band-Aids, adhesive tapes Bite blocks, mouth props, orthodontic splints Elastic in scrubs and clothing (underwear, sneakers) Face mask coating and face mask elastic band Gloves (latex), rubber utility gloves Gutta-percha points Instrument banding materials Ice wraps Mixing bowls for alginate impressions/models Nitrous oxide/oxygen mask, tubing Orthodontic "Alastic" materials, guards for brackets Orthodontic power chains and threads Prophy cups Rubber dental dams Rubber-based impression materials Rubber polishing wheels and disks Tubing to dental equipment WHAT ELSE?

Reprinted with permission, Turbyne & Associates, P.O. Box 738, Auburn, ME 04212-0738.

BOX 19-2   PREPARATION FOR A "LATEX-SAFE" DENTAL VISIT

1. The patient should be your first appointment of the day. Update the medical History. Ask the patient if he or she has taken any antihistamines (may increase blood pressure). Document.
2. The office should have been cleaned the night before. All counters, walls, and equipment washed to remove any latex powder, with non-latex gloves. Rugs in the office vacuumed. Remove any latex-containing decorations.
3. All latex equipment in the treatment room removed or covered (tubing, instrument bands, glove boxes, masks). Anticipate treatment; be prepared to use all non-latex materials. Minimize the risk of latex contamination of injected fluids.
4. The air system should remain turned off until after the patient has left the premises, to minimize airborne contact
5. Dental staff have washed their hair and showered before coming to work. Don clean uniforms; no sneakers. Do not touch or rub against any latex materials prior to patient treatment.
6. The patient should be informed to wear clothing that covers arms and legs and has a high neck. He or she should be given a latex-free mask and gloves upon arrival.
7. Have a latex-free emergency resuscitation kit and emergency medications in case of patient reaction in the treatment room. Have a Latex Free Emergency Response Team telephone number handy.
8. Place a "Warning: Latex Allergy" sign outside the treatment room to warn staff who may be using or are in contact with latex not to enter the room.
9. Be able to close the treatment room door once the patient is seated.
10. Watch the patient carefully for any signs of allergic reaction.
11. Update the patient's medical history; note any premedication for the visit, especially amount of preventive antihistamines if taken.
12. Wash your hands thoroughly; then take a blood pressure with latex-free cuff and stethoscope.

Reprinted with permission, Turbyne & Associates, P.O. Box 738, Auburn, ME 04212-0738.

is a list of dental office products that contain latex, and Box 19-2 is a list of measures that can be taken to prepare for a "latex-safe" dental visit for an allergic patient. Box 19-3 is a list of measures to be taken for the protection of employees.

Latex allergy has been documented in medical literature and recognized by experts in this area since 1979. Severe reactions have been reported in medical literature since 1986. In March 1991, the Food and Drug Administration issued a "medical alert" regarding latex-containing medical devices.

BOX 19-3   EMPLOYEE PROTECTION

1. Develop a policy for the management of latex-allergic employees.
2. Medical history
3. Consider latex allergy screening.
4. Provide latex-safe (powder-free) or latex-free personal protective equipment.
5. Inform, educate, about latex allergy/asthma for early prevention/ intervention.
6. Review how/when office is cleaned: rugs, floors, walls, air filtration.
7. Inform and protect contractors, especially facility housekeeping personnel.
8. Investigate contact dermatitis or skin irritations immediately through medical evaluation and testing.
9. Inventory all latex products and schedule replacement or SOP to cover.
10. Have on hand a Latex Free Emergency Kit
11. Make sure your staff can react correctly to an anaphylactic reaction.
12. Coach teammates who are in denial to seek care.

Reprinted with permission, Turbyne & Associates, P.O. Box 738, Auburn, ME 04212-0738.

A number of lawsuits regarding latex allergies have been initiated. They are difficult to win and have produced mixed results for the health care provider.[1]

We can expect to see further research relating to the cause and prevention of latex allergies, as well as additional guidelines from OSHA.

Issues relating to the ergonomics of the dental setting in general, as well as those related to the specific tasks we perform as dental health care providers, are of significance to our physical health and well-being. Dental health care providers are particularly at risk because of their sustained body postures and repetitive motions, which produce fatigue, pain, and injury.

We can expect to see additional research and recommendations relating to the design and placement of dental equipment, as well as the movement and positioning of the body while we are working, to reduce stress on the muscles, tendons, ligaments, and joints.

FINAL COMMENTS

We must keep in mind the fact that the great majority of federal laws and many state laws do not pertain to or protect the employees of small businesses. Dental health care providers need to concentrate their efforts on amending those federal and state laws to include and protect the employees of the small dental office.

The future of all health professionals lies in the continued involvement of the members of each profession. Laws can be changed, but not without a great deal of

---

[1]*Bishop v. Farhat*, 489 S.E.2d 323 (1997).

time and effort. It should be a goal for each of us to amend and create laws related to dental health care that are responsive to increasing changes in the health care system. This goal can be accomplished in a manner that creates advantages for the patient, the dental assistant, the dental hygienist, and the dentist.

SUGGESTED READINGS

Kushman J, Perry D, Freed J: Practice characteristics of dental hygienists operating independently of dental supervision, *Journal of Dental Hygiene* 70(5):194-205, September-October 1996.

Nathe C, Posler B: A spirit of cooperation and, yes, independence, *RDH* 19(7):20-22, 63, July 1999.

Wolfe FW: California's sweet taste of freedom, *RDH* 19(5):16-20, 61, May 1999.

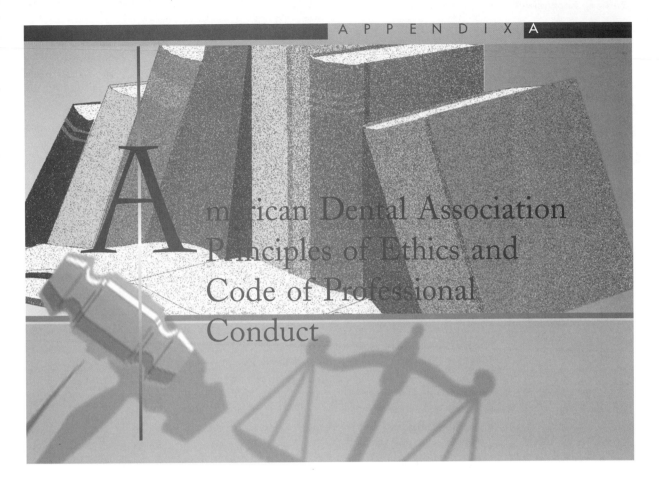

American Dental Association Principles of Ethics and Code of Professional Conduct

The ethical statements that have historically been subscribed to by the dental profession have had the benefit of the patient as their primary goal. Recognition of this goal, and of the education and training of a dentist, has resulted in society affording to the profession the privilege and obligation of self-government. The Association calls upon members of the profession to be caring and fair in their contact with patients. Although the structure of society may change, the overriding obligation of the dentist will always remain the duty to provide quality care in a competent and timely manner. All members must protect and preserve the high standards of oral health care provided to the public by the profession. They must strive to improve the care delivered through education, training, research and, most of all, adherence to a stringent code of ethics, structured to meet the needs of the patient.

PRINCIPLE—SECTION 1

SERVICE TO THE PUBLIC AND QUALITY OF CARE

The dentist's primary professional obligation shall be service to the public. The competent and timely delivery of quality care within the bounds of the clinical circumstances presented by the patient, with due consideration being given to the needs and desires of the patient, shall be the most important aspect of that obligation.

Code of Professional Conduct
Patient Selection

While serving the public, dentists may exercise reasonable discretion in selecting patients for their practices, dentists shall not refuse to accept patients into their practice or deny dental service to patients because of the patient's race, creed, color, sex, or national origin.

Patient Records

Dentists are obliged to safeguard the confidentiality of patient records.

Dentists shall maintain patient records in a manner consistent with the protection of the welfare of the patient. Upon request of a patient or another dental practitioner, dentists shall provide any information that will be beneficial for the future treatment of that patient.

Advisory Opinion

A dentist has the ethical obligation on request of either the patient or the patient's new dentist to furnish, either gratuitously or for nominal cost, such dental records or copies or summaries of them, including dental X-rays or copies of them, as will be beneficial for the future treatment of that patient.

Community Service

Since dentists have an obligation to use their skills, knowledge, and experience for the improvement of the dental health of the public and are encouraged to be leaders in their community, dentists in such service shall conduct themselves in such a manner as to maintain or elevate the esteem of the profession.

Emergency Service

Dentists shall be obliged to make reasonable arrangements for the emergency care of their patients of record. Dentists shall be obliged when consulted in an emergency by patients not of record to make reasonable arrangements for emergency care. If treatment is provided, the dentist, upon completion of such treatment, is obliged to return the patient to his or her regular dentist unless the patient expressly reveals a different preference.

Consultation and Referral

Dentists shall be obliged to seek consultation, if possible, when the welfare of patients will be safeguarded or advanced by utilizing those who have special skills, knowledge, and experience. When patients visit or are referred to specialists or consulting dentists for consultation:

1. The specialists or consulting dentists upon completion of their care shall return the patient, unless the patient expressly reveals a different preference, to the referring dentist, or if none, to the dentist of record for future care.
2. The specialists shall be obliged when there is no referring dentist and upon a completion of their treatment to inform patients when there is a need for further dental care.
3. A dentist who has a patient referred by a third party for a "second opinion" regarding a diagnosis or treatment plan recommended by the patient's treat-

ing dentist should render the requested second opinion in accordance with the Code of Ethics. In the interest of the patient afforded quality care, the dentist rendering the second opinion should not have a vested interest in the ensuing recommendation.

Use of Auxiliary Personnel

Dentists shall be obliged to protect the health of their patient by only assigning to qualified auxiliaries those duties that can be legally delegated. Dentists shall be further obliged to prescribe and supervise the work of all auxiliary personnel working under their direction and control.

Justifiable Criticism

Dentists shall be obliged to report to the appropriate reviewing agency as determined by the local component or constituent society instances of gross or continual faulty treatment by other dentists.

Patients should be informed of their present oral health status without disparaging comment about prior services.

Dentists issuing a public statement with respect to the profession shall have a reasonable basis to believe that the comments made are true.

Advisory Opinion

A dentist's duty to the public imposes a responsibility to report instances of gross or continual faulty treatment. However, the heading of this section is "Justifiable Criticism." Therefore, when informing a patient of the status of his/her oral health, the dentist should exercise care that the comments made are justifiable. For example, a difference of opinion as to preferred treatment should not be communicated to the patient in a manner that would imply mistreatment. There will necessarily be cases where it will be difficult to determine whether the comments made are justifiable. Therefore, this section is phrased to address the discretion of dentists and advises against disparaging statements against another dentist. However, it should be noted that where comments are made which are obviously not supportable and therefore unjustified, such comments can be the basis for the institution of a disciplinary proceeding against the dentist making such statements.

Expert Testimony

Dentists may provide expert testimony when that testimony is essential to a just and fair disposition of a judicial or administrative action.

Rebate and Split Fees

Dentists shall not accept or tender "rebates" or "split fees."

Representation of Care and Fees

Dentists shall not represent the care being rendered to their patients or the fees being charged for providing such care in a false or misleading manner.

Advisory Opinion

1. A dentist who accepts a third party* payment under a co-payment plan as payment in full without disclosing to the third party* payer that the patient's payment portion will not be collected, is engaged in over-billing. The essence of this ethical impropriety is deception and misrepresentation; an over-billing dentist makes it appear to the third party* payer the charge to the patient for services rendered is higher than it actually is.

2. It is unethical for a dentist to increase a fee to a patient solely because the patient has insurance.

3. Payments accepted by a dentist under a governmentally funded program, a component or constituent dental society sponsored access program, or a participating agreement entered into under a program of a third party* shall not be considered as evidence of over-billing in determining whether a charge to a patient, or to another third party* in behalf of a patient not covered under any of the aforecited programs constitutes over-billing under this section of the Code.

4. A dentist who submits a claim form to a third party* reporting incorrect treatment dates for the purpose of assisting a patient in obtaining benefits under a dental plan, which benefits would otherwise be disallowed, is engaged in making an unethical, false, or misleading representation to such third party.*

5. A dentist who incorrectly describes on a third party* claim form a dental procedure in order to receive a greater payment or reimbursement or incorrectly makes a non-covered procedure appear to be a covered procedure on such a claim form is engaged in making an unethical, false, or misleading representation to such third party.*

6. A dentist who recommends and performs unnecessary dental services or procedures is engaged in unethical conduct.

PRINCIPLE—SECTION 2

EDUCATION

The privilege of dentists to be accorded professional status rests primarily in the knowledge, skill, and experience with which they serve their patients and society. All dentists, therefore, have the obligation of keeping their knowledge and skill current.

PRINCIPLE—SECTION 3

GOVERNMENT OF A PROFESSION

Every profession owes society the responsibility to regulate itself. Such regulation is achieved largely through the influence of the professional societies. All dentists, therefore, have the dual obligation. of making themselves a part of a professional society and of observing its rules of ethics.

---

*A third party is any party to a dental prepayment contract that may collect premiums, assume financial risks, pay claims, and/or provide administrative services.

PRINCIPLE—SECTION 4

RESEARCH AND DEVELOPMENT

Dentists have the obligation of making the results and benefits of their investigative efforts available to all when they are useful in safeguarding or promoting the health of the public.

Code of Professional Conduct

Devices and Therapeutic Methods

Except for formal investigative studies, dentists shall be obliged to prescribe, dispense, or promote only those devices, drugs, and other agents whose complete formulae are available to the dental profession. Dentists shall have the further obligation of not holding out as exclusive any device, agent, method, or technique.

Patents and Copyrights

Patents and copyrights may be secured by dentists provided that such patents and copyrights shall not be used to restrict research or practice.

PRINCIPLE—SECTION 5

PROFESSIONAL ANNOUNCEMENT

In order to properly serve the public, dentists should represent themselves in a manner that contributes to the esteem of the profession. Dentists should not misrepresent their training and competence in any way that would be false or misleading in any material respect.*

Code of Professional Conduct

Advertising

Although any dentist may advertise, no dentist shall advertise or solicit patients in any form of communication in a manner that is false or misleading in any material respect.*

Advisory Opinion

1. If a dental health article, message, or newsletter is published under a dentist's byline to the public without making truthful disclosure of the source and authorship or is designed to give rise to questionable expectations for the purpose

---

*Advertising, solicitation of patients or business, or other promotional activities by dentists or dental care delivery organizations shall not be considered unethical or improper, except for those promotional activities which are false or misleading in any material respect. Notwithstanding any ADA Principles of Ethics and Code of Professional Conduct or other standards of dentist conduct that may be differently worded, this shall be the sole standard for determining the ethical propriety of such promotional activities. Any provision of an ADA constituent or component society's code of ethics or other standard of dentist conduct relating to dentists' or dental care delivery organizations' advertising, solicitation, or other promotional activities which is worded differently from the above standard shall be deemed to be in conflict with the ADA Principles of Ethics and Code of Professional Conduct.

of inducing the public to utilize the services of the sponsoring dentist, the dentist is engaged in making a false or misleading representation to the public in a material respect.

2. The Council on Ethics, Bylaws and Judicial Affairs believes it would be of service to the members to provide some insight into the meaning of the term "false or misleading in a material respect." Therefore, the following examples are set forth. These examples are not meant to be all-inclusive. Rather by restating the concept in alternative language and giving general examples, it is hoped that the membership will gain a better understanding of the term. With this in mind, statements shall be avoided which would:

   (a) Contain a material misrepresentation of fact.
   (b) Omit a fact necessary to make the statement considered as a whole not materially misleading.
   (c) Contain a representation or implication regarding the quality of dental services which would suggest unique or general superiority to other practitioners which are not susceptible to reasonable verification by the public.
   (d) Be intended or be likely to create an unjustified expectation about results the dentist can achieve.

3. The use of an unearned or non-health degree in any general announcements to the public by a dentist may be a representation to the public which is false or misleading in a material respect. A dentist may use the title Doctor, Dentist, DDS, or DMD, or any additional earned advanced degrees in health service areas. The use of unearned or non-health degrees could be misleading because of the likelihood that it will indicate to the public the attainment of a specialty or diplomate status. It may also suggest that the dentist using such is claiming superior dental skills.

   For purposes of this advisory opinion, an unearned academic degree is one that is awarded by an educational institution not accredited by a generally recognized accrediting body or is an honorary degree. Generally, the use of honorary degrees or non-health degrees should be limited to scientific papers and curriculum vitae. In all instances state law should be consulted. In any review by the council of the use of non-health degrees or honorary degrees, the council will apply the standard of whether the use of such is false or misleading in a material respect.

4. A dentist using the attainment of a fellowship in a direct advertisement to the general public may be making a representation to the public that is false or misleading in a material respect. Such use of a fellowship status may be misleading because of the likelihood that it will indicate to the dental consumer the attainment of a specialty status. It may also suggest that the dentist using such is claiming superior dental skills. However, when such use does not conflict with state law, the attainment of fellowship status may be indicated in scientific papers, curriculum vitae, third party payment forms, and letterhead and stationery which is not used for the direct solicitation of patients. In any review by the council of the use of the attainment of fellowship status, the council will apply the standard of whether the use of such is false or misleading in a material respect.

5. There are two basic types of referral services for dental care; not-for-profit and the commercial.

   The not-for-profit is commonly organized by dental societies or community services. It is open to all qualified practitioners in the area served. A fee is sometimes charged the practitioner to be listed with the service. A fee for such referral services is for the purpose of covering the expenses of the service and has no relation to the number of patients referred.

   In contrast, experience has shown that commercial referral services generally limit access to the referral service to one dentist in a particular geographic area. Prospective patients calling the service are referred to the single subscribing dentist in the geographic area and the respective dentist is commonly billed for each patient referred. Commercial referral services often advertise to the public stressing that there is no charge for use of the service and the patient is not informed of the referral fee paid by the dentist. There is a connotation to such advertisements that the referral that is being made is in the nature of a public service.

   A dentist is allowed to pay for any advertising permitted by the Code, but is generally not permitted to make payments to another person or entity for the referral of a patient for professional services. While the particular facts and circumstances, relating to an individual commercial referral service will vary, the council believes that the aspects outlined above for commercial referral services violate the Code in that it constitutes advertising which is false or misleading in a material respect and violate the prohibitions in the Code against fee splitting.

Name of Practice

Since the name under which a dentist conducts his practice may be a factor in the selection process of the patient, the use of a trade name or an assumed name that is false or misleading in any material respect is unethical.

Use of the name of a dentist no longer actively associated with the practice may be continued for a period not to exceed one year.*

Announcement of Specialization and Limitation of Practice.

This section and Section 5 D are designed to help the public make an informed selection between the practitioner who has completed an accredited program beyond the dental degree and a practitioner who has not completed such a program.

The special areas of dental practice approved by the American Dental Association and the designation for ethical specialty announcement and limitation of practice are: dental public health, endodontics, oral pathology, oral and maxillofacial surgery, orthodontics, pediatric dentistry, periodontics, and prosthodontics.

Dentists who choose to announce specialization should use "specialist in" or "practice limited to" and shall limit their practice exclusively to the announced special area(s) of dental practice, provided at the time of the announcement such dentists have met in each approved specialty for which they announce the existing educational requirements and standards set forth by the American Dental Association.

Dentists who use their eligibility to announce as specialists to make the public believe that specialty services rendered in the dental office are being rendered by qualified specialists when such is not the case are engaged in unethical conduct. The burden of responsibility is on specialists to avoid any inference that general practitioners, associated with specialists, are qualified to announce themselves as specialists.

General Standards

The following are included within the standards of the American Dental Association for determining the education, experience, and other appropriate requirements for announcing specialization and limitation of practice:

1. The special area(s) of dental practice and an appropriate certifying board must be approved by the American Dental Association.
2. Announcing dentists as specialists must have successfully completed an educational program accredited by the Commission on Dental Accreditation, two or more years in length, as specified by the Council on Dental Education, or be diplomates of an American Dental Association recognized certifying board. The scope of the individual specialist's practice shall be governed by the educational standards for the specialty in which the specialist is announcing.
3. The practice carried on by dentists who announce as specialists shall be limited exclusively to the special area(s) of dental practices announced by the dentist.

Standards for Multiple-Specialty Announcements

Educational criteria for announcement by dentists in additional recognized specialty areas are the successful completion of an educational program accredited by the Commission on Dental Accreditation in each area for which the dentist wishes to announce.

Dentists who completed their advanced education in programs listed by the Council on Dental Education prior to the initiation of the accreditation process in 1967 and who are currently ethically announcing as specialists in a recognized area may announce in additional areas provided they are educationally qualified or are certified diplomates in each area for which they wish to announce. Documentation of successful completion of the educational program(s) must be submitted to the appropriate constituent society. The documentation must assure that the duration of the program(s) is a minimum of two years except for oral and maxillofacial surgery which must have been a minimum of three years in duration.*

Advisory Opinion

1. A dentist who announces in any means of communication with patients or the general public that he or she is certified or a diplomate in an area of dentistry not recognized by the American Dental Association or the law of the jurisdiction where the dentist practices as a specialty area of dentistry is engaged in making a false or misleading representation to the public in a material respect.

General Practitioner Announcement of Services

General dentists who wish to announce the services available in their practices are permitted to announce the availability of those services so long as they avoid any communications that express or imply specialization. General dentists shall also state that the services are being provided by general dentists. No dentist shall announce available services in any way that would be false or misleading in any material respect.*

INTERPRETATION AND APPLICATION OF "PRINCIPLES OF ETHICS AND CODE OF PROFESSIONAL CONDUCT"

The preceding statements constitute the Principles of Ethics and Code of Professional Conduct of the American Dental Association. The purpose of the Principles and Code is to uphold and strengthen dentistry as a member of the learned professions. The constituent and component societies may adopt additional provisions or interpretations not in conflict with these Principles of Ethics and Code of Professional Conduct that would enable them to serve more faithfully the traditions, customs, and desires of the members of these societies.

Problems involving questions of ethics should be solved at the local level within the broad boundaries established in these Principles of Ethics and Code of Professional Conduct and within the interpretation by the component and/or constituent society of their respective codes of ethics. If a satisfactory decision cannot be reached, the question should be referred on appeal to the constituent society and the Council on Ethics, Bylaws and Judicial Affairs of the American Dental Association, as provided in Chapter XI of the Bylaws of the American Dental Association. Members found guilty of unethical conduct as prescribed in the American Dental Association Code of Professional Conduct or codes of ethics of the constituent and component societies are subject to the penalties set forth in Chapter XI of the American Dental Association Bylaws.

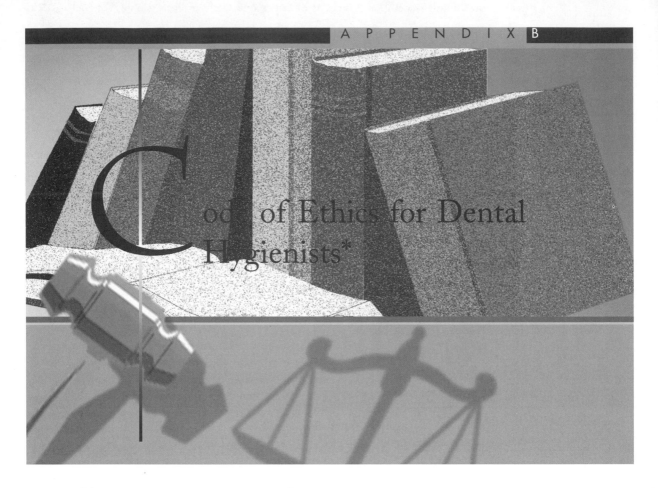

Code of Ethics for Dental Hygienists*

1. Preamble

As dental hygienists, we are a community of professionals devoted to the prevention of disease and the promotion and improvement of the public's health. We are preventive oral health professionals who provide educational, clinical, and therapeutic services to the public. We strive to live meaningful, productive, satisfying lives that simultaneously serve us, our profession, our society, and the world. Our actions, behaviors, and attitudes are consistent with our commitment to public service. We endorse and incorporate the Code into our daily lives.

2. Purpose

The purpose of a professional code of ethics is to achieve high levels of ethical consciousness, deci-

sion making, and practice by the members of the profession. Specific objectives of the Dental Hygiene Code of Ethics are

- to increase our professional and ethical consciousness and sense of ethical responsibility.
- to lead us to recognize ethical issues and choices and to guide us in making more informed ethical decisions.
- to establish a standard for professional judgement and conduct.
- to provide a statement of the ethical behavior the public can expect from us.

The Dental Hygiene Code of Ethics is meant to influence us throughout our careers. It stimulates our continuing study of ethical issues and challenges us to explore our ethical responsibilities. The Code establishes concise standards of behavior to

*From the American Dental Hygienists' Association.

guide the public's expectations of our profession and supports dental hygiene practice, laws and regulations. By holding ourselves accountable to meeting the standards stated in the Code, we enhance the public's trust on which our professional privilege and status are founded.

3. Key Concepts

Our beliefs, principles, values and ethics are concepts reflected in the Code. They are the essential elements of our comprehensive and definitive code of ethics, and are interrelated and mutually dependent.

4. Basic Beliefs

We recognize the importance of the following beliefs that guide our practice and provide context for our ethics:

- The services we provide contribute to the health and well being of society.
- Our education and licensure qualify us to serve the public by preventing and treating oral disease and helping individuals achieve and maintain optimal health.
- Individuals have intrinsic worth, are responsible for their own health, and are entitled to make choices regarding their health.
- Dental hygiene care is an essential component of overall health care and we function interdependently with other health care providers.
- All people should have access to health care, including oral health care.
- We are individually responsible for our actions and the quality of care we provide.

5. Fundamental Principles

These fundamental principles, universal concepts and general laws of conduct provide the foundation for our ethics.

Universality

The principle of universality expects that, if one individual judges an action to be right or wrong in a given situation, other people considering the same action in the same situation would make the same judgement.

Complementarity

The principle of complementarity recognizes the existence of an obligation to justice and basic human rights. In all relationships, it requires considering the values and perspectives of others before making decisions or taking actions affecting them.

Ethics

Ethics are the general standards of right and wrong that guide behavior within society. As generally accepted actions, they can be judged by determining the extent to which they promote good and minimize harm. Ethics compel us to engage in health promotion/disease prevention activities.

Community

This principle expresses our concern for the bond between individuals, the community, and society in general. It leads us to preserve natural resources and inspires us to show concern for the global environment.

Responsibility

Responsibility is central to our ethics. We recognize that there are guidelines for making ethical choices and accept responsibility for knowing and applying them. We accept the consequences of our actions or the failure to act and are willing to make ethical choices and publicly affirm them.

6. Core Values

We acknowledge these values as general for our choices and actions.

Individual Autonomy and Respect for Human Beings

People have the right to be treated with respect. They have the right to informed consent prior to treatment, and they have the right to full disclosure of all relevant information so that they can make informed choices about their care.

Confidentiality

We respect the confidentiality of client information and relationships as a demonstration of the value we place on individual autonomy. We acknowledge our obligation to justify any violation of a confidence.

Societal Trust

We value client trust and understand that public trust in our profession is based on our actions and behavior.

Nonmaleficence

We accept our fundamental obligation to provide services in a manner that protects all clients and minimizes harm to them and others involved in their treatment.

Beneficence

We have a primary role in promoting the well being of individuals and the public by engaging in health promotion/disease prevention activities.

Justice and Fairness

We value justice and support the fair and equitable distribution of health care resources. We believe all people should have access to high-quality, affordable oral healthcare.

Veracity

We accept our obligation to tell the truth and expect that others will do the same. We value self-knowledge and seek truth and honesty in all relationships.

7. Standards of Professional Responsibility

We are obligated to practice our profession in a manner that supports our purpose, beliefs, and values in accordance with the fundamental principles that support our ethics. We acknowledge the following responsibilities:

To Ourselves as Individuals . . .

- Avoid self-deception, and continually strive for knowledge and personal growth.
- Establish and maintain a lifestyle that supports optimal health.
- Create a safe work environment.
- Assert our own interests in ways that are fair and equitable.
- Seek the advice and counsel of others when challenged with ethical dilemmas.
- Have realistic expectations for ourselves and recognize our limitations.

To Ourselves as Professionals . . .

- Enhance professional competencies through continuous learning in order to practice according to high standards of care.
- Support dental hygiene peer-review systems and quality-assurance measures.
- Develop collaborative professional relationships and exchange knowledge to enhance our own lifelong professional development.

To Family and Friends . . .

- Support the efforts of others to establish and maintain healthy lifestyles and respect the rights of friends and family.

To Clients . . .

- Provide oral health care utilizing high levels of professional knowledge, judgement, and skill.
- Maintain a work environment that minimizes the risk of harm.
- Serve all clients without discrimination and avoid action toward any individual or group that may be interpreted as discriminatory.
- Hold professional client relationships confidential.
- Communicate with clients in a respectful manner.
- Promote ethical behavior and high standards of care by all dental hygienists.
- Serve as an advocate for the welfare of clients.
- Provide clients with the information necessary to make informed decisions about their oral health and encourage their full participation in treatment decisions and goals.
- Refer clients to other healthcare providers when their needs are beyond our ability or scope of practice.
- Educate clients about high-quality oral heath care.

To Colleagues . . .

- Conduct professional activities and programs, and develop relationships in ways that are honest, responsible, and appropriately open and candid.

- Encourage a work environment that promotes individual professional growth and development.
- Collaborate with others to create a work environment that minimizes risk to the personal health and safety of our colleagues.
- Manage conflicts constructively.
- Support the efforts of other dental hygienists to communicate the dental hygiene philosophy and preventive oral care.
- Inform other health care professionals about the relationship between general and oral health.
- Promote human relationships that are mutually beneficial, including those with other health care professionals.

To Employees and Employers . . .

- Conduct professional activities and programs, and develop relationships in ways that are honest, responsible, open, and candid.
- Manage conflicts constructively.
- Support the right of our employees and employers to work in an environment that promotes wellness.
- Respect the employment rights of our employers and employees.

To the Dental Hygiene Profession . . .

- Participate in the development and advancement of our profession. Avoid conflicts of interest and declare them when they occur.
- Seek opportunities to increase public awareness and understanding of oral health practices.
- Act in ways that bring credit to our profession while demonstrating appropriate respect for colleagues in other professions.
- Contribute time, talent, and financial resources to support and promote our profession.
- Promote a positive image for our profession.
- Promote a framework for professional education that develops dental hygiene competencies to meet the oral and overall health needs of the public.

To the Community and Society . . .

- Recognize and uphold the laws and regulations governing our profession.
- Document and report inappropriate, inadequate, or substandard care and/or illegal activities by a health care provider, to the responsible authorities.
- Use peer review as a mechanism for identifying inappropriate, inadequate, or substandard care provided by dental hygienists.
- Comply with local, state, and federal statutes that promote public health and safety.
- Develop support systems and quality-assurance programs in the workplace to assist dental hygienist in providing the appropriate standard of care.
- Promote access to dental hygiene services for all, supporting justice and fairness in the distribution of healthcare resources.

- Act consistently with the ethics of the global scientific community of which our profession is a part.
- Create a healthful workplace ecosystem to support a healthy environment.
- Recognize and uphold our obligation to provide pro bono service.

To Scientific Investigation . . .

We accept responsibility for conducting research according to the fundamental principles underlying our ethical beliefs in compliance with universal codes, governmental standards, and professional guidelines for the care and management of experimental subjects. We acknowledge our ethical obligations to the scientific community:

- Conduct research that contributes knowledge that is valid and useful to our clients and society.
- Use research methods that meet accepted scientific standards.
- Use research resources appropriately.
- Systematically review and justify research in progress to insure the most favorable benefit-to-risk ratio to research subjects.
- Submit all proposals involving human subjects to an appropriate human subject review committee.
- Secure appropriate institutional committee approval for the conduct of research involving animals.
- Obtain informed consent from human subjects participating in research that is based on specification published in Title 21 Code of Federal Regulations Part 46.
- Respect the confidentiality and privacy of data.
- Seek opportunities to advance dental hygiene knowledge through research by providing financial, human, and technical resources whenever possible.
- Report research results in a timely manner.
- Report research findings completely and honestly, drawing only those conclusions that are supported by the data presented.
- Report the names of investigators fairly and accurately.
- Interpret the research and the research of others accurately and objectively, drawing conclusions that are supported by the data presented and seeking clarity when uncertain
- Critically evaluate research methods and results before applying new theory and technology in practice.
- Be knowledgeable concerning currently accepted preventive and therapeutic methods, products, and technology and their application to our practice.

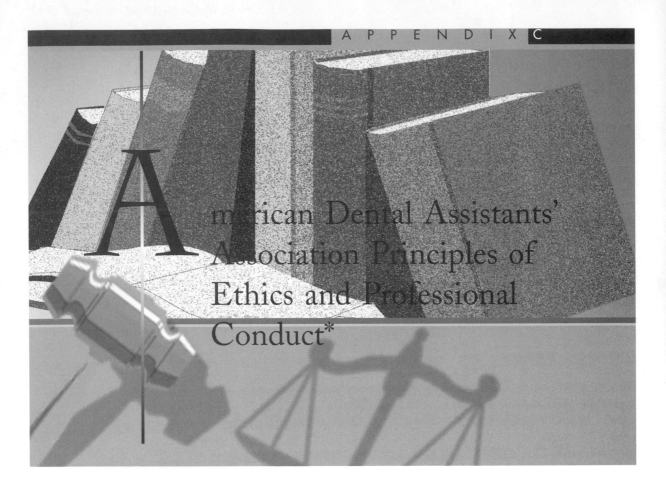

American Dental Assistants' Association Principles of Ethics and Professional Conduct*

Each individual involved in the practice of dentistry assumes the obligation of maintaining and enriching the profession. Each member shall choose to meet this obligation according to the dictates of personal conscience. This is based on the needs of the general public that the profession of dentistry is committed to serve.

The member shall refrain from performing any professional service which is prohibited by state law and has the obligation to prove competence prior to providing services to any patient. The member shall constantly strive to upgrade and expand technical skills for the benefit of the consumer public and employer. The member should additionally seek to sustain and improve the local organization, state association, and the American Dental Assistants' Association through active participation and personal commitment.

CODE OF PROFESSIONAL CONDUCT
- Abide by the bylaws of the Association
- Maintain loyalty to the Association
- Pursue the objectives of the Association
- Hold in confidence the information entrusted to me by the Association
- Maintain respect for the members and employees of the Association
- Serve all members of the Association in an impartial manner
- Recognize and follow all laws and regulations relating to activities of the Association
- Exercise and insist on sound business principles in the conduct of the affairs of the Association

*Provisional approval, 1998.

- Use legal and ethical means to influence legislation or regulation affecting members of the Association
- Issue no false or misleading statements to fellow members of the public
- Refrain from disseminating malicious information concerning the Association or any member or employee of the Association
- Maintain high standards of personal conduct and integrity
- Do not imply Association endorsement of personal opinions or positions
- Cooperate in a reasonable and proper manner with staff and members
- Accept no personal compensation from fellow members, except as approved by the Association
- Promote and maintain the highest standards of performance in service to the Association
- Assure public confidence in the integrity and service of the Association

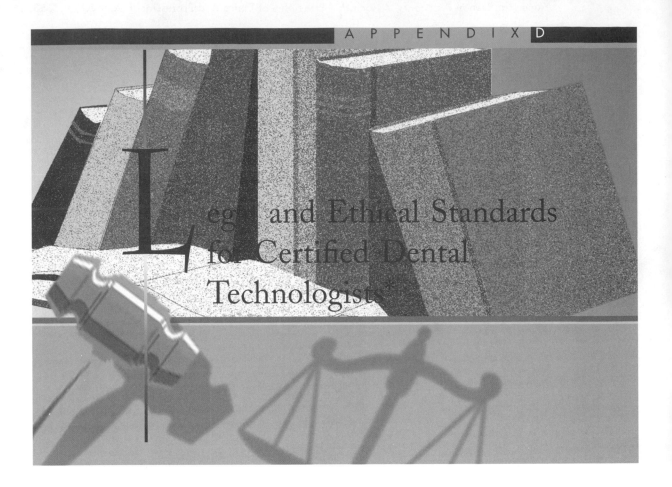

Legal and Ethical Standards for Certified Dental Technologists*

The National Board for Certification (NBC) believes that the guidelines stated in its legal and ethical standards are fair and reasonable and represent a desirable code of professional conduct for dental technology. The objective of these requirements is to enhance and preserve the professionalism and integrity that certification represents.

In those instances where non-compliance is evident and is reported with documentation to an NBC Trustee or the National Headquarters Office, the Board will seek correction or appropriate disciplinary action. Inquiries and reports are handled in strictest confidence.

Guidelines from the National Board for Certification.

LEGAL STANDARD

The NBC encourages compliance with and enforcement of state dental practice acts and all other relevant laws. NBC shall rely upon a Federal or state enforcement agency's determination that a CDT has violated federal or state law. It is proper for NBC to refer any charges brought to its attention to the proper authority, but it shall not be the function of NBC to commence its own investigation into specific activities of a CDT based upon such charges. Such investigation and any resulting determination are the responsibility of the appropriate federal or state enforcement agency.

NBC has the authority to revoke or suspend the certification of any CDT who has been found guilty, by the proper authority, of violating applicable state dental practice acts. NBC shall have the discretion to revoke or suspend the certification of any CDT who has committed a felony, as determined by the proper authority. NBC may postpone consideration of a renewal application if official charges are pending against a CDT. However, NBC shall not revoke certification based solely on official charges brought against a CDT; there must be a subsequent conviction.

ETHICAL STANDARD

The Board intends that certification reflect the highest ethical standards in dental technology. While the Board reserves the right to issue opinions on individual cases of alleged unethical performance, it has specifically identified certain acts as being contrary to the ethical requirements of certification. The Board intends to penalize persons reasonably proven to be engaged in unethical practices including, but not limited to, the following:

1. Obtaining or attempting to obtain certification or certification renewal by deliberate fraud, deception, omission or artifice;
2. Claiming or inferring, or allowing oneself or one's laboratory to be represented, in any manner, to be certified when such is not the case, including the unauthorized use of the CDT title or logo and claims to laboratory certification (CDL);
3. Unauthorized possession and/or distribution or NBC testing materials, including the possession and/or reproduction of any part of the NBC written examinations or portions thereof, current or otherwise;
4. Claiming to possess or offering to distribute any information represented to be confidential NBC examination material;
5. Neglecting or failing to enforce reasonable practices and procedures prescribed by the NBC to assure validity of the NBC's system of documenting continuing education credits, or incorrect or incomplete disclosure to registrants about program approval(s);
6. Making public statements of fact, oral or in writing, that willfully misrepresent the objectives, policies and practices of the Certified Dental Technician program, the National Board for Certification or its parent organization, the National Association of Dental Laboratories;
7. Making statements that falsely and willfully malign another Certified Dental Technician; or
8. Knowingly permitting, abetting or failing to report to NBC any of the foregoing practices by other persons.

PENALTIES

Penalties may be assessed against certifees, Recognized Graduates, candidates for Board testing, or sponsors or hosts of Board-approved continuing education programs based on demonstrated failure to support and maintain either the legal or ethical standards of certification. Penalties may include:

1. Suspension or denial of certification or certification eligibility.
2. Suspension or cancellation of NBC speaker approval or similar authorization to distribute CDT "Attendance Verification" forms.

3. Formal letters of warning, disapproval or censure for any of the above.
4. Other sanctions as may be deemed by majority vote of the Trustees, to be appropriate to the offense.

The Board reserves the right—and announces its intent—to publish factual information about its final ruling in any disciplinary case and its subsequent exercise of disciplinary procedures.

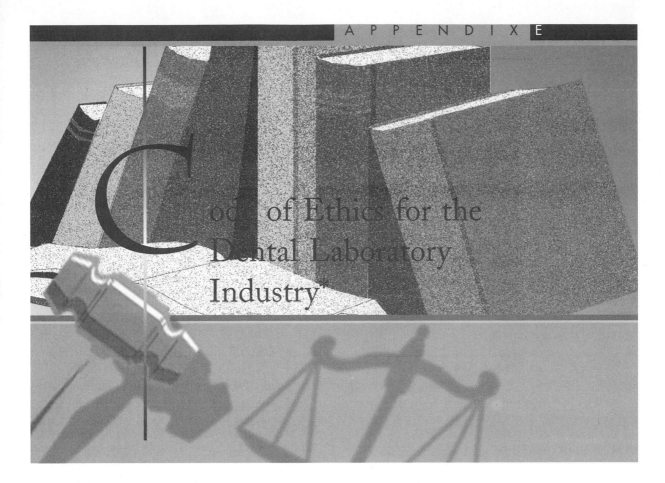

Code of Ethics for the Dental Laboratory Industry*

It shall be incumbent upon every member of this Association to govern his department in accordance with the following prescribed principles. It is not to be presumed that this code covers the whole field of moral and ethical conduct; many duties and obligations not specifically mentioned herein are expected of every member. People of good character will understand and conscientiously apply the Golden Rule.

SERVICE

The service of the dental laboratory shall be to members of the dental profession only, direct to the dentist, and no such service shall be rendered for a

*Outlined by the American Dental Association and the Federal Trade Commission.

dentist employed by a dental laboratory; this does not cancel the right of the dental laboratory to construct special appliances for dental dealers or dental manufacturers or dental laboratories if same are to be used only as samples or on authority of a licensed dentist.

MATERIALS

No materials other than those specified by the licensed dentist shall be used in the construction of any case, except with the knowledge of the licensed dentist.

Should the choice of materials be left to the discretion of the laboratory, the laboratory shall accurately inform the licensed dentist respecting the type or kind of material used.

It shall be incumbent upon each member to furnish with every new completed dental appliance,

(1) a fully itemized invoice, (2) the name of manufacturer or trade name, and (3) the kind and quality of all material that is a part of the finished product.

PRICES

No laboratory shall sell or offer to sell any service, merchandise or dental appliance at less than the cost of making, building, constructing or replacing the same.

Excepting only to remake, adjust or repair to the satisfaction of the licensed dentist a defective dental appliance previously constructed by that laboratory.

No special price, or prices other than those published or usually charged shall be offered, promised, given or allowed to any dentist that is not available to every dentist.

DISCOUNTS AND REBATES

The secret payment or allowance of rebates, refunds, commissions, credits or discounts, whether in the form of money, or otherwise, or the extension to certain licensed dentists of special services or privileges not extended to all licensed dentists on like terms and conditions are prohibited.

No laboratory shall issue checks, vouchers, credit memos or use any other means of price discrimination in order to obtain new business or to introduce new materials.

ADVERTISING

It shall be unethical for any laboratory to:
1. Advertise services, techniques or to quote prices in any newspaper, magazine, periodical or any other publication available to the general public.
2. Advertise prices in any publication usually read only by dentists.
3. Advertise prices in any way other than by enclosure in a sealed envelope addressed to a member of the dental profession.
4. No laboratory shall offer gratis any service which is usually or customarily charged for.
5. No advertising shall contain statements or implications of a deceptive or misleading nature.

SIGNS

Inasmuch as the services of association members are offered exclusively to the dental professional, it is unethical to display window or outside signs, large enough to attract the attention of the general public.

UNFAIR PRACTICES

A. FALSE BRANDING: The false marking or branding of any product of the industry which has the tendency to mislead or deceive dentists, whether as of the grade, quality, quantity, substance, character, nature, origin, size, finish or preparation of any product of the Industry, is prohibited.
B. GUARANTEES: No guarantee shall be used in advertising or sales work, as an inducement to obtain business.

C. PIRATING: Imitating, simulating, or pirating any design, mark, style, brand, drawing, sketch or dummy used by any other person in the dental laboratory industry without authorization is prohibited.

D. SUBSTITUTION OF MATERIALS with intent to defraud: Using, submitting or billing any material superior or inferior in quality to that specified by the licensed dentist of any dental laboratory product, which would represent a price discrimination, is prohibited.

E. DEFAMATION: The defamation of competitors by falsely imputing to them dishonorable conduct, inability to perform contracts, questionable credit standing, or by other false representations or by the false disparagement of the grade or quality of their goods is prohibited.

F. CONSPIRACY: Aiding or abetting any person in the dental laboratory industry in any unfair competitive practice is prohibited. Conspiracy to fix prices in violation of Anti-Trust Laws is prohibited.

G. ALSO PROHIBITED is: 1. Selling samples for less that cost of production. 2. Employing free goods or service in connection with sales transactions. 3. The use or participation in publishing or broadcasting of any statement or representation which lays claim to a policy or continuing practice of generally underselling competitors.

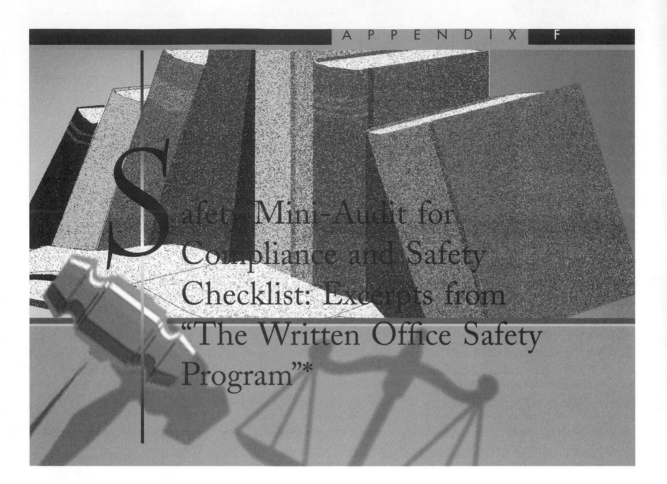

Safety Mini-Audit for Compliance and Safety Checklist: Excerpts from "The Written Office Safety Program"*

SAFETY MINI-AUDIT FOR COMPLIANCE

1. Safety Team/Self Inspection Concept
2. Posted Information for Offices/Facilities: Signs, Labels, Posters, Reports, etc.
   OSHA 2203
   Fire Exit Diagrams/Emergency Evacuation Plans
   Hazardous Chemical Communication Program
   Biohazard Signs/Tags
   Video Display Terminal Poster
   Radiation Safety Rules, Label, Certification
   Elevator/Chair Lift Certification
   Emergency Telephone Numbers
   Signs
   Lighted Exit Signs
   Fire Extinguisher
   Accident Warning Signs & Tape
   Hallway Rooms & Doors That Are Not Exits
   No Smoking
   Microwaves in Use
   Radiation Used on the Premises
   Eye Wash Station
   Bureau of Labor
     Minimum Wage
     Child Labor Laws
     Polygraph Protection Act
     Handicapped Law
     Workers' Compensation
     Sexual Harassment
3. Recordkeeping (All Standard)
   OSHA 200 Form

*Developed by Turbyne & Associates, P.O. Box 738, Auburn, ME 04212-0738.

Training Records
Written Programs/Policies for Required Standards/Laws
Confidential Medical Records
   Accident/Injury
   Medical Evaluations
   Hepatitis vaccine
   TB Screening
   Exposure Incidents
   Other Immunizations
Inspection Reports
   General Safety
   Fire Extinguishers
   Sprinkler Systems
   Electrical
   Eye Wash Stations
   First Aid Kits
   Autoclaves/Heat Sterilizers
Safety Agendas, Meetings, Minutes, Action Plans
List of Safety Team Leaders and Members
List of All Contractors, Volunteers, Students
Job Descriptions/Job Classification for Bloodborne Standard

4. Medical Services/First Aid
5. Ionizing Radiation & Lasers
6. Personal Protective Equipment & Clothing
7. General Work Environment: Lighting, Ventilation, Step Stools, Good Overhead Storage, etc.
8. Exits/Egress/Access
9. Fire Extinguishers, Alarms, Sprinklers
10. Walkways/Floors/Stairways (Steepness, Low Ceilings, Surfaces, Handrails, Repairs, Clutter)
11. Machine Guarding, Portable Power Tools
12. Compressed Gas Cylinders
13. Confined Spaces/Respiratory Protection
14. Environmental Controls: Temperature/Air Flow
15. Storage of Flammable, Combustible Materials
16. Electrical Wires, Fixtures, Cords, Outlets.
17. Boiler Chemicals
18. Video Display Terminals
19. Smoking Regulations
20. Noise
21. Violence in the Workplace

SAFETY:

_____ Written Program, Policy
_____ Professional Licenses Posted

_____ X-Ray Inspection, Registration Posted, a Radiation Warning Sticker is on the Machine

_____ Accident/Injury Records, Form 200

_____ First Aid Kit, Fire Extinguisher Monthly Inspection

_____ Fire Extinguisher Training

_____ Video Display Terminal Training

_____ First Aid Training if Office Over 5 Miles From a Hospital

_____ Laws on File: OSHA Act, CFR 29

SAFETY EQUIPMENT:

_____ Fire Extinguishers/Signs/Tags

_____ First Aid Kit Tag

_____ Exit/Egress/Fire/No Smoking/Microwave in Use/X-Rays Taken on the Premises Signs

_____ Signs on All Doors That Are Not Exits

_____ Fire Exit Diagram in Each Room

_____ Good Lighting and Ventilation

_____ Electrical Outlet Covers

_____ Nitrous/Oxygen Tank Security

_____ 2203 OSHA Poster

_____ Emergency Telephone #'s Posted At Each Phone

_____ Accident Prevention Signs/Tags

_____ Labeling of Circuit Breaker Switches

_____ Stairway Railing Security

_____ Fire Evacuation Policy

CHECKLIST RECORD KEEPING/REGISTRATIONS/ON-FILE ITEMS:

_____ Hazardous Chemical:

_____ Written Program/Policy

_____ Hazardous Chemical List

_____ Annual Report to Bureau of Labor Statistics

_____ SDS Request Letters

_____ Training Program, Records, Labeling Systems (Employee, Contractor, New Hire)

_____ Laws, 1910.1200

REQUIRED EQUIPMENT CHECKLIST:

_____ Eye Wash Station, Cold Water Plumbed, Has a Sign, Within 10 Seconds of Every Exposure Potential, Inspected Monthly

_____ Impervious Apron

_____ Goggles

_____ Impervious Gloves

_____ Metal Storage Cabinets (Fire/Explosion Proof)

_____ Labels/Posters

_____ MSDS Book/List/Sheets

_____ Emergency Spill Equipment

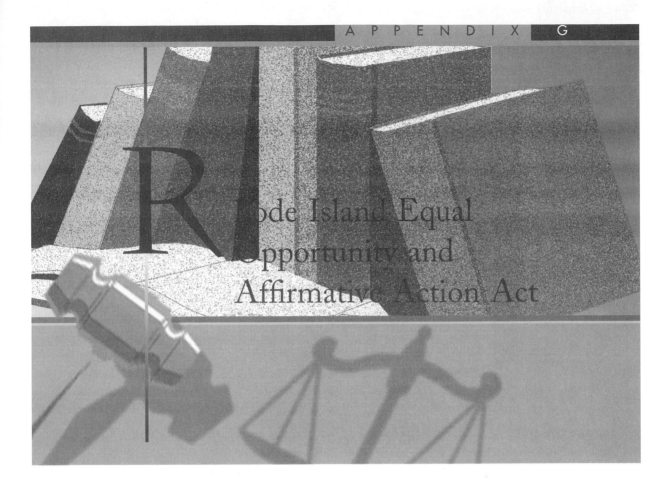

Rhode Island Equal Opportunity and Affirmative Action Act

28-5.1-1. Declaration of policy.-(a) Equal opportunity and affirmative action toward its achievement is the policy of all units of Rhode Island state government, including all public and quasi-public agencies, commissions, boards and authorities; and in the classified, unclassified, and nonclassified services of state employment. This policy shall apply in all areas where the state dollar is spent, in employment, public service, grants and financial assistance, and in state licensing and regulation. All policies, programs, and activities of state government shall be periodically reviewed and revised to assure their fidelity to this policy. Each department head shall make a report to the governor and the general assembly not later than September 30 of each year on the statistical results of the implementation of this chapter and to the state equal opportunity office; provided, that the mandatory provisions of this section shall not apply to the legislative branch of state government.

(b) The provisions of this chapter shall in no way impair any contract or collective bargaining agreement currently in effect. Any contract or collective bargaining agreements entered into or renewed after July 6, 1994 shall be subject to the provisions of this chapter.

28-5.1-2. State equal opportunity office.-(a) There shall be a state equal opportunity office. This office, under the direct administrative supervision of the director of administration/human resources, shall report to the governor and to the general assembly on state equal opportunity programs. The state equal opportunity office shall be responsible for assuring compliance with the requirements of all federal agencies for equal opportunity and shall provide training and technical assistance as may be requested by any company doing business in Rhode Island and all state departments as is necessary to comply with the intent of this chapter.

(b) The state equal opportunity office shall issue such guidelines, directives or instructions as are necessary to effectuate its responsibilities under this chapter, and is hereby authorized to investigate possible discrimination, hold hearings, and direct corrective action thereto.

28-5.1-3. Affirmative action.-(a) The state equal opportunity office shall assign an equal opportunity officer as a liaison to agencies of state government.

(b) Each state department or agency, excluding the legislative branch of state government, shall annually prepare an affirmative action plan. These plans shall be prepared in accordance with the criteria and deadlines set forth by the state equal opportunity office. These deadlines shall provide, without limitation, that affirmative action plans for each fiscal year be submitted to the state equal opportunity office and the house fiscal advisor no later than March 31. These plans shall be submitted to and shall be subject to review and approval by the state equal opportunity office.

(c) Any affirmative action plan required under this section deemed unsatisfactory by the state equal opportunity office shall be withdrawn and amended according to equal opportunity office criteria, in order to attain positive measures for compliance. The state equal opportunity office shall make every effort by informal conference, conciliation and persuasion to achieve compliance with affirmative action requirements.

(d) The state equal opportunity office shall effect and promote the efficient transaction of its business and the timely handling of complaints and other matters before it, and shall make recommendations to appropriate state officials for affirmative action steps towards the achievement of equal opportunity.

(e) The state equal opportunity administrator shall serve as the chief executive officer of the state equal opportunity office, and shall be responsible for monitoring and enforcing all equal opportunity laws, programs, and policies within state government.

(f) No later than July I each state department or agency, excluding the legislative branch of state government, shall submit to the state equal opportunity office and the house fiscal advisor sufficient data to enable the state equal opportunity office and the house fiscal advisor to determine whether the agency achieved the hiring goals contained in its affirmative action plan for the previous year. If the hiring goals contained in the previous year's plan were not met, the agency shall also submit with the data a detailed explanation as to why the goals were not achieved.

(g) Standards for review of affirmative action plans shall be established by the state equal opportunity office, except where superseded by federal law.

(h) For purposes of this section, "agency" shall include, without limitation, all departments, public and quasi-public agencies, authorities, boards, and commissions of the state, excluding the legislative branch of state government.

(i) The state equal opportunity office shall continually review all policies, procedures, and practices for tendencies to discriminate and for institutional or systemic barriers for equal opportunity, and it shall make recommendations with reference to any tendencies or barriers in its annual reports to the governor and the general assembly.

(j) Relevant provisions of this section shall also apply to expanding the pool of applicants for all positions wherein no list exists. The equal opportunity administrator is hereby authorized to develop and implement recruitment plans to assure that adequate consideration is given to qualified minority applicants in those job categories where a manifest imbalance exists, excluding those job categories in the legislative branch of state government.

28-5.1-3.1. Appointments to state boards, commissions, public authorities, and quasi-public corporation.-(a) The general assembly finds that, as a matter of public policy, the effectiveness of each appointed state board, commission, and the governing body of each public authority and quasi-public corporation is enhanced when it reflects the diversity, including the racial and gender composition, of Rhode Island's population. Consequently, each person responsible for appointing one or more individuals to serve on any board or commission or to the governing body of any public authority or board shall endeavor to assure that, to the fullest extent Possible, the composition of the board, commission, or governing body reflects the diversity of Rhode Island's population.

(b) During the month of January in each year the boards, agencies, commissions, or authorities are hereby requested to file with the state equal opportunity office a list of its members. designating their race, gender, and date of appointment.

28-5.1-3.2. Enforcement.-(a) The state equal opportunity administrator is hereby authorized to initiate complaints against any agencies, administrators, or employees of any department or division within state government, excluding the legislative branch, who or which willfully fail to comply with the requirements of any applicable affirmative action plan or of this chapter or who or which fail to meet the standards of good faith effort, reasonable basis, or reasonable action, as defined in guidelines promulgated by the federal Equal Employment Opportunity Commission as set forth in 29 CFR 1607.

(b) Whenever the equal employment opportunity administrator initiates a complaint, he or she shall cause to be issued and served in the name of the equal employment opportunity office a written notice, together with a copy of the complaint, requiring that the agency, administrator, agent, or employee respond thereto and appear at a hearing at a time and place specified in the notice. The equal employment opportunity office shall follow its lawfully adopted rules and regulations concerning hearings of discrimination complaints.

(c) The equal employment opportunity office shall have the power, after hearing, to issue an order requiring a respondent to a complaint to cease and desist from any unlawful discriminatory practice and/or to take such affirmative action, including, but not limited to, hiring, reinstatement, transfer, or upgrading employees, with or without back pay, or dismissal, as may be necessary to secure compliance with any applicable affirmative action plan or with state or federal law.

(d) A final order of the equal employment opportunity office shall constitute an "order" within the meaning of § 42-35-1(j); shall be enforceable as such; shall be rendered in accordance with § 42-35-12; and shall be subject to judicial review in accordance with § 42-35-15.

EQUAL OPPORTUNITY AND AFFIRMATIVE ACTION

28-5.1-4. Employment policies of state agencies.-Each appointing authority shall review the recruitment, appointment, assignment, upgrading, and promotion policies and activities for state employees without regard to race, color, religion, sex, age, national origin, or disability. All appointing authorities shall hire and promote employees without discrimination. Special attention shall be given to the parity of classes of employees doing similar work and the training of supervisory personnel in equal opportunity/affirmative action principles and procedures. Annually, each appointing authority shall include in its budget presentation such necessary programs, goals and objectives as shall improve the equal opportunity aspects of their department's employment policies. Each appointing authority shall make a monthly report to the state equal opportunity office on persons hired, disciplined, terminated, promoted, transferred, and vacancies occurring within their department.

28-5.1-5. Department of administration.-(a) The office of personnel administration of the department of administration shall prepare a comprehensive plan indicating the appropriate steps necessary to maintain and secure the equal opportunity responsibility and commitment of that division. The plan shall set forth attainable goals and target dates based upon a utilization study for achievement of the goals, together with operational assignment for each element of the plan to assure measurable progress. The office of personnel administration shall take positive steps to insure that the entire examination and testing process, including the development of job specifications and employment qualifications, is free from either conscious or inadvertent bias, and shall review all recruitment procedures for all state agencies covered by this chapter for compliance with federal and state law, and bring to the attention of the equal opportunity administrator matters of concern to its jurisdiction. The division of budget shall indicate in the annual personnel supplement progress made toward the achievement of equal employment goals. The division of purchases shall cooperate in administering the state contract compliance programs. The division of statewide planning shall cooperate in assuring compliance from all recipients of federal grants.

(b) The office of labor relations shall propose in negotiations the inclusion of affirmative action language suitable to the need for attaining and maintaining a diverse workforce.

(c) There is hereby created a five (5) member committee which shall monitor negotiations with all collective bargaining units within state government specifically for equal opportunity and affirmative action interests. The members of that committee shall include the director of the Rhode Island commission for human rights, the equal opportunity administrator, the personnel administrator one member of the house of representatives appointed by the speaker, and one member of the senate appointed by the senate majority leader.

28-5.1-6. Commission for human rights.-The Rhode Island commission for human rights shall exercise its enforcement powers as defined in chapter 5 of this title and in this chapter, and shall have the full cooperation of all state agencies. Wherever necessary, the commission shall, at its own initiative or upon a complaint, bring charges of discrimination against those agencies and the personnel thereof who fail to comply with the applicable state laws and this chapter. This commission shall also have the power to order discontinuance of any departmental or division employment pattern or practice deemed discriminatory in intent by the commission, after a hearing on the record, and may seek court enforcement of such an order. The commission shall utilize the state equal opportunity office as its liaison with state government. The Rhode Island commission for human rights is authorized to make such rules and regulations as it deems necessary to carry out its responsibilities under this chapter, and to establish such sanctions as may be appropriate within the rules and regulations of the state.

28-5.1-7. State services and facilities.-(a) Every state agency shall render service to the citizens of this state without discrimination based on race, color, religion, sex, sexual orientation, age, national origin, or disability. No state facility shall be used in furtherance of any discriminatory practice nor shall any state agency become a party to any agreement, arrangement, or plan which has the effect of sanctioning such patterns or practices.

(b) At the request of the state equal opportunity office, each appointing authority shall critically analyze all of its operations to ascertain possible instances of noncompliance with this policy and shall initiate sustained, comprehensive programs based on the guidelines of the state equal opportunity office to remedy any defects found to exist.

28-5.1-8. Education, training, and apprenticeship programs.-(a) All educational programs and activities of state agencies, or in which state agencies participate, shall be open to all qualified persons without regard to race, color, religion, sex, sexual orientation, national origin, or handicap. Such programs shall be conducted to encourage the fullest development of the interests, aptitudes, skills, and capacities of all participants.

(b) Those state agencies responsible for educational programs and activities shall take positive steps to insure that all programs are free from either conscious or inadvertent bias, and shall make quarterly reports to the state equal opportunity office with regard to the number of persons being served and to the extent to which the goals of the chapter are being met by the programs.

(c) Expansion of training opportunities shall also be encouraged with a view toward involving larger numbers of participants from those segments of the labor force where the need for upgrading levels of skill is greatest.

28-5.1-9. State employment services.-All state agencies, including educational institutions, which provide employment referral or placement services to public or private employees, shall accept job orders, refer for employment, test, classify, counsel and train only on a nondiscriminatory basis. They shall refuse to fill any job order which has the effect of excluding any persons because of race, color, religion, sex, sexual orientation, age, national origin, or disability. The agencies shall advise the commission for human rights promptly of any employers, employment agencies, or unions suspected of practicing unlawful discrimination, They shall assist employers and unions seeking to broaden their recruitment programs to include qualified applicants from minority groups. In addition, the department of labor and training, the governor's commission on disabilities, the advisory commission on women, and the Rhode Island economic development corporation shall fully utilize their knowledge of the labor market and economic conditions of the state, and their contacts with job applicants, employers, and unions to promote equal employment opportunities, and shall require and assist all persons within their jurisdictions to initiate actions which shall remedy any situations or programs which have a negative impact on protected classes within the state.

28-5.1-10. State contracts.-The division of purchases shall prepare such rules, regulations, and compliance reports as shall require of contractors of this state the same commitment to equal opportunity as prevails under federal contracts controlled by federal executive orders 11246, 11625 and 11375. Affirmative action plans prepared pursuant to such rules and regulations shall be reviewed by the state equal opportunity office. The state equal opportunity office shall prepare a comprehensive plan to provide compliance reviews for state contracts. A contractor's failure to abide by the rules, regulations, contract terms, and compliance reporting provisions as established shall be ground for forfeitures and penalties as shall be established by the department of administration in consultation with the state equal opportunity office.

28-5.1-11. Law enforcement.-The attorney general, the department of corrections, and the governor's justice commission shall stress to state and local law enforcement officials the necessity for nondiscrimination in the control of criminal behavior. These agencies shall develop and publish formal procedures for the investigation of citizen complaints of alleged abuses of authority by individual peace officers. Employment in all state law enforcement and correctional agencies and institutions shall be subject to the same affirmative action standards applied under this chapter to every state unit of government, in addition to applicable federal requirements.

28-5.1-12. Health care.-The state equal opportunity office shall review the equal opportunity activity of all private health care facilities licensed or chartered by the state, including hospitals, nursing homes, convalescent homes, rest homes, and clinics. These state licensed or chartered facilities shall be required to comply with the state policy of equal opportunity and nondiscrimination in patient admissions, employment, and health care service. The compliance shall be a condition of continued participation in any state program, or in any educational program licensed or accredited by the state, or of eligibility to receive any form of assistance.

28-5.1-13. Private education institutions.-The state equal opportunity office shall review all private educational institutions licensed or chartered by the state, including professional, business, and vocational training schools. These state licensed or chartered institutions shall at the request of the board of regents of elementary and secondary education be required to show compliance with the state policy of nondiscrimination and affirmative action in their student admissions, employment, and other practices as a condition of continued participation in any state program or of eligibility to receive any form of state assistance.

28-5.1-14. State licensing and regulatory agencies.-State agencies shall not discriminate by considering race, color, religion, sex, age, national origin, or handicap in granting, denying, or revoking a license or charter, nor shall any person, corporation, or business firm which is licensed or chartered by the state unlawfully discriminate against or segregate any person on such grounds. All businesses licensed or chartered by the state shall operate on a nondiscriminatory basis, according to equal employment treatment and access to their services to all persons, except unless otherwise exempted by the laws of the state. Any licensee, charter holder, or retail sales permit holder who fails to comply with this policy shall be subject to such disciplinary action as is consistent with the legal authority and rules and regulations of the appropriate licensing or regulatory agency. State agencies which have the authority to grant, deny, or revoke licenses or charters will cooperate with the state equal opportunity office to prevent any person, corporation, or business firm from discriminating because of race, color, religion, sex, age, national origin, or handicap or from participating in any practice which may have a disparate effect on any protected class within the population. The state equal opportunity office shall monitor the equal employment opportunity activities and affirmative action plans of all such organizations.

28-5.1-15. State financial assistance.-State agencies disbursing financial assistance, including, but not limited to, loans and grants, shall hereafter require recipient organizations and agencies to undertake affirmative action programs designed to eliminate patterns and practices of discrimination. At the request of the state equal opportunity office, state agencies disbursing assistance shall develop, in conjunction with the state equal opportunity office, regulations and procedures necessary to implement the goals of nondiscrimination and affirmative action and shall be reviewed for compliance according to state policy.

28-5.1-16. Prior executive orders-Effect.-All executive orders shall, to the extent that they are not inconsistent with this chapter, remain in full force and effect.

28-5.1-17. Utilization analysis.-(a) The personnel administrator, in consultation with the equal employment opportunity administrator within the department of administration, shall annually conduct a utilization analysis of positions within state government based upon the annual review conducted pursuant to §§ 28-5.1-3 and 28-5.1-4. To the extent the analysis determines that minorities as currently defined in federal employment law as Blacks, Hispanics, American Indians (including Alaskan natives), Asians (including Pacific Islanders), are being underrepresented and/or underutilized, the personnel administrator shall, through the director of administration, direct the head of the department where the underrepresentation and/or underutilization exists to establish precise goals and timetables and assist in the correction of each deficiency, to the extent permitted by law and by collective bargaining agreements. The initial analysis shall be directed toward service oriented departments of the state, state police, employment and training, corrections, children, youth, and families, courts, transportation, and human services. The equal employment opportunity administrator shall be consulted in the selection process for all positions certified as underrepresented and/or underutilized and shall report the results of progress toward goals to the governor and to the general assembly by January 31 and July 31 of each year.

In the event of a reduction in force, the personnel administrator, in consultation with the equal employment opportunity administrator and director of the department(s) where the reduction is proposed, shall develop a plan to ensure that affirmative action gains are preserved to the extent permitted by law and by collective bargaining agreements. The equal employment opportunity administrator shall report the results of the plans and their subsequent actions to the governor and to the general assembly by January 31 and July 31 of each year. Consistent with § 28-5.1-6, the Rhode Island commission for human rights shall have the power to order discontinuance of any department or division employment pattern or practice deemed discriminatory in intent or result by the commission. The equal opportunity administrator shall notify the commission of reports and results under this chapter and shall act as the commission's liaison with state government.

28-5-2. Statement as to results of discriminatory practices.-The practice or policy of discrimination against individuals because of their race or color, religion, sex, sexual orientation, disability, age, or country of ancestral origin is a matter of state concern. Such discrimination foments domestic strife and unrest, threatens the rights and privileges of the inhabitants of the state, and undermines the foundations of a free democratic state. The denial of equal employment opportunities because of such discrimination and the consequent failure to utilize the productive capacities of individuals to their fullest extent deprive large segments of the population of the state of earnings necessary to maintain decent standards of living, necessitates their resort to public relief, and intensifies group conflicts, thereby resulting in grave injury to the public safety, health, and welfare.

28-5-3. Public policy.-It is hereby declared to be the public policy of this state to foster the employment of all individuals in this state in accordance with their fullest capacities, regardless of their race or color, religion, sex, sexual orientation, disability, age, or country of ancestral origin, and to safeguard their right to obtain and hold employment without such discrimination.

28-5-4. Exercise of police power. This chapter shall be deemed an exercise of the police power of the state for the protection of the public welfare, prosperity, health, and peace of the people of the state.

28-5-5. Right to equal employment opportunities.-The right of all individuals in this state to equal employment opportunities, regardless of race or color, religion, sex, sexual orientation, disability, age, or country of ancestral origin, is hereby recognized as and declared to be a civil right.

28-5-6. Definitions.-When used in this chapter:

(1) "Age" means anyone who is at least forty (40) years of age.

(2) "Because of sex" or "on the basis of sex" include, but are not limited to, because of or on the basis of pregnancy, childbirth, or related medical conditions, and women affected by pregnancy, childbirth, or related medical conditions shall be treated the same for all employment related purposes, including receipt of benefits under fringe benefit programs, as other persons not so affected but similar in their ability or inability to work, and nothing in this chapter shall be interpreted to permit otherwise.

(3) "Commission" means the Rhode Island commission against discrimination created by this chapter.

(4) "Discriminate" includes segregate or separate.

(5) "Employee" does not include any individual employed by his or her parents, spouse, or child, or in the domestic service of any person.

(6)(i) "Employer" includes the state and all political subdivisions thereof and any person in this state employing four (4) or more individuals, and any person acting in the interest of an employer directly or indirectly.

(ii) Nothing herein shall be construed to apply to a religious corporation, association, educational institution, or society with respect to the employment of individuals of its religion to perform work connected with the carrying on of its activities.

(7) "Employment agency" includes any person undertaking with or without compensation to procure opportunities to work, or to procure, recruit, refer, or place employees,

(8) "Firefighter" means an employee the duties of whose position includes work connected with the control and extinguishment of fires or the maintenance and use of firefighting apparatus and equipment, including an employee engaged in this activity who is transferred or promoted to a supervisory or administrative position.

(9) "Disability" means any physical or mental impairment which substantially limits one or more major life activities, has a record of an impairment, or is regarded as having an impairment by any person, employer, labor organization or employment agency subject to this chapter, and shall include any disability which is provided protection under the Americans with Disabilities Act, 42 U.S.C~ §12101 et seq. and federal regulations pertaining to the act, 28 CFR 35 and 29 CFR 1630. As used in this subdivision, the phrase:

(i) "Physical or mental impairment" means any physiological disorder or condition, cosmetic disfigurement, or anatomical loss affecting one or more of the following body systems: neurological; musculoskeletal; special sense organs; respiratory, including speech organs; cardiovascular; reproductive; digestive; genitourinary; hemic and lymphatic, skin; and endocrine; or any mental or psychological disorder, such as mental retardation, organic brain syndrome, emotional or mental illness, and specific learning disabilities.

(ii) "Major life activities" means functions such as caring for one's self, performing manual tasks, walking, seeing, hearing, speaking, breathing, learning, and working.

(iii) "Has a record of an impairment" means has a history of, or has been misclassified as having, a mental or physical impairment that substantially limits one or more major life activities.

(iv) "Regarded as having an impairment" means has a physical or mental impairment that does not substantially limit major life activities but that is treated as constituting a limitation; has a physical or mental impairment that substantially limits major life activities only as a result of the attitudes of others toward such impairment; or has none of the impairments but is treated as having such an impairment.

(10) "Labor organization" includes any organization which exists for the purpose, in whole or in part, of collective bargaining or of dealing with employers concerning grievances, terms or conditions of employment, or of other mutual aid or protection in relation to employment.

(11) "Law enforcement officer" means an employee the duties of whose position include investigation, apprehension, or detention of individuals suspected or convicted of offenses against the criminal laws of the state, including an employee engaged in such activity who is transferred or promoted to a supervisory or administrative position. For the purpose of this subdivision, "detention" includes the duties of employees assigned to guard individuals incarcerated in any penal institution.

(12) "Person" includes one or more individuals, partnerships, associations, organizations, corporations, legal representatives, trustees, trustees in bankruptcy, or receivers.

(13) "Sexual orientation" means having or being perceived as having an orientation for heterosexuality, bisexuality, or homosexuality. This definition is intended to describe the status of persons and does not render lawful any conduct prohibited by the criminal laws of this state nor impose any duty on a religious organization. This definition does not confer legislative approval of said status, but is intended to as-

sure the basic human rights of persons to obtain and hold employment, regardless of such status.

28-5-7. Unlawful employment practices.-It shall be an unlawful employment practice:

(1) For any employer:

(i) To refuse to hire any applicant for employment because of his or her race or color, religion, sex, disability, age, sexual orientation, or country of ancestral origin, or

(ii) Because of such reasons, to discharge an employee or discriminate against him or her with respect to hire, tenure, compensation, terms, conditions or privileges of employment, or any other matter directly or indirectly related to employment, provided however, if an insurer or employer extends insurance related benefits to persons other than or in addition to the named employee, nothing herein shall require those benefits to be offered to unmarried partners of named employees; or

(iii) In the recruiting of individuals for employment or in hiring them, to utilize any employment agency, placement service, training school or center, labor organization, or any other employee referring source which the employer knows, or has reasonable cause to know, discriminates against individuals because of their race or color, religion, sex, sexual orientation, disability, age, or country of ancestral origin, or

(iv) To refuse to reasonably accommodate an employee's or prospective employee's disability unless the employer can demonstrate that the accommodation would pose a hardship on the employer's program, enterprise, or business;

(2) For any employment agency:

(i) To fail or refuse to classify properly or refer for employment or otherwise discriminate against any individual because of his or her race or color, religion, sex, disability, age, sexual orientation, or country of ancestral origin, or

(ii) For any employment agency, placement service, training school or center, labor organization, or any other employee referring source to comply with an employer's request for the referral of job applicants if the request indicates either directly or indirectly that the employer will not afford full and equal employment opportunities to individuals regardless of their race or color, religion, sex, sexual orientation, disability, age, or country of ancestral origin;

(3) For any labor organization:

(i) To deny full and equal membership rights to any applicant for membership because of his or her race or color, religion, sex, sexual orientation, disability, age, or country of ancestral origin, or

(ii) Because of such reasons, to deny a member full and equal membership rights, expel him or her from membership, or otherwise discriminate in any manner against him or her with respect to his or her hire, tenure, compensation, terms, conditions or privileges of employment, or any other matter directly or indirectly related to membership or employment, whether or not authorized or required by the constitution or bylaws of the labor organization or by a collective labor agreement or other contract, or

(iii) To fail or refuse to classify properly or refer for employment, or otherwise to discriminate against any member because of his or her race or color, religion, sex, sexual orientation, disability, age, or country of ancestral origin, or

(iv) To refuse to reasonably accommodate a member's or prospective member's disability unless the labor organization can demonstrate that the accommodation would pose a hardship on the labor organization's program, enterprise, or business;

(4) Except where based on a bona fide occupational qualification certified by the commission or where necessary to comply with any federal mandated affirmative action programs, for any employer or employment agency, labor organization, placement service, training school or center, or any other employee referring source, prior to employment or admission to membership of any individual, to:

(i) Elicit or attempt to elicit any information directly or indirectly pertaining to his or her race or color, religion, sex, disability, age, sexual orientation, or country of ancestral origin;

(ii) Make or keep a record of his or her race or color, religion, sex, disability, age, sexual orientation, or country of ancestral origin;

(iii) Use any form of application for employment, or personnel or membership blank containing questions or entries directly or indirectly pertaining to race or color, religion, sex, disability, age, sexual orientation, or country of ancestral origin;

(iv) Print or publish or cause to be printed or published any notice or advertisement relating to employment or membership indicating any preference, limitation, specification, or discrimination based upon race or color, religion, sex, disability, age, sexual orientation, or country of ancestral origin;

(v) Establish, announce, or follow a policy of denying or limiting, through a quota system or otherwise, employment or membership opportunities of any group because of the race or color, religion, sex, disability, age, sexual orientation, or country of ancestral origin of that group;

(5) For any employer or employment agency, labor organization, placement service, training school or center, or any other employee referring source to discriminate in any manner against any individual because he or she has opposed any practice forbidden by this chapter, or because he or she has made a charge, testified, or assisted in any manner in any investigation, proceeding, or hearing under this chapter;

(6) For any person, whether or not an employer, employment agency, labor organization, or employee, to aid, abet, incite, compel, or coerce the doing of any act declared by this section to be an unlawful employment practice, or to obstruct or prevent any person from complying with the provisions of this chapter or any order issued thereunder, or to attempt directly or indirectly to commit any act declared by this section to be an unlawful employment practice;

(7) For any employer to include on any application for employment, except applications for law enforcement agency positions, or positions related thereto, a question inquiring or to otherwise inquire either orally or in writing whether the applicant has ever been arrested or charged with any crime; provided, however, that nothing herein shall prevent an employer from inquiring whether the applicant has ever been convicted of any crime;

(8) For any person who, on June 7, 1988, is providing either by direct payment or by making contributions to a fringe benefit fund or insurance program, benefits in violation with §§ 28-5-6, 28-5-7 and 28-5-38, until the expiration of a period of one year from June 7, 1988 or if there is an applicable collective bargaining agreement in effect on June 7, 1988, until the termination of that agreement, in order to come into compliance with §§ 28-5-6, 28-5-7 and 28-5-38, to reduce the benefits or the compensation provided any employee on June 7, 1988, either directly or by failing to provide sufficient contributions to a fringe benefit fund or insurance program; provided, that where the costs of such benefits on June 7, 1988 are apportioned between employers and employees, the payments or contributions required to comply with §§ 28-5-6, 28-5-7 and 28-5-38 may be made by employers and employees in the same proportion, and provided further, that nothing in this section shall prevent the readjustment of benefits or compensation for reasons unrelated to compliance with §§ 28-5-6, 28-5-7 and 28-5-38.

28-5-7.2. Proof of unlawful employment practices in disparate impact cases.- (a) An unlawful employment practice prohibited by § 28-5-7 may be established by proof of disparate impact. An unlawful employment practice by proof of disparate impact is established when:

(1) A complainant demonstrates that an employment practice results in a disparate impact on the basis of race, color, religion, sex, sexual orientation, disability, age, or country of ancestral origin, and the respondent fails to demonstrate that the practice is required by business necessity; or

(2) A complainant demonstrates that a group of employment practices results in disparate impact on the basis of race, color, religion, sex, sexual orientation, disability, age, or country of ancestral origin, and the respondent fails to demonstrate that the practices are required by business necessity; provided that:

(i) If a complainant demonstrates that a group of employment practices results in a disparate impact, the complainant shall not be required to demonstrate which specific practice or practices within the group results in the disparate impact, and

(ii) If the respondent demonstrates that a specific employment practice within such group of employment practices does not contribute to the disparate impact, the respondent shall not be required to demonstrate that the practice is required by business necessity

(b) A demonstration that an employment practice is required by business necessity may be used as a defense only against a claim under this section.

(c) As used in this section:

(1) The terms "complainant" and "respondent" mean those individuals or entities defined as such in § 28-5-17;

(2) The term "demonstrates" means meets the burdens of production and persuasion;

(3) The term "group of employment practices" means a combination of employment practices or an overall employment process; and

(4) The term "required by business necessity" means essential to effective job performance.

(d) Nothing contained herein shall be construed as limiting the methods of proof of unlawful employment practices under § 28-5-7 to the methods set in this section.

28-5-7.3. Discriminatory practice need not be sole motivating factor.-An unlawful employment practice may be established in an action or proceeding under this chapter when the complainant demonstrates that race, color, religion, sex, sexual orientation, disability, age, or country of ancestral origin was a motivating factor for any employment practice, even though the practice was also motivated by other factors. Nothing contained herein shall be construed as requiring direct evidence of unlawful intent or as limiting the methods of proof of unlawful employment practices under § 28-5-7.

28-5-13. Powers and duties of commission.-The commission shall have the following powers and duties:

(1) To establish and maintain a principal office in the city of Providence, Rhode Island, and such other offices within the state as it may deem necessary.

(2) To meet and function at any place within the state.

(3) To appoint such attorneys, clerks, and other employees and agents as it may deem necessary, fix their compensation within the limitations provided by law, and prescribe their duties. Provided, however, that the provisions of chapter 4 of title 36 shall not apply to this chapter.

(4) To adopt, promulgate, amend, and rescind rules and regulations to effectuate the provisions of this chapter, and the policies and practice of the commission in connection therewith.

(5) To formulate policies to effectuate the purposes of this chapter.

(6) To receive, investigate, and pass upon charges of unlawful employment practices.

(7)(i) In connection with any investigation or hearing held pursuant to the provisions of this chapter, to hold hearings, subpoena witnesses, compel their attendance, administer oaths, take the testimony of any person under oath, and, in connection therewith, to require the production for examination of any books and papers relating to any matter under investigation or in question before the -commission.

(ii) The commission may make rules as to the issuance of subpoenas by individual commissioners.

(iii) Contumacy or refusal to obey a subpoena issued pursuant to this section shall constitute a contempt punishable, upon the application of the commission, by the superior court in the county in which the hearing is held or in which the witness resides or transacts business.

(8) To utilize voluntary and uncompensated services of private individuals and organizations as may from time to time be offered and needed.

(9)(i) To create such advisory agencies and conciliation councils, local or statewide, as will aid in effectuating the purposes of this chapter. The commission may itself, or it may empower these agencies and councils to:

(A) Study the problems of discrimination in all or specific fields of human relationships when based on race or color, religion, sex, sexual orientation, disability, or country of ancestral origin, and

(B) Foster through community effort or otherwise good will among the groups and elements of the population of the state.

(h) The agencies and councils may make recommendations to the commission for the development of policies and procedure in general.

(iii) Advisory agencies and conciliation councils created by the commission shall be composed of representative citizens serving without pay, but with reimbursement for actual and necessary traveling expenses.

(10) To issue such publications and such results of investigations and research as in its judgment will tend to promote good will and minimize or eliminate discrimination based on race or color, religion, sex, sexual orientation, disability, age, or country of ancestral origin.

(11) From time to time, but not less than once a year, to report to the legislature and the governor, describing the investigations, proceedings, and hearings the commission has conducted and their outcome, the decisions it has rendered, and the other work performed by it, and make recommendations for such further legislation, concerning abuses and discrimination based on race or color, religion, sex, sexual orientation, disability, age or country of ancestral origin, as may be desirable.

28-5-14. Educational program.-In order to eliminate prejudice among the various ethnic groups in this state and to further good will among those groups, the commission and the state department of education are jointly directed to prepare a comprehensive educational program, designed for the students of the public schools of this state and for all other residents thereof, calculated to emphasize the origin of prejudice based on race or color, religion, sex, sexual orientation, disability, age or country of ancestral origin, its harmful effects, and its incompatibility with American principles of equality and fair play.

28-5-17. Conciliation of charges of unlawful practices. Upon the commission's own initiative or whenever an aggrieved individual or an organization chartered for the purpose of combating discrimination, racism, or of safeguarding civil liberties, or of promoting full, free, or equal employment opportunities, such individual or organization being hereinafter referred to as the complainant, makes a charge to the commission that any employer, employment agency, labor organization, or person, hereinafter referred to as the respondent, has engaged or is engaging in unlawful employment practices and that the unlawful employment practices have occurred, have terminated, or have been applied to affect adversely the person aggrieved, whichever is later, within one (1) year, the commission may initiate a preliminary investigation; and if it shall determine after the investigation that it is probable that unlawful employment practices have been or are being engaged in, it shall endeavor to eliminate the unlawful employment practices by informal methods of conference, conciliation, and persuasion, including a conciliation agreement. The terms of the conciliation agreement shall include provisions requiring the respondent to refrain from the commission of unlawful discriminatory practices in the future and may contain such further provisions as may be agreed upon by the investigating commissioner and the respondent, including a provision for the entry in superior court of a consent decree embodying the terms of the conciliation agreement. Nothing said or done during such endeavors may be used as evidence in any subsequent proceeding. If, after an investigation and conference, the commission is satisfied that any unlawful employment practice of the respondent will be eliminated, it may, with the consent of the complainant, treat the charge as conciliated, and entry of such disposition shall be made on the records of the commission; provided, however, that the commission shall not enter a consent order or conciliation agreement settling claims of discrimination in an action or proceeding under this chapter unless the parties and their counsel attest that a waiver of all or substantially all attorneys' fees was not compelled as a condition of the settlement.

28-5-18. Complaint and notice of hearing.-If the commission fails to effect the elimination of the unlawful employment practices and to obtain voluntary compliance with this chapter, or, if the circumstances warrant, in advance of any preliminary investigation or endeavors, the commission shall have the power to issue and cause to be served upon any person or respondent a complaint stating the charges in that respect and containing a notice of hearing before the commission, a member thereof, or a hearing examiner at a place therein fixed to be held not less than ten (10) days after the service of the complaint. Any complaint issued pursuant to this section must be so issued within two (2) years after a signed and notarized charge has been filed with the Commission pursuant to § 28-5-17.

No proceeding which was pending under this chapter on April 5, 1996 shall be subject to dismissal on the basis of the Commission's failure to issue a complaint within one (1) year after the alleged unfair employment practice occurred or has been applied to affect adversely the person aggrieved, where such charge was filed with the Commission within one (1) year after the alleged unfair employment practice occurred or has been applied to affect adversely the person aggrieved, whichever is later, and the respondent had agreed to extend or waive the one (1) year period of limitations.

28-5-20.1. Proceedings before other state administrative agencies.-(a) The commission shall not be precluded from investigating, taking evidence, considering claims or issuing findings on matters which could have been presented to any other state administrative agency, but which were not actually presented and decided in a contested case as defined under the Administrative Procedures Act, chapter 35 of title 42.

(b) To the extent the commission is bound by findings of fact and conclusions of law of another state administrative agency, the commission shall be entitled to grant any relief authorized under this chapter in accordance with those findings to the extent that such relief was not available to, or within the authority of, the other agency to provide.

28-5-22. Evidence of predetermined pattern.-The commission shall, in ascertaining the practices followed by the respondent, take into account all evidence, statistical or otherwise, which may tend to prove the existence of a predetermined pattern of employment or membership; provided, that nothing herein contained shall be construed to authorize or require any employer or labor organization to employ or admit applicants for employment or membership in the proportion to which their race or color, religion, sex, sexual orientation, disability, age, or country of ancestral origin bears to the total population or in accordance with any criterion other than the individual qualifications of the applicant.

28-5-38. Liberal construction.-The provisions of this chapter shall be construed liberally for the accomplishment of the purposes thereof, and any law inconsistent with any provision hereof shall not apply. Nothing contained in this chapter shall be deemed to repeal any of the provisions of any law of this state relating to discrimination because of race or color, religion, sex, sexual orientation, disability, age or country of ancestral origin. Nothing contained in this chapter shall be deemed to repeal any of the provisions of any law of this state relating to parental leave.

28-5-40. Affirmative action report.-On February 1 of each year the governor shall, in conjunction with the state equal opportunity office, submit to the general assembly a report documenting the status of affirmative action programs for women, persons with disabilities, and minorities in each department and state agency. At a minimum, the report shall include statistics for each department and state agency, indicating the employment by race, disability, and sex of workers in each job category in the department or agency, and containing a comparison of those statistics with those of the previous year, and shall include the plans each department or state agency has adopted for the forthcoming year to correct any continuing deficiencies in the employment of women, persons with disabilities, and minorities in the workforce.

28-5-41. Right to fair employment practices.-Whenever in this chapter there shall appear the terms, "race or color, religion, sex, disability, age or country of ancestral origin" there shall be inserted immediately thereafter the words "sexual orientation".

28-5-42. Receipt of assistance-No estoppel effect.-The fact that an individual has applied for, received or continues to receive private insurance or government assistance on the basis of a physical or mental impairment shall not, by itself, relieve or excuse any employer, employment agency or labor organization from its obligations under this chapter, but may be considered as evidence by the commission or court in its determination, nor shall such a fact serve as an estoppel or otherwise preclude an individual with a disability from obtaining the protections of this chapter.

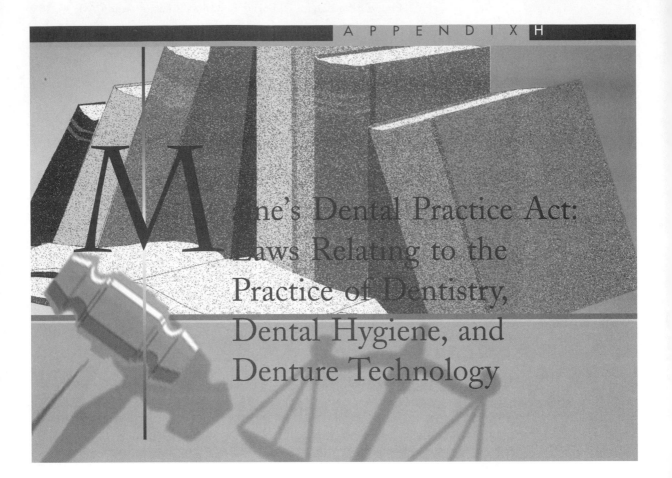

Maine's Dental Practice Act: Laws Relating to the Practice of Dentistry, Dental Hygiene, and Denture Technology

(TITLE 32)
(PROFESSIONS AND OCCUPATIONS)

(CHAPTER 16)
(DENTISTS AND DENTAL HYGIENISTS)

(SUBCHAPTER I)
(GENERAL PROVISIONS)
32 § 1061. Addresses and Change of Address
1. Furnish to board. Every licensee under this chapter shall:
A. Furnish the secretary of the board with the place or places of practice.
B. Upon a change of name or registered address or addresses, furnish the secretary-treasurer of the board with the new address within 30 days of the change.

2. Failure; fee. For failure to comply with this section, a licensee is subject to a fee imposed by the board of not more than $25.

32 § 1062-A. Penalties; Injunction
1. Penalties. A person who practices or falsely claims legal authority to practice dentistry, dental hygiene, denture technology (denturism) or dental radiography in this State without first obtaining a license as required by this chapter, or after the license has expired, has been suspended or revoked or has been temporarily suspended or revoked, commits a Class E crime.

2. Injunction. The State may bring an action in Superior Court to enjoin a person for violating this chapter, regardless of whether proceedings have been or may be instituted in the Administrative Court or whether criminal proceedings have been or may be instituted.

(SUBCHAPTER II)
(BOARD OF DENTAL EXAMINERS)
32 § 1071. Membership; Appointment; Vacancies; Removal; Nominations; Compensation

The Board of Dental Examiners, established by Title 5, section 12004-A, subsection 10, and in this chapter called the "board," consists of 7 members, appointed by the Governor as follows: five members of the dental profession, one dental hygienist and one representative of the public.

1. Membership. A person is not eligible for appointment to the board who has been convicted of a violation of the provisions of this or any other prior dental practice act, or who has been convicted of a crime punishable by more than one year's imprisonment. A person is not eligible for appointment to the board who has served 10 years or more on a dental examining board in this State. Appointment of members must comply with section 60. The Governor may remove a member of the board on proven charges of inefficiency, incompetence, immorality or unprofessional conduct.

2. Dentists. The Governor may accept nominations from the Maine Dental Association and from other organizations and individuals.

Members of the dental profession must hold a valid dental license and must have been in the actual practice of dentistry in this State for at least 10 years immediately preceding the appointment. The term for a member who is a dentist is 5 years. A dentist is not eligible to serve as a member of the board while employing a dental hygienist who is a member of the board.

3. Dental hygienist. The dental hygienist must be qualified pursuant to subchapter IV, must be a legal resident of the State and must have practiced in the State for at least 6 years immediately preceding appointment. The dental hygienist member of the board is a full-voting member of the board. The term of the dental hygienist is 5 years. The Governor may accept nominations from the Maine Dental Hygienists Association and from other organizations and individuals before the appointment of a hygienist to the board. A dental hygienist is not eligible to serve as a member of the board while employed by a dentist who is a member of the board.

4. Public member. The public member is appointed to a 5-year term.

5. Compensation. The members of the board are entitled to compensation according to the provisions of Title 5, chapter 379. Expenses of the board members must be certified by the secretary of the board.

32 § 1072. Elections; Quorum; Reports; Records; Treasurer; Expenses

At its annual meeting, the board shall elect from among its members a president, a vice-president and a secretary-treasurer. Five members constitute a quorum. The board shall have a common seal. At a time and place to be fixed by the board, the board shall hold at least one regular meeting each year and special meetings as necessary. The board may recognize nationally or regionally administered examinations given at least annually for applicants to practice dentistry in the State. The board may make rules, not contrary to law, necessary for the performance of its duties. On or before August 1st, the board shall annually make a report of its proceedings to the Commissioner of Professional and Financial Regulation. The secretary-treasurer of the board shall keep records of all proceedings of the board and be the custodian of these records. Records that constitute and are recognized as the official records of the board must be open for public inspection at reasonable times.

The secretary-treasurer of the board shall collect all fees, charges and assessments payable to the board and account for and pay them according to law. The secretary-treasurer is entitled to receive an annual salary, to be fixed by the board, in lieu of per diem compensation. The secretary-treasurer is entitled to necessary expenses incurred in the discharge of official duties, including clerical and stenographic assistance, printing and postage. The allowance for expenses must be certified by the president of the board.

32 § 1073. Powers

The board may:

1. Employees and offices; funds. Employ persons to assist in carrying out its duties in the administration and enforcement of this chapter; provide offices, furniture, fixtures, supplies or printing; and expend funds as determined necessary;

2. Rules. Adopt rules in accordance with the Maine Administrative Procedure Act that are necessary for the implementation of this chapter. The rules may include, but need not be limited to, requirements for licensure, interviews for licensing and renewal, continuing education, inactive licensure status, use of general anesthesia and fees for providing a list of addresses of licensed professionals upon request.

3. False advertising. Establish rules relating to false, deceptive or misleading advertising, except that no rules may be inconsistent with any rule promulgated pursuant to Title 5, section 207, subsection 2.

32 § 1074. Affiliation with American Association of Dental Examiners

The board may affiliate with the American Association of Dental Examiners as an active member and pay regular dues to that association and may send one or more delegates to the meetings of the American Association of Dental Examiners. These delegates are entitled to receive compensation provided for in section 1071.

32 § 1075. Liaison; Limitations

On or before August 1st of each year, the board shall submit to the Commissioner of Professional and Financial Regulation, for the preceding fiscal year ending June 30th, its annual report of its operations and financial position, together with comments and recommendations the board considers essential.

The commissioner shall act as a liaison between the board and the Governor.

The commissioner may not exercise or interfere with the exercise of discretionary, regulatory or licensing authority granted by law to the board.

The commissioner may not exercise or interfere with the exercise of discretionary, regulatory or licensing authority granted by statute to the board. The commissioner may require the board to be accessible to the public for complaints and questions during regular business hours and to provide any information the commissioner requires in order to ensure that the board is operating administratively within the requirements of this chapter.

32 § 1076. Budget

The board shall submit to the Commissioner of Professional and Financial Regulation its budgetary requirements in the same manner as is provided in Title 5, section 1665, and the commissioner shall in turn transmit these requirements to the Bureau of the Budget without any revision, alteration or change, unless alterations are mutually agreed upon by the department and the board or the board's designee. The budget submitted by the board to the commissioner must be sufficient to enable the board to comply with this subchapter.

32 § 1077. Disciplinary Actions

1. Disciplinary proceedings and sanctions.

Regarding noncompliance with or violation of this chapter or of rules adopted by the board, the board shall investigate a complaint on its own motion or upon receipt of a written complaint filed with the board.

The board shall notify the licensee of the content of a complaint filed against the licensee as soon as possible, but no later than 60 days from receipt of this information. The licensee shall respond within 30 days. If the licensee's response to the complaint satisfies the board that the complaint does not merit further investigation or action, the matter may be dismissed, with notice of the dismissal to the complainant, if any.

If, in the opinion of the board, the factual basis of the complaint is or may be true, and the complaint is of sufficient gravity to warrant further action, the board may request an informal conference with the licensee. The board shall provide the licensee with adequate notice of the conference and of the issues to be discussed. The conference must be conducted in executive session of the board, pursuant to Title 1, section 405, unless otherwise requested by the licensee. Statements made at the conference may not be introduced at a subsequent formal hearing unless all parties consent.

If the board finds that the factual basis of the complaint is true and is of sufficient gravity to warrant further action, it may take any of the following actions it considers appropriate:

A. With the consent of the licensee, enter into a consent agreement that fixes the period and terms of probation best adapted to protect the public health and safety and to rehabilitate or educate the licensee. A consent agreement may be used to terminate a complaint investigation, if entered into by the board, the licensee and the Attorney General's office;

B. In consideration for acceptance of a voluntary surrender of the license, if a consent agreement is signed by the board, the licensee and the Attorney General's office, negotiate stipulations, including terms and conditions for reinstatement, that ensure protection of the public health and safety and that serve to rehabilitate or educate the licensee;

C. If the board concludes that modification or nonrenewal of the license is in order, the board shall hold an adjudicatory hearing in accordance with the provisions of the Maine Administrative Procedure Act, Title 5, chapter 375, subchapter IV.

D. If the board concludes that suspension or revocation of the license is in order, the board shall file a complaint in the Administrative Court in accordance with Title 4, chapter 25.

2. Grounds for discipline. The board may suspend or revoke a license pursuant to Title 5, section 10004. The following are grounds for an action to refuse to issue, modify, suspend, revoke or refuse to renew the license of a person licensed under this chapter:

A. The practice of fraud or deceit in obtaining a license under this chapter or in connection with service rendered within the scope of the license issued;

B. Habitual substance abuse that has resulted or is foreseeably likely to result in the licensee performing services in a manner that endangers the health or safety of patients;

C. A professional diagnosis of a mental or physical condition that has resulted or may result in the licensee performing services in a manner that endangers the health or safety of patients;

D. Aiding or abetting the practice of a dental profession by an individual who is not licensed under this chapter and who claims to be legally licensed;

E. Incompetence in the practice for which the licensee is licensed. A licensee is considered incompetent in the practice if the licensee has:
   (1) Engaged in conduct that evidences a lack of ability or fitness to perform the duties owed by the licensee to a client or patient or the general public; or
   (2) Engaged in conduct that evidences a lack of knowledge or inability to apply principles or skills to carry out the practice for which the licensee is licensed;

F. Unprofessional conduct. A licensee is considered to have engaged in unprofessional conduct if the licensee violates a standard of professional behavior that has been established in the practice for which the licensee is licensed;

G. Subject to the limitations of Title 5, chapter 341, conviction of a crime that involves dishonesty or false statement or that relates directly to the practice for which the licensee is licensed, or conviction of a crime for which incarceration for one year or more may be imposed;

H. A violation of this chapter or a rule adopted by the board; or

I. Engaging in false, misleading or deceptive advertising.

(SUBCHAPTER III)
(DENTISTS)
32 § 1081. Definitions; Persons Excepted

1. Practicing dentistry. A person is considered to be practicing dentistry when that person performs, or attempts or professes to perform, a dental operation or oral surgery or dental service of any kind, gratuitously or for a salary, fee, money or other remuneration paid, or to be paid, directly or indirectly to the person or to any other person or agency who is a proprietor of a place where dental operations, oral surgery or dental services are performed. A person who directly or indirectly, by any means or method, takes impressions of a human tooth, teeth, jaws or performs a phase of an operation incident to the replacement of a part of a tooth; or supplies artificial substitutes for the natural teeth, or who furnishes, supplies, constructs, reproduces or repairs a prosthetic denture, bridge, appliance or any other structure to be worn in the human mouth, except on the written prescription of a duly licensed dentist; or who places dental appliances or structures in the human mouth, or adjusts or attempts or professes to adjust the same, or delivers the same to a person other than the dentist upon whose prescription the work was performed; or who professes to the public by any method to furnish, supply, construct, reproduce or repair a prosthetic denture, bridge, appliance or other structure to be worn in the human mouth, or who diagnoses or professes to diagnose, prescribes for or professes to prescribe for, treats or professes to treat, disease, pain, deformity, deficiency, injury or physical condition of the human teeth or jaws or adjacent structure, or who extracts or attempts to extract human teeth, or corrects or attempts to correct malformations of teeth or of the jaws is also considered to be practicing dentistry. A person who repairs or fills cavities in the human teeth; or who diagnoses, makes and adjusts appliances to artificial casts or malposed teeth for treatment of the malposed teeth in the human mouth, with or without instruction; or who uses an x-ray machine for the purpose of taking dental x rays, or who gives or professes to give interpretations or readings of dental x rays; or who administers an anaesthetic of any nature in connection with a dental operation; or who uses the words dentist, dental surgeon, oral surgeon or the letters D.D.S., D.M.D. or any other words, letters, title or descriptive matter that in any way represents that person as being able to diagnose, treat, prescribe or operate for a disease, pain, deformity, deficiency, injury or physical condition of the teeth or jaws or adjacent structures; or who states, or professes or permits to be stated or professed by any means or method whatsoever that the person can perform or will attempt to perform dental operations or render a diagnosis connected with dental operations is also considered to be practicing dentistry.

2. Exemptions. Nothing in this chapter applies to the following practices, acts and operations:

A. The practice of the profession by a licensed physician or surgeon under the laws of this State, unless that person practices dentistry as a specialty;

B. The giving by a qualified anesthetist or nurse anesthetist of an anesthetic for a dental operation; the giving by a certified registered nurse of an anesthetic for a dental operation under the direct supervision of either a licensed dentist who holds a valid anesthesia permit or a licensed physician; and the removing of sutures, the dressing of wounds, the application of dressings and bandages and the injection of drugs subcutaneously or intravenously by a certified registered nurse under the direct supervision of a licensed dentist or physician;

C. The practice of dentistry in the discharge of their official duties by graduate dentists or dental surgeons in the United States Army, Navy, Public Health Service, Coast Guard or Veterans Bureau;

D. The practice of dentistry by a licensed dentist of other states or countries at meetings of the Maine State Dental Association or its affiliates or other like dental organizations approved by the board, while appearing as clinicians;

E. The filling of prescriptions of a licensed dentist by any person, association, corporation or other entity for the construction, reproduction or repair of prosthetic dentures, bridges, plates or appliances to be used or worn as substitutes for natural teeth, provided that this person, association, corporation or other entity does not solicit nor advertise, directly or indirectly, by mail, card, newspaper, pamphlet, radio or otherwise, to the general public to construct, reproduce or repair prosthetic dentures, bridges, plates or other appliances to be used or worn as substitutes for natural teeth; and

F. The taking of impressions by dental hygienists or dental assistants for study purposes only.

3. Proprietor. The term proprietor, as used in this chapter, includes a person who:

A. Employs dentists or dental hygienists or other dental auxiliaries in the operation of a dental office;

B. Places in possession of a dentist or a dental hygienist or other dental auxiliary or other agent dental material or equipment that may be necessary for the management of a dental office on the basis of a lease or any other agreement for compensation for the use of that material, equipment or office; or

C. Retains the ownership or control of dental equipment or material or a dental office and makes the same available in any manner for the use by dentists or dental hygienists or other agents, except that nothing in this subsection applies to bona fide sales of dental equipment or material secured by a chattel mortgage or retain title agreement. A person licensed to practice dentistry may not enter into arrangements with a person who is not licensed to practice dentistry.

4. Corporations; names. A corporation may not practice, offer or undertake to practice or hold itself out as practicing dentistry. Every person practicing dentistry as an employee of another shall cause that person's name to be conspicuously displayed and kept in a conspicuous place at the entrance of the place where the practice is conducted. This subsection does not prohibit a licensed dentist from practicing dentistry as an employee of another licensed dentist in this State, as an employee of a nonprofit corporation, as an employee of a state hospital or state institution where the only remuneration is from the State or from a corporation that provides dental service for its employees at no profit to the corporation. This subsection does not prohibit the practice of dentists who have incorporated their practices as permitted by Title 13, chapter 22.

5. Dentist of record; office manager. Each patient in a multidentist practice must be provided with a dentist of record. The patient entering a multidentist practice, at the onset of treatment, must be informed as to the identity of the patient's dentist of record. The identity must at least consist of the name and telephone number.

Each office established or maintained in this State for the practice of dentistry by a person or persons subject to this chapter must be under the general supervision of a licensed dentist.

32 § 1082. Qualifications

Before receiving a license to practice dentistry in this State, a person must be at least 18 years of age and must be a graduate of or have a diploma from a dental college, school or dental department of a university accredited by an agency approved by the board.

32 § 1083. Application for Examination; Subjects; Reexamination

The board may at its discretion recognize the results of an examination given by the National Board of Dental Examiners or an accredited clinical testing agency approved by the board in lieu of or in addition to the examination or examinations that it may require. The board may require as part of the examination a clinical demonstration of the candidate's skill in dentistry. An applicant who fails to pass the first examination to the satisfaction of the board is entitled to one reexamination. Applicants for licensure shall pay a fee set by the board for the examination.

32 § 1084. Licenses; Fees

The board shall issue under its seal to any person who successfully meets all licensure requirements a license to practice dentistry in this State, signed by the members of the board. A dentist shall publicly exhibit the dentist's license. The license is prima facie evidence of authority to practice dentistry in this State, except that it is unlawful for a person to practice dentistry in this State after the expiration date that appears on the license unless the practitioner pays to the board on or before January 1st of even-numbered years a fee of not more than $200 to be determined by the board, and meets other conditions that the board may require. Upon receipt of the required fee, the board shall issue a renewal of the practitioner's license, which the practitioner shall place beside or attach to the practitioner's initial license. Practitioners who have not paid as provided and who otherwise qualify for renewal may be reinstated upon payment of a fee to be determined by the board of not more than $100 if paid before February 1st. A license to practice is automatically suspended on February 1st for nonpayment of the license renewal fee and may be reinstated, if approved by the board, on payment of a fee to be determined by the board of not more than $200. A new applicant having paid the application fee shall pay either the biennial licensure fee, if the applicant applies on an even-numbered year, or half the biennial licensure fee if the applicant applies in an odd-numbered year.

32 § 1084-A. Continuing Education

As a condition of renewal of a license to practice, a dentist must provide evidence of having successfully completed 40 hours of continuing education during the 2 years prior to application for renewal. To meet this requirement, the education must relate to professional competency and relate to those aspects of the profession in which the practitioner is currently engaged. The board shall specify the desired content of the program of continuing education, establish criteria for approving providers of continuing education and approve those providers. The board shall specify the criteria for successful completion of a continuing education requirement. All actions by the board in the implementation of this program must be by rule and follow the provisions of the Maine Administrative Procedure Act.

The board may indicate to an individual practitioner specific subject areas on which that practitioner's continuing education is to focus in the future. Providers are required to obtain and retain for 3 years a written course assessment from each student, which must be reviewed periodically by the board.

32 § 1085. Endorsement; Fees

The board is authorized, at its discretion, without the examination as provided, to issue a license to an applicant who furnishes proof, satisfactory to the board, that the applicant has been licensed to practice dentistry in another state after full compliance with the requirements of its dental laws. If an applicant is licensed to practice dentistry in another state, that applicant's professional education may not be less than is required in this State and the applicant must have been at least 5 years in actual practice in the state in which the license was granted. Every license of this type issued by the board must state upon its face the grounds upon which it is issued and the applicant may be required to furnish proof upon affidavit. The fee for the license is determined by the board, but may not be more than $300.

32 § 1086. Permits for Internship

The board has the authority, upon presentation of satisfactory credentials under the rules as the board may prescribe, to issue permits to a graduate of an approved dental school or college who has not been licensed to practice dentistry in this State, who has passed an examination for licensure in this State and who, in the board's judgment, has not violated a provision of this chapter or rules adopted by the board to serve as a dental intern in a licensed hospital, providing the hospital maintains a dental staff of at least one licensed dentist. Permits expire at the end of one month and may be renewed by the board. The intern functions under the supervision and direction of the dental staff of the hospital, and the intern's work is limited to patients admitted to the hospital. The intern is not eligible to receive a fee or compensation in addition to the salary or other remuneration received from the hospital.

A special permit may be issued by the board to a licensed dentist practicing outside this State when the request for the dentist comes from a charitable or social organization within the State and when the purpose for that permit is to provide free dental care for the public when resident dental service is not available. The board may provide an expiration date for a permit issued, except that a permit may not be valid for more than one year.

The board has the authority, upon presentation of satisfactory proof of academic affiliation and good academic standing, and providing, in the board's judgment, a violation of a provision of this chapter or of the board's rules has not occurred, to issue a permit to a bona fide dental student of a school or university acceptable to the board, after the completion of satisfactory training to perform limited dental service in institutional and public health service programs within the State, commensurate with the student's level of training under the supervision and control of a licensed dentist or a teaching school. The board must, prior to the issuance of this permit, determine that the supervision and control of the services to be performed by the student are adequate and that the performance of these services by the student adds to the student's knowledge and skill in dentistry. Permits expire at the end of each month and may be renewed by the board.

Specialists in particular fields of dentistry practicing outside the State may be issued a permit to practice within the State for a period not to exceed 6 months.

The board may charge a fee up to $50 for licenses issued pursuant to this section.

32 § 1087. Fee for Duplicate License

An applicant for a duplicate license granted upon proof of loss of the original shall pay a fee of $15.

32 § 1089. Drugs and Dental Procedure

A dentist has the right to prescribe drugs or medicines, perform surgical operations, administer general and local anesthetics and use appliances as may be necessary for proper dental treatment. A dentist is authorized to take case histories and perform physical examinations to the extent the activities are necessary in the exercise of due care in conjunction with the provision of dental treatment or the administration of general or local anesthetics. A dentist is not permitted to perform physical examinations within a hospital licensed by the Department of Human Services unless this activity is permitted by the hospital.

32 § 1090. Prescription Required for Dental Laboratory

1. Prescription. A dentist who uses the services of a person not licensed to practice dentistry in this State to construct, alter, repair or duplicate a denture, plate, partial plate, bridge, splint, orthodontic or prosthetic appliance shall first furnish the unlicensed person with a written prescription, which must contain:

A. The name and address of the unlicensed person;

B. The patient's name or number. In the event the number is used, the name of the patient must be written upon the duplicate copy of the prescription retained by the dentist;

C. The date on which it was written;

D. A prescription of the work to be done, with diagrams if necessary;

E. A specification of the type and quality of materials to be used; and

F. The signature of the dentist and the number of the dentist's state license.

The unlicensed person shall retain the original prescription and the dentist shall retain for 2 years a duplicate copy for inspection by the board or its agent. For purposes of this subsection, "unlicensed person" includes all legal entities.

32 § 1092. Unlawful Practice

Whoever practices dentistry without obtaining a license, or whoever practices dentistry under a false or assumed name, or under the license of another person of the same name, or under the name of a corporation, company, association, parlor or trade name, or whoever, being manager, proprietor, operator or conductor of a place for performing dental operations, employs a person who is not a lawful practitioner of dentistry of this State to do dental operations as defined in section 1081, or permits persons to practice dentistry under a false name, or assumes a title or appends or prefixes to that person's name the letters that falsely represent the person as having a degree from a dental college, or who impersonates another at an examination held by the board, or who knowingly makes a false application or false representation in connection with the examination, or whoever practices as a dental hygienist without having a license, or whoever employs a person as a dental hygienist who is not licensed to practice commits a Class E crime.

32 § 1092-A. Confidentiality

1. Definitions. As used in this section, unless the context otherwise indicates, the following terms have the following meanings.

A. "Confidential communication" means a communication not intended to be disclosed to 3rd persons other than those present to further the interest of the patient in the consultation, examination or interview or persons who are participating in the diagnosis and treatment under the direction of the dentist, including members of the patient's family.

B. "Patient" means a person who consults or is examined or interviewed by a dentist or dental auxiliary.

2. General rule of privilege. A patient has a privilege to refuse to disclose and to prevent another person from disclosing confidential communications made for the purpose of diagnosis or treatment of the patient's physical, mental or emotional conditions, including alcohol or drug addiction, among the patient, the patient's dentist and persons who are participating in the diagnosis or treatment under the direction of the dentist, including members of the patient's family.

3. Who may claim the privilege. The privilege may be claimed by the patient, by the patient's guardian or conservator or by the personal representative of a deceased patient. The dentist or dental auxiliary at the time of the communication is presumed to have authority to claim the privilege, but only on behalf of the patient.

4. Exceptions. Notwithstanding any other provisions of law, the following are exceptions.

A. If the court orders an examination of the physical, mental or emotional condition of a patient, whether a party or a witness, communications made in the course of the examination are not privileged under this section with respect to the particular purpose for which the examination is ordered unless the court orders otherwise.

B. There is not any privilege under this section as to communications relevant to an issue of the physical, mental or emotional condition of the patient in a proceeding in which the condition of the patient is an element of the claim or defense of the patient, or of a party claiming through or under the patient or because of the patient's condition or claiming as a beneficiary of the patient through a contract to which the patient is or was a party, or after the patient's death, in a proceeding in which a party puts the condition in issue.

C. There is not any privilege under this section as to information regarding a patient that is sought by the Chief Medical Examiner or the Chief Medical Examiner's designee in a medical examiner case, as defined by Title 22, section 3025, in which the Chief Medical Examiner or the Chief Medical Examiner's designee has reason to believe that information relating to dental treatment may assist in determining the identity of a deceased person.

D. There is not any privilege under this section as to disclosure of information concerning a patient when that disclosure is required by law and nothing in this section may modify or affect the provisions of Title 22, sections 4011 to 4015 and Title 29, section 1312-E.

32 § 1093. Fraudulent Sale or Alteration of Diplomas

A person who sells or offers to sell a diploma conferring a dental degree or a license granted pursuant to the laws of this State, or who procures a license or diploma with intent that it be used as evidence of the right to practice dentistry by a person other than the one upon whom the diploma or license was conferred, or who with fraudulent intent alters the diploma or license, or uses or attempts to use the same when altered, or who attempts to bribe a member of the board by the offer or use of money or other pecuniary reward or by other undue influence commits a Class E crime.

32 § 1094. Penalties

A person who violates a provision of this chapter, for the violation of which a penalty has not been prescribed, commits a Class E crime. The several prosecuting officers of this State, on notice from a member of the board, shall institute prosecutions for offenses under this chapter.

32 § 1094-A. Review Committee Immunity

Any dentist who is a member of a peer review committee of a state or local association or society composed of doctors of dentistry, any staff member of such an association or society assisting a peer review committee and any witness or consultant appearing before or presenting information to the peer review committee is immune from civil liability for, without malice, undertaking or failing to undertake any act within the scope of the function of the committee.

32 § 1094-B. Removable Dental Prostheses; Owner Identification

1. Identification required. Every complete upper and lower denture and removable dental prosthesis fabricated by a dentist licensed under this chapter, or fabricated pursuant to the dentist's work order or under the dentist's direction or supervision, must be marked with the name and social security number of the patient for whom the prosthesis is intended. The markings must be done during fabrication and must be permanent, legible and cosmetically acceptable. The exact location of the markings and the methods used to apply or implant the markings must be determined by the dentist or dental laboratory fabricating the prosthesis. If, in the professional judgment of the dentist or dental laboratory, this identification is not practical, identification must be provided as follows:

 A. The social security number of the patient may be omitted if the name of the patient is shown;

 B. The initials of the patient may be shown alone, if use of the name of the patient is impracticable; or

 C. The identification marks may be omitted in their entirety if none of the forms of identification specified in paragraphs A and B are practicable or clinically safe.

2. Dentures already in existence. A removable dental prosthesis in existence prior to the effective date of this section that was not marked in accordance with subsection 1 at the time of its fabrication must be marked in accordance with subsection 1 at the time of a subsequent rebasing.

3. Violations. Failure of a dentist to comply with this section is a violation for which the dentist is subject to proceedings pursuant to section 1077, provided that the dentist is charged with the violation within 2 years of initial insertion of the dental prosthetic device.

(SUBCHAPTER IV)
(DENTAL HYGIENISTS)
32 § 1095. Definition

The dental hygienist who practices under the supervision of a dentist of record may perform duties as defined and set forth in the rules of the Board of Dental Examiners, except that nothing in this subchapter may be construed to affect the practice of medicine or dentistry or to prevent students of a dental college, university or school of dental hygiene from practicing dental hygiene under the supervision of their instructors.

32 § 1096. Qualifications

A person 18 years old or over who has successfully completed 2 years' training in a school of dental hygiene approved by the board, or who is a full-time dental student who has satisfactorily completed at least half of the prescribed course of study in an accredited dental college, but who has not graduated from a dental college, is eligible to apply for examination.

32 § 1097. Application; Fee
An eligible person desiring to practice dental hygiene must make written application to the Board of Dental Examiners to take the examination. The application must be accompanied by a fee to be determined by the board not to exceed $100. Applicants for licensure shall pay a fee set by the board for the examination. The board may recognize a nationally or regionally administered examination for applicants to practice dental hygiene in the State.

32 § 1098. License; Biennial Fee
The board shall issue a license to practice as a dental hygienist in this State to an individual who has met the licensure requirements. The license must be exhibited publicly at the person's place of employment. The license authorizes practice as a dental hygienist in this State for the year in which it is issued until the expiration date that appears on the license. On or before January 1st of each odd-numbered year, the dental hygienist must pay to the board a license renewal fee of not more than $100 to be determined by the board or 1/2 of the biennial licensure fee if the applicant applies in an even-numbered year. Dental hygienists who have not paid as provided must be reinstated upon payment of a fee of not more than $50 to be determined by the board if paid before February 1st of the year in which license renewal is due. Failure to be properly licensed by February 1st results in automatic suspension of a license to practice dental hygiene. Reinstatement may be made, if approved by the board, by payment to the secretary-treasurer of the board of a fee determined by the board of not more than $100.

The board may issue temporary licenses to dental hygienists who present credentials satisfactory to the board. The board may charge a fee of up to $25 for a temporary license.

32 § 1098-A. Fee for Duplicate License
An applicant for a duplicate license granted upon proof of loss of the original shall pay a fee of $15.

32 § 1098-B. Continuing Education
As a condition of renewal of a license to practice, a dental hygienist must submit evidence of successful completion of 20 hours of continuing education consisting of board-approved courses in the 2 years preceding the application for renewal. The board and the dental hygienist shall follow and are bound by the provisions of section 1084-A in the implementation of this section.

32 § 1099. Endorsement
The board may at its discretion, without examination, issue a license to an applicant to practice dental hygiene who furnishes proof satisfactory to the board that

the dental hygienist has been duly licensed to practice in another state after full compliance with the requirements of its dental laws, except that the professional education may not be less than is required in this State. The board may require letters of reference as to ability. Every license so given must state upon its face that it was granted on the basis of endorsement. The fee for that license must be determined by the board, but may not be more than $100.

32 § 1100. Use of Former Employers' Lists; Scope of Duties

A dental hygienist may not use or attempt to use in any manner whatsoever any prophylactic lists, call lists, records, reprints or copies of those lists, records or reprints, or information gathered from these materials, of the names of patients whom the hygienist might have served in the office of a prior employer, unless these names appear on the bona fide call or prophylactic list of the present employer and were caused to so appear through the legitimate practice of dentistry as provided for in this chapter. A dentist may not aid or abet or encourage a dental hygienist in the dentist's employ to make use of a so-called prophylactic call list, or to call by telephone or to use written letters transmitted through the mails to solicit patronage from patients formerly served in the office of a dentist formerly employing the hygienist.

A dentist may not permit a dental hygienist operating under the dentist's supervision to perform an operation other than that permitted under section 1095.

(SUBCHAPTER V)
(DENTAL AUXILIARIES)
32 § 1100-A. Definition

Duties of dental auxiliaries other than dental hygienists must be defined and governed by the rules of the Board of Dental Examiners. Dental auxiliaries include, but are not limited to, dental hygienists, dental assistants, dental laboratory technicians and denturists.

(SUBCHAPTER VI)
(DENTURISTS)
32 § 1100-B. Definitions

As used in this subchapter, unless the context otherwise indicates, the following words and phrases shall have the following meanings.

1. Board. "Board" means the Board of Dental Examiners.

2. Denturist. "Denturist" means a person licensed under this subchapter to engage in the practice of denture technology under the supervision of a dentist of record.

3. Practice of denture technology. "Practice of denture technology" means only:

A. The taking of denture impressions and bite registration for the purpose of or with a view to the making, producing, reproducing, construction, finishing, supplying, altering or repairing of a complete upper or complete lower prosthetic denture, or both, to be fitted to an edentulous arch or arches;

B. The fitting of a complete upper or lower prosthetic denture, or both, to an edentulous arch or arches, including the making, producing, reproducing, constructing, finishing, supplying, altering and repairing of dentures; and

C. Other procedures incidental to the procedures specified in paragraphs A and B, as defined by the board.

32 § 1100-C. Rules and Regulations

1. Rules and regulations required. Not later than 90 days after the effective date of this subchapter, the board shall adopt rules and regulations relating to the licensing of denturists.

   2. Contents. These rules and regulations shall pertain, but need not be limited, to the following:

A. The administrative procedures relating to the issuance, refusal to issue, suspension and revocation of licenses;

B. The procedures and requirements relating to the issuance of temporary denturist licenses;

C. The methods by which and the conditions under which denturists are required to practice denture technology;

D. The establishment of educational requirements for the purpose of eligibility for licensing;

E. The specification of other procedures incidental to the practice of denture technology, which may be delegated to a denturist.

32 § 1100-D. Examinations

1. Authority. The board is authorized to prepare and give examinations in the area of denture technology for the purpose of licensing denturists. All examinations prepared and given under this subchapter may be prepared and given by the full board or by an appointed subcommittee of the board. The board may also recognize a nationally or regionally administered examination given at least annually for applicants to practice denture technology in the State.

   2. Eligibility for examination. A person is eligible to take the examination pursuant to subsection 1 who:

A. Is 18 years of age or older;

B. Is a high school graduate; and

C. Has successfully completed a minimum of 2 years of training in denture technology and related areas, as approved by the board, or has demonstrated equivalent training and experience, as determined by the board.

   3. Application for examination; fee. An eligible person desiring to take the examination in order to become licensed as a denturist shall make a written application to the board to take the examination. This application must be accompanied by a fee to be determined by the board but not to exceed $100.

   4. Additional examinations; fee. An applicant failing to pass the examination is entitled to at least one additional examination and shall pay a fee set by the board.

32 § 1100-E. Licenses; Reciprocity

1. Authority. The board has the authority to issue licenses to qualified persons to practice denture technology pursuant to this subchapter.

2. License issued. The board shall issue a license for the practice in this State to each person who has passed the examination under section 1100-D. This license authorizes the licensee to practice as a denturist in the State for the year in which it is issued until the expiration date that appears on the license.

3. Fee. After a license has been issued under subsection 2, and on or before January 1st of odd-numbered years, a denturist must pay to the board a license fee of not more than $100 to be determined by the board in order to renew the license and to continue to be authorized to practice as a denturist in the State or 1/2 the biennial licensure fee if application is made in an even-numbered year.

After the requirements for a license renewal have been met, a renewal card of the denturist's license for that year must be issued, which the denturist shall place beside or attach to the denturist's initial license. Denturists who have not paid as provided by January 1st must be reinstated upon payment of a fee, to be determined by the board, of not more than $50 if paid by February 1st. A license to practice is automatically suspended on February 1st and may be reinstated, if approved by the board, on payment of a fee to be determined by the board of not than $100.

4. Endorsement. The board may, at its discretion, without examination, issue a license to an applicant to practice as a denturist who furnishes proof satisfactory to the board that the denturist has been licensed to practice and has actively practiced for a period of 5 years in another state or Canadian province after full compliance with the requirements of its dental laws, if the licensure requirements are, in all essentials, at least equivalent to those of this State. The board may require letters of reference about the denturist. Every license so given must state upon its face that it was granted on the basis of endorsement. The fee for the license is $100.

4-A. Duplicate license. An applicant for a duplicate license granted upon proof of loss of the original shall pay a fee of $15.

5. Additional prohibitions. A denturist may not:

A. Falsely claim to be a licensed dentist or allow another to falsely represent the denturist as a licensed dentist;

B. Perform otherwise than at the direction and under the direct supervision of a dentist licensed by the board and practicing in the State. Direct supervision requires the dentist to be on the same premises as the denturist;

C. Perform a task beyond the denturist's competence; or

D. Administer, dispense or prescribe a medication or controlled substance.

6. Mental or physical examination. For the purposes of this subsection, by the application for and acceptance of the license, a licensed denturist is deemed to have given consent to a mental or physical examination when directed by the board. The board may direct the examination whenever it determines a denturist may be suffering from a mental illness that may be interfering with the competent practice of denture technology or from the use of intoxicants or drugs to an extent that they are preventing the denturist from practicing denture technology competently and with safety to the patients. A denturist examined pursuant to an order of the board does not have the privilege to prevent the testimony of the examining individual or to prevent the acceptance into evidence of the report of an examining individual. Failure to comply with an order of the board to submit to a mental or physical exam requires the Administrative Court to immediately order the license of the denturist suspended until the denturist submits to the examination.

32 § 1100-F. Persons and Practices Not Affected

Nothing in this subchapter may be construed to prohibit a duly qualified dental surgeon, dental laboratory technician or dental hygienist from performing work or services performed by a denturist licensed under this subchapter to the extent those persons are authorized to perform the same services under existing state law.

Nothing in this subchapter may be construed to prevent students of a dental college, university or school of dental hygiene from practicing dental hygiene under the supervision of their instructors.

32 § 1100-G. Liability of Dentist for Denturist's Actions

A dentist who supervises the activities of a denturist pursuant to this subchapter is legally liable for these activities and in this relationship the denturist must be construed as the dentist's agent.

(SUBCHAPTER VII)
(DENTAL RADIOGRAPHERS)
32 § 1100-I. Definitions

As used in this subchapter, unless the context otherwise indicates, the following terms have the following meanings.

1. Dental radiography. "Dental radiography" means the use of ionizing radiation on the maxilla, mandible and adjacent structures of human beings for diagnostic purposes.

2. General supervision. "General supervision" means the supervising dentist is not required to be physically present in the dental office while procedures are being performed on a patient of record.

3. Licensed dental radiographer. "Licensed dental radiographer" means a person who practices dental radiography and holds a valid license issued by the board.

32 § 1100-J. License Required; Exceptions

1. License required. It is unlawful for any person, not otherwise authorized by law, to practice dental radiography without having a current license issued by the board.

2. Medicine, osteopathy, dentistry. Nothing in the provisions of this subchapter may limit, enlarge or affect the practice of persons licensed to practice medicine, osteopathy or dentistry in this State.

3. Exceptions. The requirement of a license does not apply to:

A. Dental hygienists licensed pursuant to subchapter IV;

B. A resident physician or a student enrolled in and attending a school or college of medicine, osteopathy, dentistry, dental hygiene and dental assisting or radiologic technology;

C. A person serving in the United States Armed Forces or public health service or employed by the Veterans' Administration or other federal agency while performing official duties, if the duties are limited to that service or employment; or

D. Those persons having a current license to perform radiologic technology pursuant to section 9854 and who are practicing dental radiography under the general supervision of a dentist or physician.

32 § 1100-K. Supervision Required

1. Supervision. A licensed dental radiographer may practice dental radiography under the general supervision of a dentist.

32 § 1100-L. Employment of Dental Radiographers

1. Dental radiographers; license. It is unlawful for a dentist to allow a person to practice dental radiography in the dentist's employment or under the dentist's supervision who does not hold a license to practice dental radiography issued by the board or who is otherwise authorized by law to practice dental radiography.

32 § 1100-M. Qualifications

1. Requirements. To qualify for a license to practice dental radiography, an applicant shall meet the following requirements:

A. Be at least 18 years of age;

B. Have a high school diploma or its equivalent, as determined by the Department of Education; and

C. Have successfully passed a test in dental radiologic technique and safety approved by the board.

32 § 1100-N. Application

To apply for a license to practice dental radiography, an applicant shall submit a written application with supporting documents to the board, on forms provided by the board, and shall pay an application fee, which may not exceed $50.

32 § 1100-O. Renewal

1. Term of license; renewal. All licenses to practice dental radiography issued by the board are valid for 5 years from the date of issuance and may be renewed upon application to the board and payment of a renewal fee, which may not exceed $50.

32 § 1100-P. Rules

1. Rules. The board may make rules in accordance with Title 5, chapter 375, which are necessary for the implementation of this subchapter. The rules may include, but need not be limited to, licensure requirements, approved courses, application and renewal procedures and fees.

32 § 1100-Q. Disciplinary Action

1. Suspension; revocation; refusal to issue or renew license. The board may suspend or revoke a license pursuant to Title 5, section 10004. In addition, the board may refuse to issue or renew a license or the Administrative Court may revoke, suspend of refuse to renew a license issued under this subchapter for the following reasons:

A. The Practice of fraud or deceit in obtaining a license under this subchapter or in connection with service rendered within the scope of the license issued;

B. Habitual substance abuse that has resulted or is foreseeable likely to result in the licensed dental radiographer being unable to perform the duties of the profession or perform those duties in a manner that would endanger the health or safety of the patients to be served;

C. Incompetenence in the practice of dental radiography. A licensed dental radiographer is considered incompetent in the practice if the dental radiographer has:

(1) Engaged in conduct that evidenced a lack of ability or fitness to discharge the duty owed to a client or patient or the general public; or

(2) Engaged in conduct that evidenced a lack of knowledge or inability to apply principles or skills to carry out the practice of dental radiography;

D. Unprofessional conduct. In this context, unprofessional conduct means the violation of a standard of professional behavior that through professional experience has been established in the practice of dental radiography;

E. Subject to the limitations of Title 5, chapter 341, conviction of a crime that involves dishonesty or false statement or that relates directly to the practice of dental radiography or conviction of a crime for which incarceration for one year or more may be imposed; or

F. A violation of this chapter or rule adopted by the board.

CHAPTER 1: RULES RELATING TO DENTAL HYGIENISTS

Summary: This chapter sets forth rules for general and direct supervision of Dental Hygienists.

Section 1. Definitions

A. *General Supervision:* "General Supervision" shall mean that the dentist is not required to be in the dental office at the time the procedures are being performed on a patient of record.

B. *Direct Supervision:* "Direct Supervision" shall mean that the dentist must be in the dental office at the time the duties under his/her supervision are being performed. In order to provide direct supervision of patient treatment, the dentist must at least diagnose the condition to be treated, authorize the treatment procedure prior to implementation, and examine the condition after treatment and prior to the patient's discharge.

C. *Public Health Supervision:* "Public Health Supervision" means that the dentist provides general supervision to a dental hygienist who is practicing in a public health supervision status that has been approved by the Board under Section 4 of this Chapter.

Section 2. General Supervision of Dental Hygienists

Dental Hygienists may perform the following duties under the general supervision of a dentist:

A. Interview patients and record complete medical and dental histories.

B. Take and record the vital signs of blood pressure, pulse and temperature.

C. Perform oral inspections, recording all conditions that should be called to the attention of the dentist.

D. Perform complete periodontal and dental restorative charting.

E. Expose and process radiographs, permitted pursuant to Title 32 MRSA Section 1100-J (3) (Supp. 1985)

F. Perform pulp tests pursuant to the direction of the dentist.

G. Perform all procedures necessary for a complete prophylaxis including root planing and curettage.

H. Apply fluoride to control caries.

I. Apply desensitizing agents to teeth.

J. Apply liquids, pastes or gel topical anesthetics.

K. Apply sealants, provided that a licensed dentist first makes the determination and diagnosis as to the surfaces on which the sealants shall be applied. In public health or school sealant programs only, determination and diagnosis of the sealant site by a dentist need not occur.

L. Smooth and polish amalgam restorations.

M. Cement pontics and facings outside the mouth.

N. Take impressions for study casts.

O. Take impressions for single-arch athletic mouth guards and for custom fluoride trays.

P. Place and remove rubber dams.

Q. Remove sutures and periodontal dressings.

R. Perform post operative irrigation of surgical sites.

S. Place temporary restorations as an emergency procedure, provided that the patient is informed of the temporary nature of the filling.

T. Isolate operative fields.

U. Perform any other duties that may be performed by a dental assistant under Chapter 2, Sections 2 and 4 of these rules.

Section 3. Direct Supervision of Dental Hygienists

A dental hygienist may perform the following duties only when under direct supervision of a dentist:

A. Place periodontal dressings.

B. Remove socket dressings.

C. Place gingival retraction cords.

D. Apply identification microdisks.

E. Take cytological smears as requested by the dentist.

F. During nitrous oxide administration by the dentist, the dental hygienist may observe the gauges and advise the dentist of any changes in gauge indicies or readings, but by no means shall this be intended or construed as permitting adjusting or controlling the machines or as permitting administration of nitrous oxide by the dental hygienist.

G. Perform any other duties that may be performed by a dental assistant under Chapter 2, Section 3 of these rules.

Section 4. Public Health Supervision Status.

The Board may grant "Public Health Supervision" status to a hygienist in situations the Board deems appropriate in its discretion, giving due consideration to the protection of the public. "Public Health Supervision" means that a dental hygienist with an active Maine license practices in a public or private school, hospital, custodial care institution or other non-traditional practice setting provided that the service is rendered under the general supervision of a dentist with an active Maine license. In each program the dentist should have specific standing orders or policy guidelines for procedures which are to be carried out, although the dentist need not be present when the procedures are being performed. A written plan for referral or an agreement for follow-up shall be provided by the public health hygienists, recording all conditions that should be called to the attention to the dentist. A summary report at the completion of a program or once a year shall be reviewed by the supervising dentist. The hygienist shall keep the Board informed of each location at which the hygienist is practicing under public health supervision.

A dental hygienist wishing to practice under public health supervision status must apply to the board for approval, providing such information as the Board may deem necessary. In deciding whether to grant this status, the Board shall consider the following criteria:

A. The proposed program is necessary to fulfill a need not currently being met;

B. The particular proposed practice setting, including the proposed supervisor, will be adequate to accomplish the goal;

C. Appropriate public health guidelines can be followed in the proposed setting;

D. Adequate standards of care can be maintained in the proposed practice setting; and

E. A supervising dentist is available.

AUTHORITY: 21 M.R.S.A. § 1073.

CHAPTER 2: RULES RELATING TO DENTAL ASSISTANTS

Summary: This chapter sets forth rules for general and direct supervision of dental assistants and certified dental assistants.

Section 1. Definitions

A. *General Supervision:* "General supervision" shall mean that the dentist is not required to be in the dental office at the time the procedures are being performed on a patient of record.

B. *Direct Supervision:* "Direct supervision" shall mean that the dentist must be in the dental office at the time the duties under his/her supervision are being performed. In order to provide direct supervision of patient treatment, the dentist must at least diagnose the condition to be treated, authorize the treatment procedure prior to implementation, and examine the condition after treatment and prior to the patient's discharge.

C. A "dental assistant" is a person who assists the dentist and performs the duties listed in Sections 2 and 3 of this chapter.

D. A "certified dental assistant" (C.D.A.), is a dental assistant who has successfully passed a certification examination administered by the Dental Assistants' National Board

Section 2. General Supervision of Dental Assistants.

A dental assistant may perform the following duties under the general supervision of a dentist:

A. Give oral health instructions.

B. Perform dietary analyses for dental disease control.

C. Take and record the vital signs of blood pressure, pulse and temperature.

D. Take intra-oral photographs.

E. Retract lips, cheek, tongue and other tissue parts.

F. Irrigate and aspirate the oral cavity.

G. Expose and process radiographs, but only if licensed as a Dental Radiographer pursuant to Title 32 M.R.S.A. Sections 1100-I through 1100-R.

H. For instruction purposes, a dental assistant may demonstrate to a patient how the patient should place and remove removable prostheses, appliances or retainers.

I. Take dental plaque smears for microscopic inspection and patient education.

J. For the purpose of eliminating pain or discomfort, remove loose, broken or irritating orthodontic appliances.

K. Take impressions for study casts.

Section 3. Direct Supervision of Dental Assistants.

A dental assistant may perform the following intra-oral procedures only, and then, only under the direct supervision of a dentist:

A. Apply liquids, pastes, and gel topical anesthetics.

B. Place and remove rubber dams.

C. Recement temporary crowns with temporary cement.

D. Place and remove matrix bands.

E. Place, hold or remove celluloid and other plastic strips prior to or subsequent to the placement of a filling by the dentist.

F. Place and remove wedges.

G. Apply cavity varnish.

H. Deliver, but not condense or pack, amalgam or composite restoration material.

I. Remove gingival retraction cord.

J. Select and try in stainless steel or other preformed crowns for insertion by the dentist.

K. Take impressions for single-arch athletic mouth guards and for custom fluoride trays.

L. Irrigate and dry root canals.

M. Remove sutures.

N. Place or remove temporary separating devices.

O. Remove orthodontic arch wires and tension devices and any loose bands or bonds, but only as directed by the dentist.

P. Prepare tooth sites and surfaces with a rubber cup and pumice for banding or bonding of orthodontic brackets. This procedure shall not be intended or interpreted as an oral prophylaxis, which is a procedure specifically reserved to be performed by dental hygienists or dentists. This procedure also shall not be intended or interpreted as a preparation for restorative material. A dentist or dental hygienist shall check and approve the procedure.

Q. Place wires, pins and elastic ligatures to tie in orthodontic arch wires that have been fitted and approved by the dentist at the time of insertion.

R. Perform preliminary selection and fitting of orthodontic bands, but final placement and cementing in the patient's mouth shall be done by the dentist.

S. Remove excess cement from the supragingival surfaces of teeth.

T. Take intra-oral measurements and make preliminary selection of arch wires and intra and extra-oral appliances, including head gear.

U. Take impressions for opposing models and retainers.

V. Place elastics and/or instruct in their use.

W. Reapply, on an emergency basis only, orthodontic brackets.

X. Isolate the operative field.

Section 4. General Supervision of Certified Dental Assistants.

In addition to the duties permitted under Chapter 2, Section 2 of these Rules, a certified dental assistant may perform the following duties under general supervision of a dentist:

A. Remove sutures.

B. Place temporary fillings on an emergency basis, provided that the patient is informed of the temporary nature of the fillings.

C. Remove excess cement from the supragingival surfaces of teeth.

AUTHORITY: 32 M.R.S.A. § 1073.

CHAPTER 5: LEAD APRONS

Summary: This chapter contains rules relating to the use of lead aprons in dental procedures involving radiation.

I. In the interest of protecting the public health and safety it is required by the Maine Board of Dental Examiners that before a dental X-ray (radiograph) is taken of a patient by a dentist or his duly authorized auxilliary, a lead apron be placed over the body of that patient.

    A. Failure to follow the above procedure is deemed by the Board to be presumptively an act of incompetence or unskillfulness.

AUTHORITY: 32 M.R.S.A. § 1073

CHAPTER 7: FALSE AND MISLEADING ADVERTISING

Summary: Any advertisement by a professional dental corporation must include the names of all licensed dentists whose services for such corporation constitute the practice of dentistry.

    1. Advertising by Professional Service Corporations: Dentists who have incorporated their practices as a professional service corporation pursuant to Title 13 M.R.S.A. Chapter 22 and Title 32 M.R.S.A. § 1081 (4) may advertise in the name of the professional service corporation provided that all such advertising shall clearly include the names of all licensed dentists affiliated with the professional service corporation who provide services which constitute the practice of dentistry as defined in 32 M.R.S.A. § 1081, and provided further that such advertising shall not include the name of any dentist who is not providing such services.

AUTHORITY: 32 M.R.S.A. §§ 1073 (3), 1081 (4) and 1092.
Effective Date: Dec. 13, 1982

CHAPTER 8: COMPLAINTS

Summary: These regulations establish a procedure for the processing of complaints concerning practices of persons licensed by the Board of Dental Examiners.

I. Complaints

The Board shall, to the extent practicable, receive and process complaints as follows:

    A. All complaints shall be submitted to the Board in writing. The Board may request that complaints be submitted on a complaint form which it provides. The Board may, on its own motion, conduct or authorize an investigation without a written complaint in any matter involving possible noncompliance with or violation of 32 M.R.S.A. Chapter 16 or any Board rule or regulation.

    B. A written complaint should set forth the facts which provide the basis for the complaint, and include all available information concerning the identification of persons involved and dates.

    C. The Board will send a letter to the complaining party acknowledging receipt of the complaint. The Board will also furnish a copy to the person against whom the complaint has been registered and a written response to the charges shall be requested.

    D. In the event of an investigation pertinent records shall be made available to the Board by a licensee at written Board request for purposes of review and/or investigation of the complaint.

E. Hearings may be conducted by the Board to assist with investigations, to determine whether cause exists for revocation or suspension of a license or for any other lawful purpose. Hearings shall be conducted in conformity with the Administrative Procedure Act, Title 5 M.R.S.A. Chapter 375, to the extent applicable. In an appropriate case, the Board may hold an informal proceeding to determine whether a matter may be disposed of by consent agreement.

F. If the Board determines that any person has violated a provision of 32 M.R.S.A. Chapter 16 or has violated a rule or regulation of the Board, it may refer the matter to the Department of the Attorney General with a recommendation for further action.

II. Definition of Unprofessional Conduct

Unprofessional conduct under 32 M.R.S.A. Section 1077 includes, but is not limited to, the following:

A. Engaging in any activity which assists, encourages or induces any person to violate this chapter or the rules of the board.

B. The obtaining of any fee by fraud or misrepresentation.

C. Division of fees or an agreement to split the fees received for dental services with any person for referring a patient or for assisting in a care of a patient, without the knowledge of the patient's representative.

D. Possession, use, prescription for use, or distribution of controlled substances or prescription drugs in any way other than for dental therapeutic purposes. Controlled substances and prescription drugs in the possession of a licensee which are prescribed for the licensee by a medical practitioner legally licensed to so prescribed and which are being used for therapeutic purposes are exempted from this rule.

E. The inappropriate prescribing or administering of drugs or treatment, or the excessive use for diagnostic procedures, or the excessive use of diagnostic or treatment facilities.

F. The advertising of either professional superiority or the advertising of the performance of professional services in a superior manner.

G. The use of threats and harassment against any patient or licensee for providing evidence in any possible or actual disciplinary action, or other legal action.

H. The alteration of a patient's record with the intent to deceive.

I. The failure of a dentist to surrender a copy of a patient's records upon appropriate request by the patient or his agent and prepayment of a reasonable duplication cost. This rule does not require a dentist to surrender original patient records.

J. Violation of sanitary and unsafe office conditions as set forth below:
1. Premises shall be kept clean and orderly and free of accumulated rubbish and similar substances;
2. Premises shall be kept free of all insects and vermin by utilizing proper control and eradication methods;
3. Water shall be piped under pressure and in an approved manner to all equipment and fixtures requiring the use of water. The water shall be

from a properly constructed ground water supply and should be tested yearly if the source of the water is not from a recognized public water source. Water from private water sources shall meet all applicable state standards;

4. All structures shall be in compliance with local and state building codes;
5. All plumbing shall be in accordance with local and state plumbing codes;
6. Evidence of violations of local and state codes referred to in D and E above which also constitute violations of these Rules may be used by the Board as the basis of a disciplinary action;
7. Sanitary conditions for patients and employees shall be maintained at all times;
8. Sewage disposal shall be in accordance with the Maine Plumbing Code;
9. Adequate toilet facilities shall be located on the premises of every dental office. Toilet facilities shall conform to standards of the State Board of Health.

K. The abandonment of the patient by the licensee before the completion of a phase of treatment.

L. Delegations by a dentist of the duties set forth below:
   1. Diagnosis and treatment planning;
   2. Surgical or cutting procedures on hard or soft tissue; except if provided under Chapter 2 of these rules;
   3. Prescription of drugs, medicaments or work authorization;
   4. Taking impressions for fabrication of fixed or removable appliances or restorations, except as provided under these rules, Chap. 1, Part II, Section J, and, Chap. 10, Part III, section A and Part IV, section A;
   5. Placing or adjusting fixed or removable appliances or restorations, except if provided by Chapter 1 and Chapter 2;
   6. Making occlusional adjustments;
   7. Performing pulp capping and pulpotomy procedures;
   8. Condensing and carving amalgam restorations;
   9. Placing and contouring composite restoration.

EFFECTIVE DATE: December 13, 1982
AMENDED: October 1, 1986—Section 2 (added)

CHAPTER 9: LICENSURE REQUIREMENTS FOR RADIOGRAPHERS

To qualify for a license to practice dental radiography, an applicant shall meet the following requirements:

1. Be at least 18 years of age;
2. Have a high school diploma or its equivalent;
3. Have successfully passed a test in dental radiologic technique and safety approved by the Board;
4. Upon successful completion of the radiologic exam, an applicant has 5 years to obtain a radiography license. After the five year period has elapsed, if the

candidate has not been issued a license, a new radiologic exam must be successfully completed.

Effective Date: June 7, 1995

CHAPTER 10: REQUIREMENTS FOR LICENSURE FOR DENTAL HYGIENISTS
A. Licensure of Graduates of a Dental Hygiene Program Approved by the American Dental Associates (ADA) Commission on Dental Accreditation (CODA)

To be licensed, candidates in this category shall meet the following requirements:

1. Have received, at least, an associate degree from a dental hygiene program accredited by CODA and provide a notarized statement from the Dean of the school affirming that the applicant has met all applicable degree requirements;
2. Have completed with a passing grade the National Board Dental Hygiene examination;
3. Have completed with a passing grade the Northeast Regional Board (NERB) Dental Hygiene examination;
4. Have complete with a passing grade the jurisprudence examination given by the Board; and
5. For any applicant who has completed NERB more than one year prior to application for licensure in Maine, have successfully completed a personal interview before the Board.

B. Licensure by Endorsement.

To be licensed, candidates in this category shall meet the following requirements:

1. Have graduated from an accredited dental hygiene program;
2. If the candidate was graduated subsequent to 1964, have completed with a passing grade the National Board Dental Hygiene examination if such examination was required;
3. Furnish proof, satisfactory to the Board, that the candidate has been duly licensed to practice dental hygiene in another state after full compliance with the requirements of its laws;
4. If the candidate was graduated subsequent to 1970, have completed with a passing grade the Northeast Regional Board Dental Hygiene examination if such examination was required;
5. Have engaged in active clinical practice for a minimum of five years prior to application;
6. Have completed with a passing grade the jurisprudence examination given by the Board; and
7. Have successfully completed a personal interview before the Board.
8. The Board may at its discretion waive the NERB exam if all other requirements have been met.

Effective Date: June 7, 1995

CHAPTER 11: REQUIREMENTS FOR DENTAL LICENSURE

A. Licensure of Graduates of an American Dental Association (A.D.A.) Accredited Undergraduate Dental School

To be licensed, candidates in this category shall meet the following requirements:

1. Have received a D.M.D. or D.D.S. degree from an undergraduate dental school accredited by the A.D.A. Council of Accreditation and shall provide a notarized statement from the Dean of the school affirming that the applicant has met all applicable degree requirements;
2. Have successfully completed, with a passing grade, Parts I and II of the National Dental Board Examination;
3. Have successfully completed, with a passing grade, all parts of the Northeast Regional Board Dental examination;
4. Have successfully completed the jurisprudence exam given by the Board; and
5. For any applicant who completed all of the above requirements more than one year prior to application for licensure in Maine, have successfully completed a personal interview before the board.

B. Licensure of Foreign Trained Dentists or Graduates of Schools Other Than A.D.A. Accredited Undergraduate Dental Schools.

To be licensed, candidates in this category shall meet the following requirements:

1. Have received a D.M.D. or D.D.S. degree from an A.D.A. accredited undergraduate dental school and shall provide a notarized statement from the dean of the school affirming that the applicant has met all degree requirements;
2. Have successfully completed, with a passing grade, parts I and II of the National Dental Board examination;
3. Have successfully completed, with a passing grade, all parts of the Northeast Regional Board dental Examination;
4. Have successfully completed the jurisprudence exam given by the Board; and
5. For any applicant who completed all of the above requirements more than one year prior to application for licensure in Maine, have successfully completed a personal interview before the Board.

C. Licensure by Endorsement.

To be licensed, candidates in this category shall meet the following requirements:

1. Have received a D.M.D. or D.D.S. degree from an A.D.A. accredited undergraduate dental school;
2. If the candidate was graduated subsequent to 1952, have successfully completed, with a passing grade, Parts I and II of the National Dental Board Examination if such examination was required;
3. Furnish proof, satisfactory to the Board, that the candidate has been duly licensed to practice dentistry in another state after full compliance with the requirements of its dental laws;
4. If the candidate was graduated subsequent to 1972, have successfully completed, with a passing grade, all parts of the Northeast Regional Board Dental Examination if such examination was required;

5. Have engaged in an active clinical practice for a minimum of five years prior to application;

6. Have successfully completed the jurisprudence exam given by the Board; and

7. Have successfully completed a personal interview before the Board.

8. The Board may at its discretion waive the NERB exam if all of the other requirements have been met.

CHAPTER 12: CONTINUING DENTAL EDUCATION

Pursuant to the provisions of 32 M.R.S.A. § 1084-A of the Maine Revised Statutes as amended in 1989, the Board of Dental Examiners herewith establishes the following rules and regulations for Continuing Dental Education required for reregistration in the year 1992 for dentists and 1993 for dental hygienists and all subsequent biennial reregistrations with this Board.

A. Requirements

1. Every dentist licensed by the Board shall complete biennially a minimum of forty (40) hours of acceptable continuing education. Every dental hygienist licensed by the Board shall complete biennially a minimum of twenty (20) hours of acceptable continuing education. This requirement must be completed during the two calendar years preceding December 31 of the year of expiration of the license.

   a. The total forty (40) or twenty (20) may be in Category 1, however at least 30 hours for dentists and 15 hours for hygienists must be in Category 1 (as defined in subsection (B) (1).

   b. No more than ten (10) hours for dentists or five (5) for hygienists may be in Category 2 (as defined in subsection (B) (2).

   c. Those courses that are directly related to the clinical practice of the dental professions will receive credit in category one, as defined below. Those courses that are not directly related to the clinical practice of the dental professions, such as business management, financial planning, or other topics not directly related to the clinical practice of the dental professions are limited to category two status, as defined below. This rule will be effective for dentists starting in January, 1996 and for dental hygienists starting in January, 1997.

B. Definitions and Categories

1. **Category 1** activities are those planned Continuing Dental Education (CDE) or Continuing Medical Education (CME) programs sponsored or co-sponsored by an organization or institutions accredited by (1) The ADA Commission of Dental Accreditation, (2) The Council on Medical Education of the AMA, (3) The ADA and its constituent societies, (4) The ADHA and its constituent societies, or (5) the Academy of General Dentistry.

   a. All Category 1 CDE programs will be properly identified as such by the approved sponsoring organization.

   b. One credit hour may be claimed for each hour of participation.

2. **Category 2**
   a. **CDE programs with non-accredited sponsorship** are those dental and hygiene meetings and CDE programs not within the definition of Category 1: Value one credit for each hour of participation.
   b. **Teaching** includes teaching of Dental/Medical students, interns, residents practicing dentists, dental hygienists and physicians and allied health professional. One credit for each hour of participation.
   c. **Papers, publications, books** as described below are acceptable. Credit may be claimed only for the first time the material is presented and should be claimed as of the date the materials were presented or published. Ten (10) credits for each presentation or publication.
      1. A paper published in a recognized professional journal.
      2. Each chapter of a book that is authorized and published in the dental/Medical field.
   d. **Presentation or exhibits** presented to a professional audience, including allied health professional. (Five hours maximum credit for a minimum of one hour presentation.)
   e. **Non-supervised individual CDE/CME** activities. One credit for each hour of activity, maximum of ten (10) credits for dentists and five (5) credits for hygienists per biennium. Credit will be given in an amount to be determined by the State Board of Dental Examiners for these self-instructional activities, provided they are sponsored by an approved organization and incorporate an approved testing mechanism.
      1. Home study or correspondence courses; self-assessment tests.
      2. Educational television, audio-tape cassettes, and other audio-visual materials accompanied by a testing mechanism provided by the sponsor.
   f. **General attendance at multi-day convention** type meetings sponsored by medical or dental organizations shall be given a maximum 5 credit hours per biennium.
   g. **Other meritorious learning experiences.**

All requests for consideration of credit in this section must be submitted to the Board of Dental Examiners in writing no later than 90 days prior of date of expiration of license.

3. **The Requirements of the following programs,** if completed during the two calendar years preceeding the registration or reregistration date may be considered as equivalent to the requirements listed in section B: Definitions and categories, (1) and (2) above.
   a. Certification or recertification by a Specialty Board within two previous years preceding registration.
   b. Completion of fellowship or mastership level in Academy of General Dentistry (AGD) within the two previous years preceding registration.

4. Each full year of completed post graduate training in one of the following programs will be considered the equivalent of the annual CDE requirements of 20 credits for a dentist and 10 credits for a hygienist:

  a. Internship or residency

  b. Graduate program in an approved specialty.

  c. Related Dental, Medical or Dental Hygiene degree program.

C. Evidence of Completion.

1. The registration application for dentists for the year 1992 and for each even numbered year thereafter, and for hygienists for the year 1993 and each odd numbered year thereafter shall include a statement certifying that the required number of CDE courses have been completed.

    On or before January 1, 1992 (1993 for hygienists) and every other year thereafter, dentists and hygienists licensed by this Board shall submit to the Board of Dental Examiners on a form provided by the Board evidence of successful completion of the CDE/CME requirements as outlined in Section A of these rules.

    The applicant shall be ultimately responsible for record keeping and proof of attendance and satisfactory completion of all courses and credit for the same.

D. Monitoring Procedure.

1. For each renewal period the Continuing Education Activity of some licensees will be audited by the Board. If the submitted data does not fulfill the requirements of these rules and regulations, the licensee shall be notified and may be called before the Board for a hearing. At this time the Board may impose additional requirements to be completed; or the license may be suspended, revoked or not renewed.

E. Exceptions/Waivers to CDE Requirements

1. The Board, at its discretion, may grant an extension of time or other waiver to a licensee who because of prolonged illness or other extenuating circumstances, has been unable to meet the requirements of CDE.

2. Dentists and hygienists who become licensed for the first time in the course of a calendar year will not be required to fulfill the CDE requirements for that calendar year.

3. Dentists and hygienists who are not actively practicing dentistry may be excused from completing CDE requirements for reregistration by submitting to the Board of Dental Examiners an affidavit certifying that he/she will render no dental services during the term of the registration biennium. Such a license will be considered not valid and the registration will be stamped INACTIVE STATUS.

    Active status will only be re-acquired by a written request to the Board of Dental Examiners who may set new exams, interviews and/or other requirements on an individual basis; this is retroactive until January 1, 1992.

CHAPTER 13: REGULATIONS FOR USE OF GENERAL ANESTHESIA/SEDATION BY DENTISTS

Definitions

As outlined in Guidelines for Teaching the Comprehensive Control of Pain and Anxiety in Dentistry approved by the American Dental Association, Council on Dental Education.

General Anesthesia—(To include Deep Sedation)—is a controlled state of depressed consciousness or unconsciousness, accompanied by partial or complete loss of protective reflexes, including inability to independently maintain an airway and respond to physical stimulation or verbal command, produced by a pharmacologic method or a non pharmacologic method, or a combination thereof.

Conscious Sedation—Is a minimally depressed level of consciousness that retains the patient's ability to independently and continuously maintain an airway and respond appropriately to physical stimulation and verbal command, produced by a pharmacologic or non-pharmacologic method, or a combination thereof.

General Anesthesia/Sedation is not meant to include nitrous oxide-oxygen analgesia with a fail-safe system; or oral premedication.

Use of General Anesthesia/Sedation

A. No dentist shall employ or use general anesthesia/sedation on an outpatient basis for dental patients, unless such dentist possesses a permit of authorization issued by the Maine State Board of Dental Examiners (The Board). The dentist holding such a permit shall be subject to review and such a permit must be renewed every five years. This rule is subject to the exception noted in Part D of this rule.

B. In order to received such permit, the dentist must apply on a prescribed application form to the Board, submit an application fee of $125.00, and produce evidence showing that he/she:

   1. Has completed a minimum of one (1) year of advanced training in anesthesiology and related academic subjects (or its equivalent) beyond the undergraduate dental school level in training program as described in Part II of the *Guidelines for Teaching the Comprehensive Control of Pain and Anxiety in Dentistry;* or

   2. Is a diplomate of the American Board of Oral and Maxillofacial Surgery, or is a fellow/member of the American Association of Oral and Maxillofacial Surgeons or has completed an ADA approved residency in Oral and Maxillofacial Surgery, or is a Fellow of the American Dental Society of Anesthesiology; in view of the fact that the training requirements as outlined in § B.1 above is a partial requirement for receiving or being eligible for these credentials; or

   3. Employs or works in conjunction with a trained M.D., D.O., D.M.D. or D.D.S. who is a permit holder under this regulation. Such anesthesiologist must remain on the premises of the dental facility until any patient given a general anesthetic regains consciousness; and

4. Has a properly equipped facility for the administration of general anesthesia/sedation staffed with a supervised team of auxiliary personnel capable of reasonably handling procedures, problems, and emergencies incident thereto. Adequacy of the facility and competence of the anesthesia/sedation team may be determined by the consultants appointed by the Board as outlined in Part C and H of this rule. The dentist is required to remain on the premises of the dental facility during administration of any anesthetic drug and until any patient given a general anesthetic regains consciousness.

C. Prior to the issuance of such permit, the Board may, at its discretion, require an onsite inspection of the facility, equipment and personnel to determine if, in fact, the aforementioned requirements have been met. This evaluation shall be carried out in a manner described by the American Society of Oral and Maxillofacial Surgeons following the published guidelines provided by the Board. The evaluation shall be carried out by a team of consultants appointed by the Board as referred to in section H in this rule. The on site evaluation team shall consist of at least two (2) members of the committee. Upon written request of the applicant, a second evaluation, shall be conducted by a different team of consultants if the applicant can substantiate just cause.

D. Each dentist who has been using or employing general anesthesia/sedation prior to adoption of these rules shall make application on the prescribed form to the Board within one year of the effective date of these rules if such dentist desires to continue to use or employ general anesthesia/sedation. If he meets the requirements of these rules, he shall be issued such a provisional permit of 1 to 3 years (the initial applicant for permits will be divided into three groups to facilitate initial and subsequent evaluation by the anesthesia consultants). An onsite evaluation of the facilities, equipment, and personnel may be, but is not necessarily required prior to issurance of such permit.

E. For new applicants who are otherwise properly qualified, a temporary provisional permit of one year duration may be granted by the Board based solely upon the credentials contained in the application, pending complete processing of the application and thorough investigation via an on-site evaluation as described in Part C of this rule.

F. The Board shall with charge renew the permit every five (5) years based on successful completion of the on-site evaluation. This evaluation to be completed within one year prior to permit renewal.

G. The board, based on formal application stating all particulars which would justify the granting of such permit, may grant a provisional permit to those dentist who have not had the benefit of the formal training requirements as outlined in this ruled but who can document their use or employment of general anesthesia/sedation in a competent and effective manner prior to implementation of this rule. Dentists applying for an anesthesia/sedation permit under this section would be required to meet all the other clinical requirements referred to in section B-4 of this rule.

H. The Board shall appoint an Anesthesia Evaluation Committee which shall be comprised of at least three licensees. To be eligible to serve on this committee, members shall meet the education and clinical requirements as set forth in this rule.

I. Anesthesia Evaluation committee members shall be reimbursed for travel expenses incurred while evaluating outpatient facilities.

J. The Board shall issue an application for renewal one year prior to permit renewal. The applicant shall pay a fee to the Board and the Anesthesia Evaluation Committee shall schedule an appointment for on-site anesthesia/sedation evaluation. When the evaluation is successfully completed the applicant shall receive a certificate which shall be kept in the office location.

K. Morbidity and Mortality Reports—A permit holder shall, within a period of fifteen days, report to the Board:

    A. Any anesthetic related death; or

    B. The determination that a permanently disabling incident has occurred, during or as a direct result of general anesthesia/sedation.

L. Penalties for Violations:

A violation of these regulations pertaining to the use of general anesthesia/sedation shall constitute unprofessional conduct and may result in disciplinary action against the dentist.

CHAPTER 14: GENERAL PROVISIONS
Mortality or Life-Threatening Situations in a Dental Office.

All licensees shall report to the Board, within thirty days from the date of the occurrance, any mortality or life threatening incidents requiring medical care as a sequela of care in a dental office.

Effective Date: June 7, 1995

TABLE OF CONTENTS
Maine Dental Practice Act (32 M.R.S.A. Chapter 16)

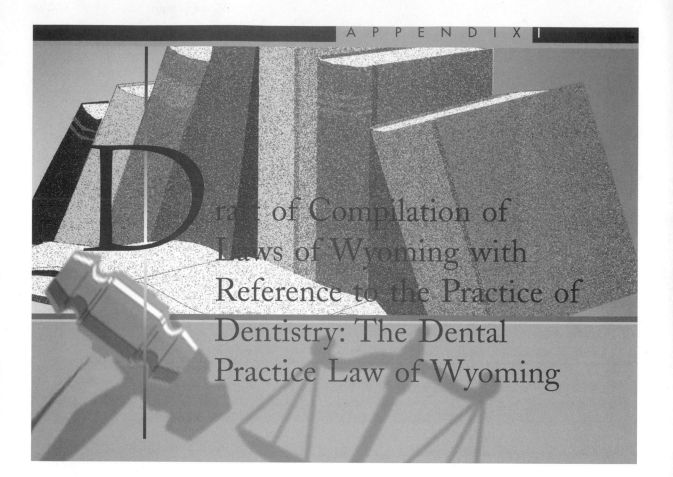

APPENDIX I

Draft of Compilation of Laws of Wyoming with Reference to the Practice of Dentistry: The Dental Practice Law of Wyoming

DENTISTS AND DENTAL HYGIENISTS
33-15-101. Board of Dental Examiners; generally.

(a) The board shall carry out the purposes and enforce the provisions of this act. The board shall consist of six (6) members appointed by the governor with the advice and consent of the state senate. Appointments made between sessions of the legislature shall be made in accordance with W.S. 28-12-101. The interim appointments are not considered a term for the purposes of subsection (c) of this section, relating to reappointment to the board.

(b) The term for board members is four (4) years, and expires on March 1. Effective July 1, 1979, appointments and terms shall be in accordance with W.S. 28-12-101 through 28-12-103.

(c) No person is eligible to membership on the board who is not legally qualified to practice; who has not engaged in the active practice of dentistry in the state of Wyoming for at least five (5) continuous years immediately prior to appointment; who does not at the time of his appointment hold a certificate entitling him to practice dentistry in the state of Wyoming; and who is not a resident of the state of Wyoming. One (1) appointed member of the board shall be a dental hygienist who has the qualifications provided in this act. No member shall succeed himself in office for more than two (2) successive terms.

(d) Any vacancy upon the board caused by resignation, death or removal of a member shall be filled by the governor by appointment for the unexpired term of that member. Any appointment to fill a vacancy shall be made within ninety (90) days after the vacancy occurs.

(e) Appointments by the governor to the board shall be made from a list of recommended names submitted by the Wyoming Dental Association and Wyoming Dental Hygiene Association as follows:

(i) The Wyoming Dental Association shall, through its secretary, present to the governor within fifteen (15) days after its regular annual meeting a list of the names of not less than ten (10) candidates from which appointments for vacancies on the board occurring during the ensuing year shall be made; and

(ii) The Wyoming Dental Hygiene Association shall, through its secretary, present to the governor within fifteen (15) days after its regular annual meeting a list of not less than three (3) candidates from which appointments for vacancies on the board occurring during the ensuing year shall be made.

(f) Each member of the board shall, before entering upon the duties of his office, take and subscribe an oath or affirmation that he will support the constitution and the laws of the United States and the state of Wyoming, and that he will faithfully perform the duties as a member of the board.

(g) The dental hygienist member of the board may act on all matters properly before the board except those matters involving the issuance, renewal or revocation of licenses of dentists in Wyoming.

33-15-102. Board of Dental Examiners; officers; seal; meeting; quorum.

(a) The board shall elect from its members a president, vice-president and a secretary-treasurer. The board shall have a common seal. The board shall meet in June each year, and more often if necessary, at such times and places designated by the president and the board. The meeting of the board shall be at the call of the president and the secretary-treasurer. Five (5) days notice shall be given by the secretary-treasurer to all board members of the time and place of the meeting. A majority of the board constitutes a quorum.

(b) Repealed by Laws 1981, ch. 172, §3.

33-15-103. Board of Dental Examiners; removal of members. The governor may remove any member as provided in W.S. 9-1-202 or for discontinued residence in Wyoming.

33-15-104. Board of Dental Examiners; indebtedness; compensation. The board shall not create any indebtedness on behalf of the state of Wyoming, except as provided in this section. Out of the funds assessed by the board, each of the members of the board shall receive as compensation the sum of seventy-five dollars ($75.00) for each day actually engaged in the duties of his office, actual expenses, and mileage in the same manner and amount as employees of the state of Wyoming. The secretary of the board shall receive compensation for his services.

33-15-105. Disposition of monies received and collected under provisions of chapter; report.

(a) All monies shall be received and collected as provided by law. The state treasurer shall place the money in an account within the earmarked revenue fund, which shall only be paid out upon an authorized voucher duly verified and signed by the president and secretary of the board, showing that the expenditure is a necessary expense and has been actually and properly incurred by the board. Upon presentation of the voucher, the auditor shall draw the warrant upon the treasurer but no warrant shall be drawn unless and until there are sufficient monies in the account to pay same and the expenses of the board shall not be charged upon any other state fund or account. Any money on hand at the dissolution of the board or the repeal of this act shall be paid to the credit of the common school permanent land fund account.

(b) The board shall report annually to the governor respecting all activities, as required by W.S. 9-2-1014.

33-15-106. Determination of fees. The board shall determine each year the fees to be collected for examinations, reexaminations and renewals.

33-15-107. Sale of license. Any member of the board who sells or offers to sell any license, or modify scoring or grading of a test to issue a license is subject to prosecution under W.S. 6-5-102.

33-15-108. Qualifications of applicants for license; examination; registration and licensing; examination and reexamination fees; notice of results of examination; reexamination; record book; rules.

(a) Any person of good moral character, who has been graduated and admitted to the degree of a doctor of dental surgery, doctor of dental medicine from a college or university accredited by the American Dental Association, or other equivalent degree by any accredited university or college authorized to grant the degree by the laws of the United States or by the laws of any state of the United States or Dominion of Canada, upon deposit of the examination fee set by the board, may make application in writing to the board to be examined by it with reference to his qualifications to practice dentistry. The applicant shall pass a written and practical examination in a manner satisfactory to the board. The written examination shall be, so far as the board deems practicable, on subjects prescribed in the curriculum in the accredited colleges and universities which offer courses of study leading to the degree of doctor of dental surgery or doctor of dental medicine. At the discretion of the board, part I and part II of the National Board of Dental Examiners' examination may be accepted in lieu of the written examination administered by the board. The clinical practical examination shall be held at a place and manner designated by the board. Upon passing the written and practical examination, the board shall register the name and residence of the person and issue to the person a license to practice dentistry. The license shall contain, along with the other necessary information, the name of the person to whom issued and the date of issuance.

(b) The examination fee shall be set by the board each year, and all reexamination fees shall be the same as the current fee for the initial examination. Fees shall be paid to the secretary of the board before examination. The fee shall be paid by money order, cashier's check or certified check, and in no case shall the fee be refunded.

(c) The applicant shall be informed in writing by certified mail of the results of his examination within thirty (30) days after the examination.

(d) An applicant who fails an examination may apply to the board for a reexamination at the next scheduled examination meeting. Application shall be made in writing and shall be accompanied by a fee as provided.

(e) If the applicant fails the board examination three (3) times, he shall show evidence of additional education to the satisfaction of the board before he may be reexamined.

(f) The board shall keep a record book in which is recorded the names and addresses of all applicants and such other matters as affords a full record of the actions of the board. The records or transcripts therefrom, duly certified by the president and secretary of the board with the seal of the board attached, is prima facie evidence before all courts of this state of the entries therein.

(g) The board shall make and prescribe all reasonable rules for its government and for the conduct of its business.

(h) The board may make and prescribe rules and regulations for the practice of dentistry in the state of Wyoming, not inconsistent with this act.

33-15-109. Renewal license certificate.

(a) On or before December 31 each year, each dentist licensed to practice dentistry in this state, upon receipt of written notice, shall transmit to the secretary of the board his signature and address, together with a fee determined by the board and the number of his license, and receive therefore a renewal license certificate. Any license granted by the board shall be cancelled after ten (10) days written notice sent to the holder by registered mail if the holder fails to secure the renewal certificate within three (3) months after December 31 each year, but any license thus cancelled may be restored by the board upon the payment of a fee as set by the board, if paid by December 31 of that year.

(b) Five (5) years after July 15, 1981, any dentist whose application for renewal indicates that he has not actively practiced dentistry or engaged in teaching dentistry for the preceding five (5) years shall be issued a renewal certificate by the board only after a hearing and upon notice to the applicant, wherein the applicant demonstrates to the board that he has maintained the qualifications set forth in this act. No reexamination is required unless the board finds good cause to believe that the person has not maintained the professional ability and knowledge required of an original licensee of this act.

(c) The board may set continuing education requirements for relicensure.

33-15-110. Certificate entitles dentist to practice in any county; lost certificates. The certificate provided for in this act entitles the holder to practice dentistry in any county in Wyoming. The board, upon satisfactory proof of loss of the certificate issued under this act, shall issue a new certificate. The cost of replacement shall be determined by the board and paid by the person requesting replacement.

33-15-111. List of licensees filed with secretary of state. A list of all dentists and dental hygienists licensed under this act shall be published by the board each year. This list shall contain the name and address of each dentist or dental hygienist and such other information as the board deems advisable. The board shall place a copy of the list on file in the office of the secretary of state who shall furnish copies to the public, upon request.

33-15-112. Grounds and procedure for revocation or suspension of license.

(a) Any dentist may have his license revoked or suspended by the board for any of the following causes:

(i) Conviction of a felony or high misdemeanor involving moral turpitude, in which case the record of conviction certified by the clerk or judge of the court in which the conviction is had is conclusive evidence;

(ii) For renting or loaning to any person his license or diploma to be used as a license or diploma for such person;

(iii) For unprofessional conduct, advertising or soliciting patients in any form of communication in a manner that is false or misleading in any material respect; or

(iv) Willful violation of any provisions of this act.

(b) The proceedings under this section may be taken by the board from matters within its knowledge or upon information from another. If the informant is a member of the board, the other members of the board shall judge the accused. All complaints shall be in writing, verified by some party familiar with the facts therein charged, and shall be filed with the secretary of the board. Upon receiving the complaint, the board, if it deem the complaint sufficient, shall proceed as in a contested case under the Wyoming Administrative Procedure Act (§§ 16-3-101 through 16-3-115). Upon revocation of any license, the fact shall be noted upon the records of the board and the license shall be marked cancelled upon the date of its revocation. The secretary of the board, upon judgment of suspension or revocation being entered, shall transmit to the secretary of state a copy of the judgement order, certified by the secretary of the board, and the same shall be kept in the same manner as the list of licensed dentists.

33-15-113. Secretary of state's certificate that no license listed by board is prima facie proof of unauthorized practice. In any prosecution for violation of any provision of this act the certificate of the secretary of state that the person accused of the violation of this act is not named in the list presented to him by the secretary of the board is prima facie proof that the person is not entitled to practice dentistry in Wyoming.

33-15-114. Persons deemed to be practicing dentistry; work authorizations from licensed dentist.

(a) Except as provided by paragraph (xii) of this subsection, any person is deemed to be practicing dentistry within the meaning of this act:

(i) Who performs, or attempts, or advertises to perform, or causes to be performed on the patient or any other person, or instructs in the performance of any dental operation or oral surgery or dental service of any kind gratuitously or for a salary, fee, money or other remuneration paid, or to be paid, directly or indirectly, to himself or to any other person or agency;

(ii) Who is a manager, proprietor, operator or a conductor of a place where dental operations, oral surgery or dental services are performed;

(iii) Who directly or indirectly by any means or method, furnishes, supplies, constructs, reproduces or repairs any prosthetic denture, bridge, appliance or other structure to be worn in the human mouth, or places such appliance or structure in the human mouth or attempts to adjust the same;

(iv) Who advertises to the public by any method to furnish, supply, construct, reproduce or repair any prosthetic denture, bridge, appliance or other structure to be worn in the human mouth;

(v) Who diagnoses or professes to diagnose, prescribes for or professes to prescribe for, treats or professes to treat disease, pain, deformity, deficiency, injury or physical condition of human teeth or jaws, or adjacent structure;

(vi) Who extracts or attempts to extract human teeth, or corrects or professes to correct malpositions of teeth or of the jaw;

(vii) Who gives or professes to give interpretations or readings of dental roentgenograms;

(viii) Who administers an anesthetic of any nature in connection with dental operations;

(ix) Who uses the words "dentist," "dental surgeon" or "oral surgeon," the letters "D.D.S.," "D.M.D." or any other words, letters, title or descriptive matter which in any way represents him as being able to diagnose, treat, prescribe or operate for any disease, pain, deformity, deficiency, injury or physical condition of human teeth or jaws, or adjacent structures;

(x) Who states or advertises or permits to be stated or advertised by a sign, card, circular, handbill, newspaper, radio or otherwise that he can perform or will attempt to perform dental operations or render a diagnosis in connection therewith; or

(xi) Who engages in any of the practices included in the curriculum of an approved dental college;

(xii) A dental laboratory or dental technician is not practicing dentistry within the meaning of this act when engaged in the construction, making, alteration or repairing of bridges, crowns, dentures or other prosthetic or surgical appliances, or orthodontic appliances if the casts or molds or impressions upon which work is constructed have been made by a regularly licensed and practicing dentist, and if all crowns, bridges, dentures or prosthetic appliances, surgical appliances, or orthodontic appliances are returned to the dentist upon whose order the work is constructed.

(b) Any licensed dentist who employs or engages the service of any person, firm or corporation to construct, reproduce, make, alter or repair bridges, crowns, dentures or other prosthetic, surgical or orthodontic appliances, shall furnish the person with a written work authorization on forms prescribed by the board, which contain:

(i) The name and address of the person to whom the work authorized is directed;

(ii) The patient's name or identification number, but if only a number is used the patient's name shall be written upon the duplicate copy of the work authorization retained by the dentist;

(iii) The date on which the work authorization was written;

(iv) A description of the work to be done, including diagrams, if necessary;

(v) A specification of the type and quality of the material to be used;

(vi) The signature of the dentist and the number of his license to practice dentistry.

(c) The person, firm or corporation receiving a work authorization from a licensed dentist shall retain the original work authorization and the dentist shall retain the duplicate copy for inspection at any reasonable time by the board or its authorized agents for two (2) years from date of issuance.

33-15-115. Persons to whom chapter inapplicable.

(a) Nothing in this act contained applies:

(i) To a legally qualified medical doctor;

(ii) To a legally qualified dental hygienist or dentist engaged in full-time duties with the United States armed forces, public health service, veterans administration or other federal agencies; or

(iii) To a legally qualified dental hygienist or dentist of another state making a clinical demonstration before a meeting of dentists or dental auxiliaries; or

(iv) To dental and dental hygiene students actively enrolled in any American Dental Association accredited dental educational program performing services as a part of the curriculum of that program under the direct supervision of a Wyoming licensed dentist or Wyoming licensed dental hygienist instructor.

33-15-116. Certain persons prohibited from soliciting patronage of general public. No person engaged in the business of constructing, altering or repairing bridges, crowns, dentures or other prosthetic appliances, surgical appliances or orthodontic appliances shall directly or indirectly solicit the patronage of the general public.

33-15-117. Dental laboratory technicians. Dentists may employ one (1) or more dental laboratory technicians who work only under the direction and supervision of the dentist and who shall not be permitted under any circumstances to do any work upon any patient. Dental laboratory technicians shall not be allowed to do laboratory work of any kind except at the direction of dentists duly licensed to practice, and then only upon written prescription issued by the dentists.

33-15-118. Repealed by Laws 1981, ch. 172, §3.

33-15-119. Dental hygienists; generally. Any dentist authorized to practice dentistry within the state may employ dental hygienists who shall be examined and possess the qualifications provided in this act. A dental hygienist may remove calcareous deposits, accretions and stains from the teeth and may perform any services for a patient which are consistent with what dental hygienists are trained to do in accredited dental hygiene schools. Hygienists shall not perform any other operation on the teeth or mouth and shall be regulated by the rules and regulations promulgated by the board. The above services shall be performed under the supervision of a licensed dentist. If the dental hygienist has been educated in expanded duties as a student in a dental hygiene program accredited by the commission on dental accreditation of the American Dental Association, or as a student in a continuing education course which had the prior approval of the board, he may be permitted to engage in those duties after the hygienist has received an expanded duties certificate from the board issued after appropriate examination to test the applicant's qualifications. Dental hygienists shall practice in the office of any licensed dentist, or in any public or private institution under the supervision of a licensed dentist. The board may revoke or suspend the license of any dental hygienist for violating any provision hereof, and may revoke or suspend the license of any dentist who permits any dental hygienist operating under his supervision to perform any operations other than those permitted under this act.

33-15-120. Dental hygienists; qualifications; examination; fees and license.

(a) Any person of good moral character who is a graduate of an American Dental Association accredited school for dental hygienists, upon payment of a fee set annually by the board, may be examined by the board on the subjects prescribed and taught in accredited colleges or universities offering courses leading to the certificate of degree of dental hygienist. At the discretion of the board, the examination of the National Board of Dental Examiners may be accepted in lieu of the written examination, together with a clinical examination approved by the board. If the applicant has received training in expanded duties and intends to perform those expanded duties he shall qualify by examination covering those expanded areas and receive an expanded duties certificate from the board listing these services. Expanded duties certificates shall be issued after the applicant has successfully completed a written examination approved by the board covering those expanded duties together with a clinical examination approved by the board. If the applicant fails to pass either examination, the applicant may take another examination at the next regular examination meeting upon payment of a fee set annually by the board.

(b) If the applicant fails the board examination three (3) times, he shall show evidence of additional education to the satisfaction of the board before he may be reexamined.

(c) If the applicant successfully passes the examinations, the applicant shall be licensed as a dental hygienist. If the expanded duties applicant has successfully passed the expanded duties examination the applicant shall be certified in those expanded duties. The certificate issued by the board shall list the expanded duties which the hygienist is qualified and permitted to perform. On or before December 31 each year, each dental hygienist licensed to practice dental hygiene, upon receipt of written notice, shall transmit to the secretary of the board his name and address, together with a fee set by the board and the number of his registration certificate, and receive a renewal license certificate. The renewal certificate shall at all times be properly displayed in the office of the one who is named as holder of the license and no person is deemed in legal practice who does not possess a renewal certificate. Any license granted by the board shall be cancelled after ten (10) days written notice by registered mail if the holder fails to secure the renewal certificate within three (3) months after December 31 each year. Any license cancelled may be restored by the board upon payment of a fee set annually by the board, if paid by December 31 of that year.

(d) Five (5) years after July 1, 1981, any dental hygienist whose application for renewal indicates that he has not actively practiced dental hygiene or engaged in teaching dental hygiene for the preceding five (5) years shall be issued a renewal certificate by the board only after a hearing and upon notice to the applicant, wherein the applicant demonstrates to the board that he has maintained the qualifications set forth in this act. No reexamination is required unless the board finds good cause to believe that the person has not maintained the professional ability and knowledge required of an original licensee of this act.

33-15-121. Grounds and proceedings for suspension of, revocation of, or refusal to renew license.

(a) The board may refuse to issue or renew, or may suspend or revoke, the license of any dental hygienist for any of the following causes:

(i) Conviction of a felony or high misdemeanor;

(ii) For unprofessional conduct, advertising or soliciting patients in any form of communication in a manner that is false or misleading in any material respect;

(iii) For renting or loaning to any person his or her license or diploma to be used as a license or diploma for that person; or

(iv) For willful violation of any provision of this act.

(b) All proceedings taken by the board in the revocation or suspension of any dental hygienist's license shall be taken under the proceedings set forth in W.S. 33-15-112 in the same manner as provided for the revocation or suspension of a dentist's license.

33-15-122. Reciprocity. The board may accept by reciprocity, upon payment of a registered fee determined by the board, the license of a dentist who was licensed in another state or territory of the United States if the license requirements of that state or territory were as great or greater than those of Wyoming when that license was granted. Reciprocity may only be granted to dentists from those states which grant reciprocity to dentists licensed in Wyoming.

33-15-123. Duties of other dental auxiliary. Duties of all other dental auxiliary personnel not mentioned in this act shall be set and governed by the rules and regulations of the board.

33-15-124. Violations. Any person who practices dentistry without being properly qualified and licensed, or who violates any provision of this act is subject to a fine, not to exceed one thousand dollars ($1,000.00), or imprisonment of not more than two (2) years in the penitentiary, or both. Each separate violation of this act constitutes a separate offense.

33-15-125. Repealed by Laws 1981, ch. 172, §3.

33-15-126. Regulation of proceedings relating to revocation or suspension of licenses. All proceedings before the board relating to the revocation or suspension of licenses shall be conducted according to the Wyoming Administrative Procedure Act (§§16-3-101 through 16-3-115).

33-15-127. Action for injunction. The board in its own name may bring an action for an injunction, and courts of this state may enjoin any person from violation of this act. Such proceedings shall be prosecuted by the attorney general's office or by private counsel.

33-15-128. Definitions; short title.

(a) As used in this act:
  (i) "Board" means the Wyoming Board of Dental Examiners established by this act;
  (ii) "Dentistry" means the healing art practiced by a dentist which is concerned with the examination, diagnosis, treatment planning and care of conditions within the human oral cavity and its adjacent tissues and structures;
  (iii) "Dentist" means a person who performs any intraoral or extraoral procedure required in the practice of dentistry and to whom is reserved:
    (A) The responsibility for final diagnosis of conditions within the human mouth and its adjacent tissues and structures;
    (B) The responsibility of the final treatment plan of any dental patient;
    (C) The responsibility for prescribing drugs which are administered to patients in the practice of dentistry;
    (D) The responsibility for overall quality of patient care which is rendered

or performed in the practice of dentistry regardless of whether the care is rendered personally by the dentist or by a dental auxiliary; and

(E) Other specified services within the scope of the practice of dentistry.

(iv) "Dental" means pertaining to dentistry;

(v) "Dental hygienist" means a person who is supervised by a dentist and licensed to render the educational, preventive and therapeutic dental services defined in this act, as well as any extraoral procedure required in the practice of a dental hygienist's duties;

(vi) "Dental assistant" means a person who is supervised by a dentist and renders assistance to a dentist, dental hygienist, dental technician or another dental assistant as described in this act;

(vii) "Dental laboratory" means an enterprise engaged in making, repairing, providing or altering oral prosthetic appliances and other artificial materials and devices which are returned to the dentist and inserted into the human mouth or which come into contact with its adjacent structures and tissues;

(viii) "Dental laboratory technician" means a person who, at the direction of the dentist, makes, provides, repairs or alters oral prosthetic appliances and other artificial devices which are inserted into the human mouth or which come into contact with the human mouth and its adjacent tissues and structures. A dental technician is a dental prosthetic auxiliary when working under the supervision of a dentist;

(ix) "Dental auxiliary" means any person who works under the supervision of a dentist and who provides dental care services to a patient;

(x) "Supervision" of a dental auxiliary means the act of directing or overseeing duties performed by a dental auxiliary, as defined by rules and regulations of the board;

(xi) "Unprofessional conduct" means conduct related to the practice of dentistry or any dental auxiliary occupation which constitutes a departure from or failure to conform to the standards of acceptable and professional practices, including but not limited to gross ignorance or inefficiency in the profession, habitual drunkenness, habitual addiction to the use of any controlled substance, employing anyone known as a capper or steerer to obtain business, the obtaining of any fee by fraud or misrepresentation, willingly betraying patient confidences, employing directly or indirectly any student or any suspended or unlicensed dentist to perform operations of any kind for the treatment of the human teeth, jaws or to correct malimposed formations thereof, the willful violation of any rule or regulation adopted by the Wyoming Board of Dental Examiners and other generally accepted codes of ethics and professional behavior as may be adopted as rules and regulations by the board;

(xii) "Proprietor" includes any person who:

(A) Employs dentists, dental hygienists or dental auxiliaries in the operation of a dental office, except as defined in the act; or

(B) Places in the possession of a dentist, dental hygienist or dental auxiliary or other agent such dental material or equipment as may be necessary for the management of a dental office on the basis of a lease or any other agreement for compensation for the use of such material, equipment or offices; or

(C) Retains the ownership or control of dental equipment or material or office and makes the same available in any manner for the use by dentists, dental hygienists, dental auxiliaries or any other agents, excepting that nothing in this subparagraph shall apply to bona fide sales of dental equipment or material secured by a chattel mortgage or retain-title agreement or the loan of articulators.

(xiii) "Expanded duties" means those patient's services which are beyond those regularly practiced by dental hygienists or dental technicians or other dental auxiliary functions and which require additional education which shall be approved by the Board of Dental Examiners of Wyoming and are to be performed under the direct supervision of a licensed dentist;

(xiv) "Specialty" means a special area of dental practice for ethical specialty announcement and limitation of practice which are dental public health, endodontics, oral pathology, oral and maxillofacial surgery, orthodontics, pediatric dentistry, periodontics, prosthodontics and any other specialty area recognized by the Board of Dental Examiners of Wyoming;

(xv) "Radiograph" means the film used with an x-ray machine and includes the product of a film exposed by an x-ray machine;

(xvi) "X-ray machine" means an assemblage of components for the controlled production of x-rays. It includes, at a minimum, an x-ray high voltage generator, an x-ray control, a tube housing assembly, a beam limiting device and the necessary supporting structures;

(xvii) "This act" means W.S. 33-15-101 through 33-15-130 and may be cited as the "Wyoming Dental Practice Act".

33-15-129. Radiograph use permits.

(a) Any dental assistant who places or exposes radiographs shall hold a radiograph use permit.

(b) Any licensed dentist using an x-ray machine shall have that machine inspected by a qualified radiation expert periodically as determined by the board.

(c) The board shall promulgate reasonable rules and regulations necessary for granting or revoking a radiograph use permit and for inspection of x-ray machines.

33-15-130. General anesthesia or parenteral sedation permit.

(a) Any dentist licensed under this act who administers general anesthesia or parenteral sedation shall apply for and receive a general anesthesia or parenteral sedation permit. The permit shall be issued to a licensed dentist who passes an appropriate examination and has the necessary equipment as defined by the board.

(b) The board shall provide for the inspection of the anesthesia and sedation equipment of permitted dentists on a regular basis to insure the equipment is of the appropriate type and is in working order.

(c) Any dentist using general anesthesia or parenteral sedation without a permit may have his license revoked or suspended.

(d) The board shall promulgate reasonable rules and regulations, including establishing examination fees, as necessary to carry out this section.

RULES AND REGULATIONS OF THE WYOMING BOARD OF DENTAL EXAMINERS RELATING TO THE PRACTICE OF DENTISTRY AND THE DUTIES AND SUPERVISION OF DENTAL AUXILIARIES.

These Rules supersede all other Rules previously filed.

Chapter I
General Provisions

Section 1. *Law Under Which Board Created and Operates.* The State Board of Dental Examiners, hereinafter referred to as the "Board," is created by and operates under and in accordance with Title 33, Chapter 15 (Sections 33-15-101 through 33-15-130) of the Wyoming Statutes, 1991, hereinafter called the "Act". In the event any rule of the board is inconsistent with any provision of the Act, the Act shall control.

Section 2. *Jurisdiction.* This board has, and the Act grants it, jurisdiction of all applicants and applications for license to practice dentistry and dental hygiene in the state of Wyoming. This board is specifically charged with the administration of the Act, including the duty to revoke or suspend any license for any of the causes specified in the Act.

Section 3. *Membership of the Board.* As provided in the Act, this board consists of five resident electors of Wyoming duly licensed to practice dentistry in this state, and one resident elector of Wyoming duly licensed to practice dental hygiene, each of whom before entering upon the duties of a board member shall subscribe an oath to support the Constitution of the United States and of the state of Wyoming and that he will faithfully perform the duties of the office to the best of his ability.

Section 4. *Officers of the Board.* The board shall, at its regular yearly session in June of each year, choose from its members a President, Vice President and a Secretary-Treasurer. The majority of the board shall constitute a quorum.

Section 5. *Purpose.* The board has been given the duty of controlling the quality of dentistry for the protection of the people of the state of Wyoming. To fulfill this purpose, the board sets forth the following Rules and Regulations to safeguard the health and welfare of the people of this state. W.S. 33-15-108(h).

Chapter II
Definitions

Section 1. *Definitions.* For the purpose of these Rules and Regulations, the following definitions in the Act shall apply:

(a) "The Board" means the Board of Dental Examiners of the state of Wyoming.

(b) "Dental Assistant" means a person who is supervised by a dentist and renders assistance to a dentist, dental hygienist, dental technician, or another dental assistant.

(c) "Dental Auxiliary" means any person who works under the supervision of a dentist and who provides dental health care services to a patient.

(d) "Dental Hygienist" means a person who is supervised by a dentist and is licensed to provide educational, preventive, and therapeutic dental services, as well as any extraoral procedures required in the practice of a dental hygienist's duties.

(e) "Dental Laboratory" means an enterprise engaged in making, repairing, providing, or altering oral prosthetic appliances and other artificial devices which are inserted into the human mouth and its adjacent tissues and structures.

(f) "Dental Laboratory Technician" means a person who, at the direction of the dentist, makes, provides, repairs, or alters oral prosthetic appliances and other artificial devices which are inserted into the human mouth and its adjacent tissues and structures. A dental laboratory technician is a dental prosthetic auxiliary when working under the supervision of a dentist.

(g) "Direct Supervision" of a dental auxiliary means that a dentist is physically present in the dental office, a dentist has diagnosed the condition to be treated, a dentist has authorized the procedure to be performed, and before dismissal of the patient, a dentist has approved the work performed by the auxiliary.

(h) "General Supervision" of a dental auxiliary means that a dentist has diagnosed and authorized the procedures which are being carried out; however, a dentist need not be present when the authorized procedures are being performed.

(i) "Indirect Supervision" of a dental auxiliary means that a dentist is physically present in the dental office, a dentist has diagnosed the condition to be treated, and a dentist has authorized the procedure to be performed.

(j) "Inefficiency" means incapable of producing the effect intended or desired; not competent, capable, or proficient.

(k) "Proficient" means one well advanced in any business, art, science, or branch of learning; an expert.

(l) "Supervision" of dental auxiliary means the act of overseeing or directing duties performed by a dental auxiliary.

Chapter III
Dental Practice

Section 1. *Practice of Dentistry.* The following rules and regulations apply to the Practice of Dentistry:

(a) The dentist has the responsibility for the quality of dentistry performed in his office, regardless of whether it is performed by him personally or by auxiliaries working under his supervision.

(b) Each dentist is responsible for maintaining a high level of proficiency in the practice of dentistry and for keeping up with current educational standards of the profession.

(c) A dentist shall not advertise in any way that is false or misleading in any material respect.

(d) A dentist should be willing to aid any of his colleagues, but should have uppermost in his mind the protection of the general public and should report gross and/or recurring improprieties to the proper board or agency.

(e) Any dentist who is suffering from a disease or condition that adversely affects the quality of his work shall notify the board through its secretary.

(f) Dentists will practice in accordance with the most recently adopted Code of Ethics and Principles of Practice of the Wyoming Board of Dental Examiners.

(g) Satellite offices: When a dentist is the proprietor of more than one (1) office, he shall designate one (1) as his main office; all others shall be termed satellite offices. Satellite offices shall abide by the same rules and regulations as the main office.

(h) Radiograph use permits: After July 1, 1991, all dental x-ray machines must be inspected by a board-approved Medical/Health Physicist qualified to inspect such machines. These units shall be inspected every five (5) years. No fee is charged by the board. Dentists are responsible to contract directly with an approved inspector who in turn will submit to the secretary of the dental board the pass/fail results of all equipment inspected. Upon notification that units have passed the safety inspection, a dated sticker will be issued from the board secretary. Machines failing inspection must have a copy of the work order showing satisfactory repair completed sent to the secretary's office.

Chapter IV
Anesthetic Administration

Section 1. *Definitions.* For the purpose of these rules relative to the administration of general anesthesia, parenteral sedation, and nitrous oxide inhalation analgesia by licensed dentists the following definitions shall apply:

(a) *General Anesthesia* means a controlled state of unconsciousness, produced by a pharmacologic agent, accompanied by a partial or complete loss of protective reflexes, including inability to independently maintain an airway and respond appropriately to physical stimulation or verbal command.

(b) *Parenteral Sedation* means a depressed level of consciousness produced by the parenteral administration of pharmacologic substances, that retains the patient's ability to independently and continuously maintain an airway and respond appropriately to physical stimulation or verbal command.

(c) *Nitrous Oxide Inhalation Analgesia* means the administration by inhalation of a combination of nitrous oxide and oxygen producing an altered level of consciousness that retains the patient's ability to independently and continuously maintain an airway and respond appropriately to physical stimulation or verbal command.

Section 2. *Prohibitions.* The following are hereby prohibited:

(a) *General Anesthesia:* Effective July 1, 1991, dentists licensed in this state shall not administer general anesthesia in the practice of dentistry unless they have complied with the provisions of this rule.

(b) *Parenteral Sedation:* Effective July 1, 1991, dentists licensed in this state shall not administer parenteral sedation in the practice of dentistry unless they have complied with the provisions of this rule.

(c) *Nitrous Oxide Inhalation Analgesia:* Effective July 1, 1991, dentists licensed in this state shall not administer nitrous oxide inhalation analgesia in the practice of dentistry unless they have complied with the following provisions:

(i) A dentist may use nitrous oxide inhalation analgesia sedation on an out-patient basis for dental patients provided the dentist:

(A) Has completed a board approved course of training; or

(B) Has training equivalent to that required of a student in an accredited school of dentistry, and

(C) Has adequate equipment with fail-safe features and a 25% minimum oxygen flow.

(ii) A dentist utilizing nitrous oxide inhalation analgesia and auxiliary personnel who monitor its use shall be trained and capable of administering basic life support. This certification must be renewed in compliance with the standards set forth by the American Heart Association.

(iii) A licensed dentist who has been utilizing nitrous oxide inhalation analgesia in a competent manner for the twelve month period preceding the effective date of this rule, but has not had the benefit of formal training outlined in subsections (A) or (B), may continue such use provided the dentist fulfills the requirements of (C) above and is trained and capable of administering basic life support.

Section 3. *Requirements for Administering Anesthesia.*

(a) *General Anesthesia:* After July 1, 1991, general anesthesia may only be administered by a licensed dentist who has received a general anesthesia permit from the board. Permits will be issued by the board only after the following requirements have been met:

(i) *Proof of Proficiency:* A licensed dentist can show proof of proficiency in administering general anesthesia by successfully passing an appropriate examination which includes:

1. Discussion and review of three surgical cases including anesthetic technique
2. Review of records
3. Demonstration of managing emergencies

In addition, a dentist must provide:

(A) Proof that he has completed a minimum of one year of advanced training in anesthesiology and related academic subjects beyond the under graduate dental school level in a training program approved by the board; or

(B) Proof that he is a diplomate of the American Board of Oral and Maxillofacial Surgery; or

(C) Proof that he is eligible for examination by the American Board of Oral and Maxillofacial Surgery; or

(D) Proof that he is a member of the American Association of Oral and Maxillofacial Surgeons; or

(E) Proof that he is a fellow of the American Dental Society of Anesthesiology; or

(F) Proof that he is a licensed dentist who has been utilizing general anesthesia in a competent manner for the five (5) year period preceding the effective date of this rule.

(ii) A dentist using general anesthesia shall provide and maintain proper equipment for the administration of general anesthesia staffed with supervised auxiliary personnel, capable of reasonable handling procedures, problems and emergencies incident thereto.

(iii) A dentist using general anesthesia shall be trained and capable of administering advanced cardiac life support. This certification shall be renewed in compliance with the standards set forth by the American Heart Association.

(iv) A dentist using general anesthesia shall employ auxiliary personnel who are trained and capable of administering basic life support. This certification shall be renewed in compliance with the standards set forth by the American Heart Association.

(v) A dentist who is performing a procedure for which general anesthesia was induced shall not administer the general anesthetic and monitor the patient without the presence and assistance of trained and capable auxiliary personnel.

(vi) A dentist qualified to administer general anesthesia under this rule may administer parenteral sedation and nitrous oxide inhalation analgesia.

(vii) General anesthetic equipment of permitted dentists shall be inspected on a regular basis as designated by the board to insure the equipment is of the appropriate type and is in working order.

(A) General Anesthesia equipment includes:
.....Oxygen and supplemental gas-delivery system and backup system
.....Suction and backup system
.....Auxiliary lighting system
.....Gas storage facilities
.....Suitable operating suite
.....Recovery areas
.....Emergency anesthetic equipment and medications
.....Monitoring equipment

(B) Inspection of offices where general anesthesia is administered shall be conducted every five (5) years.

(C) Inspections shall be done by at least two qualified experts as determined by the board.

(D) Any malfunctioning equipment shall be called to the attention of the applicant and a permit will not be issued until the experts determine all equipment is operating satisfactorily.

(E) The annual permit fee will be $45.00 which includes the parenteral sedation fee and is to be paid at the time of the license renewal. The renewal license shall indicate when the five (5) year inspection is due.

(F) A dentist shall apply to the secretary of the Board of Dental Examiners who will arrange with the qualified experts and the applicant dentist for an onsite inspection.

(G) Any permitted dentist who operates with malfunctioning equipment as determined by the board, shall cease administering general anesthesia until such equipment has been repaired. A copy of the work order showing satisfactory repair completed shall be sent to the secretary's office.

(viii) Any dentist using general anesthesia without a permit may have his license revoked or suspended.

(ix) The board shall establish examination fees as necessary to carry out this section.

(b) *Parenteral Sedation:* After July 1, 1991, parenteral sedation may only be administered by a licensed dentist who has received a parenteral sedation permit from the board. Permits will be issued by the board only after the following requirements have been met:

(i) *Proof of Proficiency:* A licensed dentist can show proof of proficiency in administering parenteral sedation by successfully passing an appropriate examination which includes:

1. Discussion and review of three surgical cases including anesthetic technique
2. Review of records
3. Demonstration of managing emergencies

In addition, a dentist must provide:

(A) Proof that he is a licensed dentist who has documented experience at the graduate level, acceptable to the board, specifying the type, the number of hours, the length of training and the number of patient contact hours, including documentation of the number of supervised parenteral sedation cases; or

(B) Proof that he is a licensed dentist who has successfully completed a formal training program, approved by the board, which included physical evaluation, IV sedation, airway management, monitoring, advanced cardiac life support and emergency management; or

(C) Proof that he is a licensed dentist who has been utilizing parenteral sedation on an out-patient basis in a competent manner for five (5) years preceding the effective date of this rule, but has not had the benefit of formal training as outlined in this rule. He may continue such use provided the licensed dentist fulfills the provisions set forth in (ii), (iii), (iv) and (v) below.

(ii) A dentist utilizing parenteral sedation shall maintain a properly equipped facility for the administration of parenteral sedation, staffed with supervised auxiliary personnel, capable of reasonable handling procedures, problems, and emergencies incident thereto.

(iii) A dentist using parenteral sedation shall be trained and capable of administering advanced cardiac life support. This certification shall be renewed in compliance with the standards set forth by the American Heart Association.

(iv) A dentist using parenteral sedation shall employ auxiliary personnel who are trained and capable of administering basic life support. This certification shall be renewed in compliance with the standards set forth by the American Heart Association.

(v) A dentist who is performing a procedure for which parenteral sedation is being employed shall not administer the pharmacologic agents and monitor the patient without the presence and assistance of trained and qualified auxiliary personnel.

(vi) Dentists qualified to administer parenteral sedation may administer nitrous oxide inhalation analgesic.

(vii) If parenteral sedation results in a general anesthetic state, the rules for general anesthesia apply.

(viii) Parenteral sedation equipment of permitted dentists shall be inspected on a regular basis as designated by the board to insure the equipment is of the appropriate type and is in working order.

(A) Parenteral Sedation equipment includes:
.....Oxygen and supplemental gas-delivery system and backup system
.....Suction and backup system
.....Auxiliary lighting system
.....Gas storage facilities
.....Suitable operating suite
.....Recovery areas
.....Emergency anesthetic equipment and medications
.....Monitoring equipment

(B) Inspection of offices where parenteral sedation is administered shall be conducted every five (5) years.

(C) Inspections shall be done by at least two qualified experts as determined by the board.

(D) Any malfunctioning equipment shall be called to the attention of the applicant and a permit will not be issued until the experts determine all equipment is operating satisfactorily.

(E) The annual permit fee will be $45.00 which includes the general anesthesia fee and is to be paid at the time of the license renewal. The renewal license shall indicate when the five (5) year inspection is due.

(F) A dentist shall apply to the secretary of the Board of Dental Examiners who will arrange with the qualified experts and the applicant dentist for an on-site inspection.

(G) Any permitted dentist who operates with malfunctioning equipment as determined by the board, shall cease administering parenteral sedation until such equipment has been repaired. A copy of the work order showing satisfactory repair completed shall be sent to the secretary's office.

(ix) Any dentist using parenteral sedation without a permit may have his license revoked or suspended.

(x) The board shall establish examination fees as necessary to carry out this section.

Section 4. *Reporting of Adverse Occurrences Related to General Anesthesia, Parenteral Sedation, and Nitrous Oxide Inhalation Analgesia.*

(a) All licensed dentists in the practice of dentistry in this state should submit a report within a period of thirty (30) days to the board of any mortality or other incident which results in temporary or permanent physical or mental injury requiring hospitalization of said patient during, or as a result of, nitrous oxide inhalation analgesia, parenteral sedation, or general anesthesia related thereto. The report shall include, at the minimum, responses to the following:

(i) Description of dental procedure.

(ii) Description of preoperative physical condition of patient.

(iii) List of drugs and dosage administered.

(iv) Description, in detail, of techniques utilized in the administration of the above listed drugs.

(v) Description of adverse occurrence.

(A) Describe in detail symptoms of any complications, to include but not limited to onset, and type of symptoms in patient.

(B) Treatment instituted on the patient.

(C) Response of patient to treatment.

(vi) Describe patient's condition on termination of any procedures undertaken.

Chapter V
Code of Ethics

Section 1. *Principle. Service to the Public and Quality of Care.* The dentist's primary obligation of service to the public shall include the delivery of care, competently and timely, within the bounds of the clinical circumstances presented by the patient. Quality of care shall be a primary consideration of the dental practitioner.

(a) *Code of Professional Conduct.*

(i) *Patient Selection.* While dentists, in serving the public, may exercise reasonable discretion in selecting patients for their practices, dentists shall not refuse to accept patients into their practice or deny dental service to patients because of the patient's race, creed, color, sex, or national origin.

(ii) *Patient Records.* Dentists are obliged to safeguard the confidentiality of patient records. Dentists shall maintain patient records in a manner consistent with the protection of the welfare of the patient. Upon request of a patient or another dental practitioner, dentists shall provide any information that will be beneficial for the future treatment of that patient.

(iii) *Community Service.* Since dentists have an obligation to use their skills, knowledge, and experience for the improvement of the dental health of the public and are encouraged to be leaders in their community, dentists in such service shall conduct themselves in such a manner as to maintain or elevate the esteem of the profession.

(iv) *Emergency Service.* Dentists shall be obliged to make reasonable arrangements for the emergency care of their patients of record.

Dentists shall be obliged when consulted in an emergency by patients not of record to make reasonable arrangements for emergency care. If treatment is provided, the dentist, upon completion of such treatment, is obliged to return the patient to his or her regular dentist unless the patient expressly reveals a different preference.

(v) *Consultation and Referral.* Dentists shall be obliged to seek consultation, if possible, whenever the welfare of patients will be safeguarded or advanced by utilizing those who have special skills, knowledge, and experience. When patients visit or are referred to specialists or consulting dentists for consultation:

(A) The specialists or consulting dentists, upon completion of their care, shall return the patient, unless the patient expressly reveals a different preference, to the referring dentist, or if none, to the dentist of record for future care.

(B) The specialists shall be obliged when there is no referring dentist and upon a completion of their treatment to inform patients when there is a need for further dental care.

(vi) *Use of Auxiliary Personnel.* Dentists shall be obliged to protect the health of their patient by only assigning to qualified auxiliaries those duties which can be legally delegated. Dentists shall be further obliged to prescribe and supervise the work of all auxiliary personnel working under their direction and control.

(vii) *Justifiable Criticism.* Dentists shall be obliged to report to the appropriate reviewing agency as determined by the local component or constituent society instances of gross and continual faulty treatment by other dentists. Patients shall be informed of their present oral health status without disparaging comment about prior services.

(viii) *Expert Testimony.* Dentists may provide expert testimony when that testimony is essential to a just and fair disposition of a judicial or administrative action.

(ix) *Rebate and Split Fees.* Dentists shall not accept or tender "rebates" or "split fees."

(x) *Representation of Care and Fees.* Dentists shall not represent the care being rendered to their patients or the fees being charged for providing such care in a false or misleading manner.

(xi) Dentists, because of their position of power and authority over both patients and staff, must exercise extreme discretion in their conduct and avoid any form of sexual coercion and/or harassment.

Section 2. *Principle. Education.* The privilege of dentists to be accorded professional status rests primarily in the knowledge, skill, and experience with which they serve their patients and society. All dentists, therefore, have the obligation of keeping their knowledge and skill current.

Section 3. *Principle. Government of a Profession.* Every profession owes society the responsibility to regulate itself. Such regulation is achieved largely through the influence of the professional societies. All dentists, therefore, have the dual obligation of making themselves a part of a professional society and of observing its rules of ethics.

Section 4. *Research and Development.* Dentists have the obligation of making the results and benefits of their investigative efforts available to all when they are useful in safeguarding or promoting the health of the public.

(a) *Devices and Therapeutic Methods.* Except for formal investigative studies, dentists shall be obliged to prescribe, dispense, or promote only those devices, drugs, and other agents whose complete formulae are available to the dental profession. Dentists shall have the further obligation of not holding out as exclusive any device, agent, method, or technique.

(b) *Patents and Copyrights*. Patents and copyrights may be secured by dentists provided that such patents and copyrights shall not be used to restrict research or practice.

Section 5. ***Principle.***

(a) *Professional Announcement*. In order to properly serve the public, dentists should represent themselves in a manner that contributes to the esteem of the profession. Dentists should not misrepresent their training and competence in any way that would be false or misleading in any material respect.*

(b) *Advertising*. Although any dentist may advertise, no dentist shall advertise or solicit patients in any form of communication in a manner that is false or misleading in any material respect.*

(c) *Name of Practice*. Since the name under which a dentist conducts his practice may be a factor in the selection process of the patient, the use of a trade name or an assumed name that is false or misleading in any material respect is unethical.

Use of the name of a dentist no longer actively associated with the practice may be continued for a period not to exceed one year.*

(d) *Announcement of Specialization and Limitation of Practice*. This section and Section 5(e) are designed to help the public make an informed selection between the practitioner who has completed an accredited program beyond the dental degree and a practitioner who has not completed such a program.

The special areas of dental practice approved by the American Dental Association and the designation for ethical specialty announcement and limitation of practice are: dental public health, endodontics, oral pathology, oral and maxillofacial surgery, orthodontics, pediatric dentistry, periodontics and prosthodontics. Dentists who choose to announce specialization should use "specialist" or "practice limited to" and shall limit their practice exclusively to the announced special area(s) of dental practice, provided at the time of the announcement such dentists have met in each approved specialty for which they announce the existing educational requirements and standards set forth by the American Dental Association.

Dentists who use their eligibility to announce as specialists to make the public believe that specialty services rendered in the dental office are being rendered by qualified specialists, when such is not the case, are engaged in unethical conduct. The burden of responsibility is on specialists to avoid any inference that general practitioners who are associated with specialists are qualified to announce themselves as specialists.

General Standards. The following are included within the standards of the American Dental Association for determining which dentists have the education, experience, and other appropriate requirements for announcing specialization and limitation of practice:

(a) The special area(s) of dental practice and an appropriate certifying board must be approved by the American Dental Association.

(b) Dentists who announce as specialists must have successfully completed an educational program accredited by the Commission on Dental Accreditation, two (2) or more years in length, as specified by the Council on Dental Education or be diplomates of nationally recognized certifying boards.

(c) The practice carried on by dentists who announce as specialists shall be limited exclusively to the special area(s) of dental practice announced by the dentist. *Standards for Multiple-Specialty Announcements.*

Educational criteria for announcement by dentists in additional recognized specialty areas are the successful completion of an educational program accredited by the Commission on Dental Accreditation in each area for which the dentist wishes to announce.

Dentists who completed their advanced education in programs listed by the Council on Dental Education prior to the initiation of the accreditation process in 1967 and who are currently ethically announcing as specialists in a recognized area may announce in additional areas, provided they are educationally qualified or are certified diplomates in each area for which they wish to announce. Documentation of successful completion of the educational program(s) must be submitted to the appropriate constituent society. The documentation must assure that the duration of the program(s) is a minimum of two (2) years, except for oral and maxillofacial surgery which must have been a minimum of three (3) years in duration.*

(e) *General Practitioner Announcement of Services.* General dentists who wish to announce the services available in their practices are permitted to announce the availability of those services so long as they avoid any communications that express or imply specialization. General dentists shall also state that the services are being provided by general dentists. No dentist shall announce available services in any way that would be false or misleading in any material respect.*

*Advertising solicitation of patients or business, or other promotional activities by dentists or dental care delivery organizations, shall not be considered unethical or improper, except for those promotional activities which are false or misleading in any material respect. Notwithstanding any ADA *Principles of Ethics and Code of Professional Conduct* or other standards of dentist conduct which may be differently worded, this shall be the sole standard for determining the ethical propriety of such promotional activities. Any provision of an ADA constituent or component society's code of ethics or other standard of dentist conduct relating to dentists' or dental care delivery organizations' advertising, solicitation, or other promotional activities which is worded differently from the above standard, shall be deemed to be in conflict with the ADA *Principles of Ethics and Code of Professional Conduct.*

Interpretation and Application of "Principles of Ethics and Code of Professional Conduct." The preceding statements constitute the *Principles of Ethics and Code of Professional Conduct* of the American Dental Association. The purpose of the *Principles and Code* is to uphold and strengthen dentistry as a member of the learned professions. The constituent and component societies may adopt additional provisions or interpretations not in conflict with these *Principles of Ethics and Code of Professional Conduct* which would enable them to serve more faithfully the traditions, customs, and desires of the members of these societies.

Problems involving questions of ethics should be solved at the local level within the broad boundaries established in these *Principles of Ethics and Code of Professional*

Conduct and within the interpretation by the component and/or constituent society of their respective codes of ethics. If a satisfactory decision cannot be reached, the question should be referred on appeal to the constituent society and the Council on Bylaws and Judicial Affairs of the American Dental Association, as provided in Chapter XI of the Bylaws of the American Dental Association. Members found guilty of unethical conduct, as prescribed in the American Dental Association *Code of Professional Conduct* or codes of ethics of the constituent and component societies, are subject to the penalties set forth in Chapter XI of the American Dental Association *ByLaws*.

Chapter VI
Dental Auxiliaries

Section 1. ***Dental Auxiliary Personnel.*** The following applies to dental auxiliary personnel generally:

(a) No irreversible procedures may be conducted by any dental auxiliary personnel unless otherwise specified.

Section 2. ***Practice of Dental Hygiene and Supervision Required.*** The following applies to the practice of Dental Hygiene:

(a) Each dental hygienist is responsible for maintaining a high degree of proficiency in the practice of dental hygiene and for keeping up with current educational standards of the profession.

(b) A dental hygienist shall work under the supervision of a qualified dentist.

(c) Dental hygienists may work in the private office of a dentist, in the Armed Forces of the United States, in federal or state institutions, and nursing or retirement facilities.

(d) Dental hygienists are encouraged to promote oral health through lectures. They may accomplish this through talks to schools, institutions, groups, or individuals when asked. In no event should these appearances be used for the purpose of advertising or soliciting patients for himself/herself or a dentist.

(e) The following is a list of procedures that may be performed by a dental hygienist and the type of supervision required:

(i) General Supervision:

(A) Community dental health activities.

(B) Functions that are authorized for dental assistants set forth in rules or prescribed duties promulgated by the board.

(C) Scaling and polishing of teeth.

(D) Polishing amalgams and composites.

(E) Conduct screening examination of the oral cavity for oral disease.

(F) Placement of temporary fillings which require no removal of tooth structure.

(G) Root planing and soft tissue curettage.

(H) Place and expose radiographs.

(I) Process radiographs.

(J) Perform any related procedures required in the practice of the above duties.

(ii) Direct Supervision:

(A) Preparing, placing, and removing periodontal packs.

(B) Place pit and fissure sealants.

(C) Removal of overhanging margins.

(D) Treatment of diagnosed dry socket.

(E) Treatment of diagnosed pericoronitis.

(F) Expanded dental duties are to be performed under the direct supervision of a qualified dentist.

Section 3. *Expanded Dental Duties.*

(a) Expanded dental duties are to be performed under the direct supervision of a qualified dentist with the exception of the administration of a local anesthetic which can be performed under indirect supervision.

(b) In order to practice expanded duties, a dental hygienist must meet educational standards and pass an examination approved by the board, in a manner satisfactory to the board, for which an expanded duty certificate will be issued in which each individual expanded duty to be performed will be listed.

(c) Training programs will be approved in advance in writing by the board. Due to the varied programs, individual courses will require individual approval after the course content is reviewed by the board.

(d) The following is a list of accepted expanded duties:

(i) Placing, carving, and finishing amalgams.

(ii) Placing and finishing composites.

(iii) Administration of local anesthetic.

(e) Thirty (30) days prior to the exam each candidate will be required to supply proof, in writing, from the course administrator of satisfactory completion of the course in the expanded functions for which he/she was trained.

(f) Examination will occur twice per year at those times that the board examines all licensure candidates. The exam will be performed on patient(s) in a clinical setting. The materials and equipment are to be supplied by the candidate. Also, the exam will include an oral interview for the purpose of ascertaining the candidate's knowledge of the duties he/she wishes to be certified to perform.

Section 4. *Dental Assistants.* The following applies to all dental assistants:

(a) A dentist holding a current Wyoming license may employ persons designated as "Dental Assistants." They may be trained by their employer or by an accredited school for dental assistants.

(b) The following is a list of procedures that may be performed by dental assistants and the type of supervision required:

(i) General Supervision:

(A) Take vital statistics and health histories.

(B) Mix dental materials to be used by the dentist.

(C) Instruct patients in proper dental health care.

(D) Process radiographs.

(ii) Indirect Supervision:

(A) Take study model impressions.

(B) Apply topical medications, excluding pit and fissure sealants.

      (C) Place and expose radiographs if the criteria set forth in Section 5 of this Chapter have been met.

(iii) Direct Supervision:

      (A) Remove sutures.

      (B) Assist the dentist in all operative and surgical procedures.

      (C) Place and remove rubber dams.

      (D) Place and remove matrices.

      (E) Remove excess cement from the coronal surfaces of the teeth.

      (F) Prepare and remove periodontal packs.

      (G) Polish the surfaces of the teeth, rubber cup only and not for the purpose of prophylaxis.

      (H) Orthodontic procedures involving the following:

            (I)   Tying ligature wires and/or elastic ties.

            (II) Removing of ligature wire and/or elastic ties.

            (III) Placement and removal of orthodontic wires and/or appliance that have been activated by the dentist.

            (IV) Take impressions for orthodontic retainers and removable orthodontic appliances.

            (V) Removal of orthodontic bands.

            (VI) Placement and removal of orthodontic separators.

      (I) The following orthodontic procedures may not be performed by dental assistants:

            (I)   Removal of tooth structure for the placement of orthodontic appliances.

            (II) Activate an orthodontic appliance.

            (III) Diagnosis for orthodontic treatment.

            (IV) Remove direct bond attachments.

Section 5. *Placement and Exposure of Radiographs by Dental Assistants.* As of July 1, 1991, no dental assistant shall place and expose radiographs under the indirect supervision of a licensed dentist unless one of the following requirements has been met:

(a) The assistant has completed an American Dental Association or board approved course in dental radiography.

(b) The assistant has at least three (3) years experience with a minimum of 1000 hours per year in the last four (4) years before July 1, 1990, and can demonstrate proficiency.

(c) The assistant is engaged in a course for radiologic technology, dental hygiene or dental assisting on July 1, 1990, who has completed the course or has completed a twenty-four (24) month course in radiologic technology within two (2) years before July 1, 1990, and can demonstrate proficiency.

(d) The assistant has been licensed by other states or certifying groups whose requirements are at least as stringent as those set forth by these rules.

(e) A dental assistant should complete a course of instruction approved in accordance with the requirements of this section. The board shall accept, in lieu of such course, the satisfactory completion of the certification examination given by the American Dental Association National Board, Inc. and any educational requirements as may be recommended by the board.

Section 6. *Code of Ethics for Dental Auxiliaries.* Each dental hygienist practicing in the state of Wyoming shall subscribe to the following:

(a) To provide oral health care utilizing highest professional knowledge, judgment, and ability.

(b) To serve all patients without discrimination.

(c) To hold professional patient relationships in confidence.

(d) To utilize every opportunity to increase public understanding of oral health practices.

(e) To generate public confidence in members of the dental health profession.

(f) To cooperate with all health professions in meeting the health needs of the public.

(g) To recognize and uphold the laws and regulations governing this profession.

(h) To participate responsibly in this professional Association and uphold its purpose.

(i) To maintain professional competence through continuing education.

(j) To exchange professional knowledge with other health professions.

(k) To represent dental hygiene with high standards of personal conduct.

Chapter VII
Revocation or Suspension of License

Section 1. *Dentists.* Any dentist may have his or her license revoked or suspended by the board for any of the causes outlined in and under the procedures set forth in the Act, or for violation of any of the rules of ethics as adopted or promulgated by this board.

Section 2. *Dental Hygienists.* Any dental hygienist may have his or her license revoked or suspended by the board for any of the causes outlined in and under the procedures set forth in the Act or for violation of any of the rules of ethics as adopted or promulgated by this board.

Section 3. *Reinstatement of License.* The following applies to any dentist or dental hygienist whose license has been revoked by the board:

(a) A person whose license has been revoked after a hearing or who has consented to revocation may not apply for reinstatement until the expiration of at least five (5) years from the effective date of the revocation.

(b) A person whose license has been suspended for a specific period may not move for reinstatement until the expiration of the period specified in the order of suspension.

(c) Motions for reinstatement by persons whose licenses have been revoked for violation of the Act and these Rules and Regulations shall be served upon the board at least two (2) months prior to the return date thereof. Upon receipt of the motion for reinstatement, the board shall cause the matter to be investigated. The board shall promptly schedule a hearing at which respondent-dentist or hygienist shall have the burden of demonstrating by clear and convincing evidence that he/she has the moral qualifications, competency, and learning in dentistry or dental hygiene required for admission to practice dentistry or dental hygiene in this state and that his/her resumption of the practice of dentistry or dental hygiene will not be detrimental to the integrity and standing of the practice of dentistry in the state of Wyoming, nor the health and welfare of the public.

At the conclusion of the hearing, the board shall promptly file a report, and issue an order concerning said reinstatement within sixty (60) days following the motion.

(d) Nothing in the above provisions of this section (Section 3) shall be construed to apply to the voluntary suspension of a license pursuant to Chapter III, Section 1.(e) of these rules.

Chapter VIII
Rules of Practice Governing Contested Cases Before the Wyoming Board of Dental Examiners

Section 1. *Authority.* These Rules of Practice are promulgated by authority of W.S. 33-15-101 through 33-15-130 and pursuant to the Wyoming Administrative Procedure Act, W.S. 16-3-101 through 16-3-115.

Section 2. *Definitions.* All of the definitions set forth in W.S. 33-15-128 and W.S. 16-3-101 are incorporated herein by reference and for the purposes of contested hearing, the following definitions of parties shall prevail:

(a) "Board" means the State Board of Dental Examiners for the state of Wyoming.

(b) "Contestee" means the person, persons, firm, or corporation licensed by law under the jurisdiction of the board and against whom the board is proceeding for alleged violation of any of the provisions of W.S. 33-15-101 through W.S. 33-15-130 or any of the Rules and Regulations of the board.

Section 3. *Notice.* Contested cases shall be commenced by a notice filed with the board. The notice shall include a statement setting forth:

(a) The name and address of each contestee.

(b) A statement in ordinary and concise language of the facts upon which the contest is based, including, whenever applicable, particular reference to the statutes, rules, and/or orders allegedly violated.

(c) A statement of the time, place, and nature of the hearing.

(d) A statement of the legal authority and jurisdiction under which the hearing is to be held.

Section 4. *Service.*

(a) Notice shall be served upon each contestee at least twenty (20) days prior to the date set for hearing.

(b) Service of the notice or of any other document or pleading required to be served may be made either personally or by mailing to the last known address of the contestee. If personal service is made, the return of service shall be made by certification of the person who made such service. Such return of service must be filed with the board prior to the commencement of the hearing.

Section 5. *Answer or Appearance.* Each contestee shall be allowed twenty (20) days from the date of service, in which time to file with the board his or her answer or other appearance. The board may, for good cause shown, grant an extension of time in which to answer and reschedule the hearing accordingly.

Section 6. *Prehearing Conference.* At any time prior to the date set for hearing, the board may direct the representative for the parties to appear before the board to consider:

(a) The simplification of the issues.

(b) The necessity or desirability of amending the pleadings.

(c) The possibility of obtaining admissions of fact and documents which will avoid unnecessary proof.

(d) Such other matters as may aid in the disposition of the case. Such conference shall be conducted informally. A memorandum will be prepared which recites the action taken at the conference.

Section 7. *Default in Answering or Appearing.* In the event of failure of any contestee to answer or otherwise appear within the time allowed, and provided that the foregoing rules as to service have been compiled with, each contestee so failing to answer or otherwise plead or to appear, shall be deemed to be in default, and the allegations of the petition or the formal notice, as the case may be, may be taken as true and the Order of the board entered accordingly.

Section 8. *Subpoenas.* Upon application of any party, the board or its designated presiding officer shall issue subpoenas requiring the appearance of witnesses for the purpose of taking evidence or requiring the production of any relevant books, papers, or other documents.

Section 9. *Motions.* Upon reasonable notice of all parties, the board or its designated presiding officer may hear orally, or otherwise, any motion filed in contested cases.

Section 10. *Hearing.* At the date, time and place of hearing set down by the board, and in accordance with the Notice given, the board shall hear all matters presented. All matters enumerated in the Notice shall be presented by an officer, agent, or representative acting on behalf of the board. Any contestee may be represented personally or by counsel, provided that such counsel be duly authorized to practice law in the state of Wyoming or otherwise associated at the hearing with a representative authorized to practice law in this state.

Section 11. *Order of Procedure at Hearing.* As nearly as may be, hearings shall be conducted in accordance with the following order of procedure:

(a) Each party may make an opening statement.

(b) The board's evidence will be presented. The board's exhibits will be marked with letters of the alphabet beginning with "A".

(c) The contestee's evidence will be presented. The contestee's exhibits will be marked with numbers beginning with "1".

(d) Any party may offer rebuttal evidence.

(e) After all proceedings have been concluded, the presiding officer shall declare the hearing closed.

Members of the board and the designated presiding officer may examine witnesses.

The presiding officer may allow evidence to be offered out of order herein prescribed.

Section 12. *Reopening Hearing.* A hearing may be reopened for good cause shown by order of the board upon motion of any party to the proceeding, or the board itself.

Chapter IX
Effective Date and Amendment of Rules

Section 1. *Effective Date.* These rules shall become effective as of April 28, 1993.

Section 2. *Amendments.* The above and foregoing rules may be amended, altered, or changed at any time by the board, provided that no amendment, alteration, or change shall be or become effective unless and until a certified copy thereof is filed in the office of the secretary of state of Wyoming as provided by W.S. 9-4-104, 9-4-105 (1977).

Glossary

abandonment Once a health care professional establishes a relationship with a patient, services must continue to be provided for the patient, or a legal action of abandonment may be commenced against the health care provider. There are specific conditions under which the relationship may be terminated and no action may be taken.

accreditation The processes of approving, certifying, or endorsing. For example, a dental education program can be accredited by the American Dental Association.

action A suit or formal complaint brought to a court of law with the proper jurisdiction.

adjudicate To make a final determination of issues through court action; to settle by judicial decree.

affidavit A written statement of facts made under oath.

affirmative defense A new matter, not brought to light in a complaint, that is a defense against the allegations, even if they are true.

allegation A claim or an assertion in the pleading of a party to a lawsuit, specifying what he or she expects to prove.

answer The formal written statement made by a defendant, stating the grounds for his or her defense.

antemortem Prior to death.

appeal To submit a lawsuit to a superior court or an appellate court to review the decision of a lower trial court or administrative agency.

appellate jurisdiction Authority of a court to hear only cases that are appealed to it in order to review or revise decisions of lower courts.

appellate review Review of a lower court's proceedings by an appellate court.

appropriation The wrongful use or reproduction of a person's name or likeness for financial gain.

arraignment The pre-trial procedure whereby an individual accused of a crime is brought before a court to plead (guilty or not guilty) to a criminal charge in the indictment or information.

asepsis The absence of microorganisms.

assault Threatening to do bodily harm to another individual. Assault can be a civil or a criminal offense.

battery   Committing bodily harm against another individual. Battery can be a civil or a criminal offense.

bellicose   Belligerent or quarrelsome.

bill   A federal or state proposed law that is introduced in a legislative body for approval. Should a bill pass in the legislative body and be signed by the appropriate executive officer, it becomes a law.

bonus   An amount paid in addition to salary or other employment benefits.

business tort   A wrongful act committed in the course of business.

causation   Derivation, basis, or origin of some specific condition or event.

cause of action   Facts that provide an individual the right to request relief in a court of law.

certification   The formal documentation of recognition. For instance, a certification of proficiency in a specific skill.

chain of custody   When an item of real evidence is offered in a court of law, the party presenting the evidence must account for the care of the evidence from the time it reaches his or her possession until the time it is presented in court.

chamber   Normally, state legislative bodies have two chambers, as does the federal government. The United States Congress is made up of the Senate and the House of Representatives. Nebraska is an exception; its legislative body is termed unicameral, as it consists of only one chamber.

citation   References to legal authority, such as reported case law or statutes.

civil action   Action brought to a court of law to protect private rights (generally, all types of actions other that criminal).

civil jurisdiction   Authority of a court to hear only civil cases.

civil tort action   A lawsuit brought in response to a wrongful act; the suit is brought to a civil court that has authority to hear the case.

common law   Judge-made law or law based on court decisions.

complaint   A claim for relief that initiates a lawsuit.

confidentiality   The principle that a health care professional must hold in strict confidence all information gained regarding a patient in the course of treatment.

conflict of interest   Discord between an individual's public duty and his or her private monetary interest.

consensual   Characterized by the mutual agreement of two parties.

consent   Approval or permission.

consent form   A signed document indicating a patient's agreement to receive treatment and acknowledging his or her understanding of the specific treatment or procedure recommended by a health practitioner.

consideration   A legal benefit received or a legal detriment suffered by one party to a contract, which represents the inducement to a contract.

contempt of court   Any act designed to obstruct the administration of justice.

contract   "A contract is a promise, or set of promises, for breach of which the law gives a remedy, or the performance of which the law in some way recognizes as a duty."

contributory negligence   The situation that exists when a plaintiff's negligent actions or omissions have contributed to his or her own injury.

controlled substance   Any substance designated as a narcotic under state or federal law. The purpose of this designation is to control the distribution, use, and sale of these drugs.

cover letter A letter of introduction usually accompanying a resume or an application for employment.

credentialing The process of conferring credentials, which can consist of accreditation, certification, licensure, and so forth.

criminal jurisdiction Authority of a court to hear only criminal cases.

defamation Written or printed matter (libel) or oral statements (slander) that damage the reputation of another.

defendant The individual or party against whom a suit for recovery is brought in a civil case, or the accused in a criminal case.

delegation The giving of authority to act for another. For example, the delegating of a duty.

dental history A record of all preventive, restorative, and aesthetic treatment that a person has received, as well as his or her dental experiences.

deposition Out-of-court testimony of a witness, conducted under oath. A transcript and/or video is made of a deposition. A deposition is conducted by one party to a lawsuit, who asks questions of another party or another party's witness to gain insight into all of the facts of the matter being litigated.

disability A condition that incapacitates an individual in some manner; an impairment that renders a person unable to work for an extended period of time.

disciplinary action Action that regulates or punishes, such as suspension of one's license to engage in a particular profession.

disclosure The act of revealing facts that had been unknown or not understood.

discovery The procedure by which a party to litigation may secure information (verbal or written). For example, depositions, interrogatories.

discrimination Bias against a group of individuals on the basis of race, gender, religion, age, physical infirmity, or sexual preference.

diversity of citizenship One of the criteria for jurisdiction of federal courts. The situation in which one party to the lawsuit is a citizen of one state and the other party is a citizen of another state or country.

doctrine of vicarious liability The principle that legal liability can be acquired through another. Vicarious liability most often exists when employers are found liable for acts of their employees. See respondeat superior, Chapter 4.

duty An obligation of care that one party owes to another; an obligation, in law, that one owes to another person or a business.

ergonomics The scientific study of human work, specifically as it relates to the use of technology for the purpose of creating a healthy work environment.

ethics Morals or standards of conduct. Each health profession defines professional ethics in written standards of professional behavior.

expert testimony Testimony offered by a specialist in a particular field. For example, a radiologist's testimony about the interpretation of radiographs.

express consent Permission given specifically by words, written or oral.

express contract A contract that is either written or verbally agreed to by the parties.

false light An "invasion of privacy" tort. A plaintiff may sue if he or she is placed in a false light before the public. The false light must be highly offensive to a reasonable person.

family leave Unpaid absence from employment for the birth, adoption, or care of a child or the care of a spouse, a parent, or oneself. The federal Family and Medical

Leave Act requires businesses of 50 or more employees to provide 12 weeks of un-paid leave for eligible employees. Any paid leave benefits from an employer would be in addition to FMLA requirements.

felony Any offense punishable by death or by imprisonment for at least one year.

forensic dentistry The science of dentistry as it relates to the law. For example, uti-lizing the human dentition to identify a deceased individual.

fraud An intentional untruth that is told for the purpose of inducing another to rely on the falsehood and surrender something of value.

Frye test Criteria used by some courts to determine whether to admit scientific evi-dence. (See Chapter 14.)

grounds for discipline The basis or the real reason for punishment.

harassment Words or actions designed to provoke another person.

health maintenance organization (HMO) An organization providing health care services for enrolled members, who pay a fixed monthly fee.

Hippocratic oath An oath, written by Hippocrates in the fourth century B.C., speci-fying standards of conduct for physicians.

human rights statute A state law prohibiting discrimination. See Appendix G, Rhode Island Equal Opportunity and Affirmative Action Act.

impanel To complete the entire process of jury selection, to final selection of the ju-rors who will sit for a specific case.

implied consent Permission that is implied by the behavior of the parties rather than written or spoken.

implied contract A contract that is assumed, under law, from the circumstances or facts of the situation.

incompetent Lacking the capacity to discharge a legal duty.

indemnity plan (or **reimbursement plan)** A contract whereby one party secures another against anticipated loss. For instance, an insurance plan that pays health care providers and health care facilities for services rendered, or the patient di-rectly for out-of-pocket medical expenses, for procedures that are covered under the plan.

independent contractor An individual with special skills whom an employer hires sporadically, such as a consultant.

indictment A charge that must be proven at trial in order to convict an individual of a crime.

informed consent A patient's consent to medical or dental treatment that is given after the patient understands the nature of his or her condition, the treatment options, the risks involved in treatment, and the risks if no treatment is sought.

injurious falsehood Defamation that causes actual damages.

insurance A written contract (policy) whereby an insured pays a stipulated sum (pre-mium) to an insurer, who agrees to compensate the insured for losses relating to the subject matter of the policy.

intentional tort A tort in which there was intent to cause physical or mental harm to another individual or the property of another.

interrogatories A discovery device. Written questions submitted by one party in a lawsuit to another party or to a witness of another party. The individual answering the interrogatories signs a sworn statement that the answers are true. (See Figure 2-4.)

intrusion upon seclusion An "invasion of privacy" tort. A plaintiff may sue if his or her solitude is intruded upon. This intrusion must be highly offensive to a reasonable person.

invalid consent Permission given with no force of law. For instance, an individual may sign an informed consent form that appears legal; however, if the person is under the age of majority or is mentally incompetent, the consent is invalid.

invitee A business visitor, such as a patient in a dental office. The business owner has the duty to protect the invitee against any known dangers and against any dangers that the owner could have discovered with reasonable care.

judgment The official decision of a court.

judicial circuit One of the thirteen judicial divisions of the federal court system. (See Figure 1-3.)

judicial review A review by a court of a finding from an administrative body, such as a state board of dental examiners.

jurisdiction The authority of a court to hear a case and enforce the judgment rendered.

leased employee An employee who is employed by a temporary-employee leasing service. An employer pays the leasing service a fee to hire one of its employees for short-term employment.

liability Responsibility for a breach of duty.

licensure The process whereby a competent authority issues permission to perform a certain act or engage in a specific business that would otherwise be unlawful.

litigant A party to a lawsuit.

litigate To settle a dispute in a court of law.

litigation A lawsuit; court proceedings to determine legal issues regarding the rights and responsibilities between parties.

lobbyist An individual who is hired by various organizations to induce legislators to vote for or against specific bills pending before the legislature.

long arm statutes State statutes that enable a state court to gain personal jurisdiction over a nonresident business or individual, for limited purposes.

malpractice Failure of a professional to exercise reasonable care, which results in harm to another; negligent conduct of professional individuals or a breach of a standard of care.

measure of damages A determination of the amount of remuneration that an injured party to a lawsuit will receive.

Medicaid A program of assistance to low-income families. Funds for Medicaid are provided jointly by the federal and state governments.

medical history A record of all past medical conditions of a patient and treatment received for them.

Medicare A federal program that provides medical insurance for the elderly.

misdemeanor A crime punishable by less than a year in prison; an offense committed in violation of the law that is less than a felony.

misrepresentation An untrue or deceptive statement of fact; a falsehood or an incorrect assertion.

motion An application to a court or judge in order to obtain a ruling or order directing an action to be done in favor of the applicant.

mutual assent The state that exists when parties agree to the terms of a contract.

negligence The failure to use such care as a reasonable and careful person would use under similar circumstances.

nondisclosure   Failure to divulge facts. Nondisclosure need not be associated with deception.

notice   This term is used in many different ways. Generally, in the law, notice is the knowledge of the existence of a fact. Often notice is intended to warn or inform a person of a proceeding in which his or her interests are involved.

offer and acceptance   Requirements of a contract. Offer and acceptance are referred to as mutual assent.

open dental practice act   A state dental practice act that permits a supervising dentist to delegate tasks to other dental personnel on the basis of his or her judgment.

overbroad language   Language that is not sufficiently specific to enable one to determine its exact meaning.

party   The plaintiff or the defendant in a lawsuit.

patient identification data   All information collected to provide medical or dental information for a specific patient.

personal jurisdiction   The authority of a court over a person (defendant), as opposed to jurisdiction of a court over the person's property.

plaintiff   The party who sues in a civil action and is named on the record of the lawsuit. In a criminal action the plaintiff would be the people—the people of the state in a state action (e.g., *Oregon v. Ray Smith)* and the people of the United States in a federal action *(*e.g., *United States v. Ray Smith).*

pleadings   Claims and defenses formally made by parties to a lawsuit. For example, complaints, answers. (See Figures 2-2 and 2-3.)

postmortem   After death.

precedent   A previous court decision that is relevant to a current case because it involves the same or a similar question of law.

preemptory challenge   The privilege or right of each party to a lawsuit to request deletion of specific jurors during jury selection, without having to give a reason.

preferred provider organization (PPO)   An organization of health care providers (doctors, hospitals, dentists, etc.). Members of a PPO discount their fees for services to member subscribers.

prima facie case   A lawsuit in which facts or evidence can be judged from first sight, unless disproved by some other, contradictory evidence.

privilege   An advantage conferred on a person. In law, a privileged communication (such as a doctor-patient communication) can be made under circumstances whereby a doctor cannot be compelled to disclose it in court.

probate   Generally, a court established to administer estates of deceased individuals, adoptions, and name changes.

process   In law, a summons and complaint and related documents served upon a defendant in a lawsuit.

progress notes   A record of all treatment provided and observable conditions pertaining to the health of a person on a continuing basis.

protected group   A group of individuals protected by a law designed to ensure fair treatment. For example, consumer laws are enacted to protect the consumer against unscrupulous business practices.

prudent   sensible, careful.

publicity of private life   An "invasion of privacy" tort. Publicizing private details of a person's private life. This invasion must be highly offensive to a reasonable person.

punitive   Characterized by or involving punishment of an individual by legal authority.

punitive damages   An amount of remuneration awarded to a plaintiff that is greater than actual damages suffered. Punitive damages are designed to punish the defendant for egregious behavior.

quasijudicial   Said of judicial action of an administrative officer or body (such as a board of dental examiners) rather than a judge.

quid pro quo   Something for something. Giving something of value for something else of value.

references   Recommendations, written or oral, attesting to another person's competencies.

referral   A practitioner's seeking of advice from another regarding a patient's medical or dental treatment or diagnosis.

registration   The process of entering or recording in some official register, record, or list.

regulatory power   The authority to issue regulations to ensure uniform application of the law and to carry out the intent of the law. Regulations are not the same as laws; however, they influence how laws are interpreted.

reimbursement plan   See indemnity plan.

requests for admissions   Requests for written statements of fact, presented to an adverse party. That party must admit or deny these statements. (See Figure 2-5.)

res ipsa loquitur   "The thing speaks for itself." That is, the instrument that caused the damage was under the defendant's exclusive control.

respondeat superior   The principle that, generally, an employer is liable for the wrongful acts of his or her employee if the employee was acting within the scope of his or her employment.

sanctions   Penalties imposed for violating the law or failure to comply with a court order.

scheduled benefits   Under workers' compensation law, a listing of benefits provided to an injured employee, with specific amounts being based on the types of injury or impairment suffered as a result of employment.

slander per se   To prevail in a lawsuit based upon slander, the plaintiff must prove that he or she sustained some special monetary harm. However, there are four types of slander, called slander per se, in which such proof is not necessary: statements that the plaintiff (1) engaged in criminal behavior, (2) suffers from a loathsome disease, (3) is unfit to conduct his or her business, or (4) engaged in serious sexual misconduct.

standard of care   The degree of care that a reasonably prudent professional should exercise.

state fair employment statute   A state law that prohibits discrimination in the work place.

statute of limitations   A state statute that specifies the time period within which a lawsuit must be filed after the event that caused the action or suit to be filed. Once this time period has passed, the right to bring the action is lost.

statutes   Laws enacted and written by federal or state legislatures.

sterilization   The process of destroying all microorganisms.

subject matter jurisdiction   The authority of a court to hear particular types of cases or cases relating to a specific subject matter. For instance, a bankruptcy court has the authority to only hear bankruptcy cases.

subpoena   A legal document commanding an individual to attend court under penalty for failure to appear.

subrogate   To substitute one person for another. The person substituted has a claim to rights of the other.

summary judgment   A motion made by either party to a lawsuit that may be granted by the court when there is no real issue of fact and the moving party is entitled to judgment.

territorial jurisdiction   The jurisdiction of a court is generally limited to cases arising within a specified geographical area or involving persons residing within a specified geographical area. For example, the geographical area may be the United States or any state.

tort   A civil wrong or injury, other than a breach of contract, for which the plaintiff is compensated monetarily (should the plaintiff prevail) for the unreasonable harm he or she has sustained. For example, see Chapter 4, negligence.

tortious   Characterized by wrongful conduct that subjects one to liability in tort. The courts are constantly changing the definition of tortious conduct through court decisions.

trial   A court's examination of facts and determination of issues between parties to a lawsuit (criminal or civil).

trial jurisdiction   The authority of a court to hear only cases at the trial stage (as opposed to appellate jurisdiction).

unemployment compensation   A state insurance program that provides benefits to persons who are terminated from employment. Former employees are generally not eligible if they left their jobs without good cause or were fired for serious misconduct.

unscheduled benefits   Under workers' compensation law, a method of salary compensation for workers who are unable to return to work after a specified time period.

venue   Geographical location where a trial is held.

vicarious   Indirect.

voir dire   A process by which the court examines jurors or witnesses to determine their ability to participate in a trial.

waive   To voluntarily forfeit a right.

wanton   Willfully cruel or malicious.

workers' compensation   Insurance (state or private) that provides employees with income and medical expenses when they are unable to work because they suffer from work-related injury or illness.

wrongful discharge   The termination of an employee for reasons that violate the law, such as race, age, religion, gender, national origin, or disability.

Index

Medical malpractice, 45; *see also* Malpractice
  choice of law for, 45
Medical practice, unauthorized, 114-115
Medical record
  duty to disclose and, 77
  of employee, 209
  wrongful disclosure of, 75-76
Medical savings account, 230
Medical treatment, emergency, 173
Medicare, 126-128
Medication, administration of, 158
MEDLINE, 48
Melcher v. Charleston Area Medical Center, 59
Mental distress, 55
Meritor Savings Bank v. Vinson, 12, 221
Minor
  consent by, 59
  consent for, 60
Minority person
  discrimination cases involving, 91-92
  refusal to treat, 82
*Mirkin v. Medical Mutual Liability Insurance Society of
  Maryland,* 160
Miscellanous tort, 53
Misconduct
  intentional
    assault and battery, 53
    defamation, 53-54
    fraud or misrepresentation, 55-56
    infliction of mental distress, 55
    interference with advantageous relations, 56
    invasion of privacy, 54-55
    wrongful discharge, 56
  unintentional, 45-51
    contributory negligence and, 51
    duty and, 46-47
    expert testimony and, 48-49
    malpractice liability and, 45-46
    negligence and, 46
    res ipsa loquitur doctrine, 49-50
    respondeat superior doctrine, 50-51
    standards of care and, 47-48
Misdemeanor
  definition of, 9, 117
  violation of practice act as, 117
Misrepresentation
  consent obtained by, 59-60, 62
  intentional, 55-56
Money, proper handling of, 2, 4, 37
Monge v. Superior Court, 222
Moore. v. Baker, 61
Motion
  definition of, 19
  for summary judgment, 23
Mutual assent, 79

N
Name, appropriation of, 54
National Board for Certification for Dental Technologists, 31
National Practitioners Data Bank, 115-116
Needle stick injury, 175
Negative defense, denial as, 22-23
Neglect statute, 60
Negligence, 42
  contributory, 51
  defamation and, 54
  duty and, 46-47
  elements of, 46
  in malpractice, 45
Negligent hiring, 207
New Mexico Dental Practice Act, 107-110
Newport News Shipbuilding & Dry Dock v. EEOC, 233
No-duty rule, 80
Nondisclosure, consent and, 61-62
Northeastern Reporter, 13
Notice, 16
Numbering system for teeth, 157

O
Oath, Hippocratic, 75
Occupational Safety and Health Act, 205
Occupational Safety and Health Administration, 124-126
Offer and acceptance of contract, 79
Office equipment, 176
Office manual, sterilization procedures in, 175
Office procedures, 172-179
  asepsis and sterilization and, 173-175
  case example of, 175-176
  case study on, 133-153
  child abuse reporting and, 178-179
  emergency medical treatment and, 173
  equipment and, 176
  housekeeping and, 176-177
  radiographic techniques and, 177-178
  recordkeeping, 154-162; *see also* Records
Office-trained dental assistant, 116
Oncale v. Sundowner Offshore Services, Inc., 222
On-call substitute, 81
Open dental practice act, 105
Oral consent, 76
Organization, professional, 122-125
Outcomes in consent statement, 60-61
Overbroad language of consent form, 62-63

P
Pacific Reporter, 13
Party, 16
Patient
  contributory negligence by, 51
  identification of, forensic, 164-168
Patient acquaintance form, 135, 138
Patient chart, 136, 137